Palgrave Studies in Science and Popular Culture

Series Editor
Sherryl Vint
Department of English
University of California
Riverside, CA, USA

This book series seeks to publish ground-breaking research exploring the productive intersection of science and the cultural imagination. Science is at the centre of daily experience in twenty-first century life and this has defined moments of intense technological change, such as the Space Race of the 1950s and our very own era of synthetic biology. Conceived in dialogue with the field of Science and Technology Studies (STS), this series will carve out a larger place for the contribution of humanities to these fields. The practice of science is shaped by the cultural context in which it occurs and cultural differences are now key to understanding the ways that scientific practice is enmeshed in global issues of equity and social justice. We seek proposals dealing with any aspect of science in popular culture in any genre. We understand popular culture as both a textual and material practice, and thus welcome manuscripts dealing with representations of science in popular culture and those addressing the role of the cultural imagination in material encounters with science. How science is imagined and what meanings are attached to these imaginaries will be the major focus of this series. We encourage proposals from a wide range of historical and cultural perspectives.

More information about this series at
http://www.palgrave.com/gp/series/15760

Bianca C. Frazer • Heather R. Walker
Editors

(Un)doing Diabetes: Representation, Disability, Culture

palgrave
macmillan

Editors
Bianca C. Frazer
Department of Disability and Human Development
University of Illinois Chicago
Chicago, IL, USA

Heather R. Walker
Medical Group Analytics
University of Utah Health
Salt Lake City, UT, USA

ISSN 2731-4359 ISSN 2731-4367 (electronic)
Palgrave Studies in Science and Popular Culture
ISBN 978-3-030-83109-7 ISBN 978-3-030-83110-3 (eBook)
https://doi.org/10.1007/978-3-030-83110-3

Cover illustration: spxChrome / Getty Images

This Palgrave Macmillan imprint is published by the registered company Springer Nature Switzerland AG.
The registered company address is: Gewerbestrasse 11, 6330 Cham, Switzerland

Dedicated to all diabetic people who have survived as many pricks as we have

Acknowledgements

(Un)doing Diabetes began when Carrie Sandahl connected our paths and ignited the creation of this volume. Many thanks to Carrie, Camille Davies at Palgrave Macmillan, and Therese (Tess) Jones at the University of Colorado Anschutz. Their editorial support and guidance throughout the development of the project made the work possible. For every answered email, bit of feedback, and general care as humans, we thank you.

This collection of essays would not have been possible without the brilliance and labor of our incredible authors who put forward this effort during a pandemic: Jeffrey A. Bennett, Lora Arduser, Clair Irwin, Valentina Sturiale & Guido Anselmi, Phyllisa Deroze, Samuel Thulin, Matt Paczkowski, G. William Zorn, Sheila Bock, Taylor Johnson, Stephen Horrocks, Elizabeth Jan Jones, Mila Clarke Buckley, Cynthia Martin, Justine Debelius, Kirsten E. Gardner, S.K. Sabada and Stephen Shaul. As this book came together, our authors navigated a pandemic, cared for family in the hospital, had babies, lost loved ones, weathered mental health challenges, survived natural disasters, moved across the country, and everything in between. We are evermore awestruck with the rigor they brought to the critiques that truly make this collection remarkable.

Extended thanks to the University of Illinois at Chicago (UIC) and specifically the Department of Disability and Human Development. Within the department, Carrie Sandahl championed the volume from its inception to finish. We extend our appreciation to the members of the Program on Disability Art Culture and the Humanities (PDACH) Writing Group: Maggie Bridger, Sydney Erlikh, Margaret Fink, Alison Kopit and

Sara Miller. Further gratitude for the joyful discussions and the sharing of recourses on the craft of editing to the Director of the Disability Cultural Center at UIC, Margaret Fink, and Sam Tynen, Research Fellow at the Czech Academy of Sciences. Also, we extend gratitude toward to the University of Utah Health, and specifically Heidi Cozart, for affording us the time and deliverance to complete this project.

This project was made possible thanks to the activism and advocacy of diabetic people who are putting in the time to dismantle diabetes stereotypes and stigma online and off. We hope this book can be a token of gratitude and recognition for everything you have done and will do.

From the bottom of our hearts, we want to thank our home teams for their care, encouragement, and overwhelming support. We thank our siblings, their partners, and our friends, Miles Gordon and Kevin Leon, Allie H. Rasmussen, Mallory Kaufman, and Brittany and Michel Estefan-Gabel; and our parents and in-laws, Jill and Steve Gordon, Mary and Richard Gabel, Tim and Melody Frazer, and Renee and Shane Walker. And, we give a particularly tender thanks to our partners, Travis Frazer and Jesse Walker, whose love and support has made it possible for us to go with abandon towards healing and liberation. You mean the world to us.

As a final acknowledgement, we express gratitude to Shawna Husdon, who reviewed and gave feedback on more drafts than a good friend should have to. For someone without diabetes, you really seem to "get it." Thank you for sharing with us how pieces of this book moved you and shifted your thinking.

As editors, we turn towards each other and offer immense gratitude. While this project came together over two years of phone calls, Zoom meetings and email exchange, we maintained a rich foundation of respect, intellectual rigor, and care. The collaboration has survived the onset of a global pandemic, the birth of a child, and the general upheaval of every aspect of our professional and personal lives. We emerge from this work as colleagues and friends with renewed passion for the wholeness and dignity of diabetic people.

Contents

Notes on Contributors

Guido Anselmi is a Lecturer in Big Data and Digital Methods. His scientific interests lie in the political economy of platforms, their intersection with capital concentration as well as in computational methods for social science. Valentina and Guido are the parents of Vittorio to whom they dedicate their chapter, in the hope that he will live in a world in which access to lifesaving therapies will be a universal right.

Lora Arduser is an associate professor in technical and professional writing at the University of Cincinnati. Her research is situated in the rhetoric of health and medicine and focuses on rhetorics of expertise and rhetoric, gender and technology. Her book *Living Chronic: Agency and Expertise in the Rhetoric of Diabetes* was published by The Ohio State University Press in 2017. Her research has also been published in *Technical Communication Quarterly*, *Journal of Technical Writing and Communication*, and *Women's Studies in Communication, Computers and Composition, and Narrative Inquiry*.

Jeffrey A. Bennett is Professor of Communication Studies at Vanderbilt University. He has published two books, *Managing Diabetes: The Cultural Politics of Disease* and *Banning Queer Blood: Rhetorics of Citizenship, Contagion, and Resistance*. He has lived with Type 1 diabetes since 2004.

Sheila Bock is Associate Professor in the Department of Interdisciplinary, Gender, and Ethnic Studies at the University of Nevada, Las Vegas. A folklorist by training, her research interests include the contested domains of illness experience, material/digital enactments of personal and community identities, the intersections between folklore and popular culture, and the values and challenges of cross-disciplinary collaboration. Her work on narrative and performative responsive to the stigmas attached to diabetes has been published in the Journal of Folklore Research, the Western Journal of Black Studies, the Journal of Medical Humanities, Diagnosing Folklore: Perspectives on Disability, Health, and Trauma, and The Oxford Handbook of American Folklore and Folklife Studies.

Mila Clarke Buckley is an author, speaker, diabetes advocate and founder of HangryWoman.com. Hangry Woman aims to take away the shame and stigma that comes with a diabetes diagnosis and covers topics like diabetes management, cooking, and self-care from the perspective of someone living with the chronic condition.

Justine Debelius PhD is a postdoctoral researcher at the Karolinska Institutet in Stockholm, Sweden. She has been writing diabetes-centric fanfiction for more than a decade.

Phyllisa Smith Deroze, PhD is a scholar in Literature, Health Humanities, and African Diaspora Feminism. She is also a global diabetes patient advocate and you can find her on LinkedIn.

Bianca C. Frazer, PhD is a Postdoctoral Research Associate at the University of Illinois Chicago. She researches the ways in which performance can generate new knowledge about living with chronic illness, specifically all forms of diabetes. Her writing has been featured in *Metanarratives of Disability: Culture, Assumed Authority, and the Normative Social Order*, *ArtsPraxis*, and *Theatre Journal.*

Kirsten E. Gardner is an Associate Professor of History at the University of Texas San Antonio. Gardner earned a PhD in history and her research focuses on gender, disease, and medical technologies. She has published her research in several book chapters and many academic journals including T*he Journal of Medical Humanities; Enterprise and Society; Literature and Medicine; Gender, Health and Popular Culture: Historical Perspectives;* and *Dreamers, Visionaries and Revolutionaries in Life Science.*

Stephen Horrocks is a Cultural Studies scholar and historian with a Ph.D. in American Studies. His research identifies and interrogates the cultural, technological, and embodied networks of insulin pump use by people with Type 1 Diabetes. More information about his research, teaching, and other work as well as links to his publications can be found at https://www.stephenhorrocks.com/.

Clair Irwin is a 2nd year PhD student at the graduate school of information sciences at University of Illinois Urbana-Champaign. Mx. Irwin's research focuses on the embodied information behavior of people with diabetes, including consideration of how healthcare advocacy affects our diabetes self-management. The founder of the Illinois #insulin4all chapter, she currently volunteers as the chapter's resource, research, and education lead.

Taylor Johnson is a mental health educator and outreach worker. She has a Master's degree in Applied Psychology from Angelo State University. Her research interests include community based mental health promotion and improving mental health outcomes for Black children and young adults diagnosed with diabetes.

Elizabeth Jan Jones is a PhD candidate at The University of North Carolina at Chapel Hill. Her research centers on representations of disability, both fictional and nonfictional, in the Hispanophone world. Elizabeth's research can be found in academic journals such as *Disability in the Global South* and the *Journal of Literary and Cultural Disability Studies* as well as the volume *Disability Experiences*.

Therese (Tess) Jones PhD is Associate Director of the Center for Bioethics and Humanities (CBH) and Director of the Arts and Humanities in Healthcare Program at the University of Colorado Anschutz Medical Campus. She is an Associate Professor in the Department of Medicine. She has published and presented extensively on HIV/AIDS and the arts; literature, film and medicine; and medical education and is the editor of the *Journal of Medical Humanities* and lead editor for the *Health Humanities Reader* published by Rutgers University Press (2014). She is currently under contract with Routledge as co-editor of *The Handbook of Health and Media* (forthcoming 2022).

Cynthia Martin, MA, Virginia Tech, is an instructor in the School of Writing, Rhetoric, & Technical Communication at James Madison University. Her advocacy and research interests encompass stigma of disease, rhetoric of diabetes, and disability and sports. When not chauffeuring her son to multiple swim practices a day, she keeps a blog about parenting a child who lives with Type 1 diabetes, which can be found at http://teachingt1d.com.

Matt Paczkowski is an adjunct Assistant Professor of English at The City College of New York and holds a Masters of Fine Arts Degree in English. He writes fiction and creative nonfiction, and his work has appeared in literary journals including *Fiction Southeast*, *Ponder Review*, *Riprap Journal*, and *South 85 Journal*.

SK Sabada is an artist and PhD student at York University. Their research focuses on the intersections between madness, disability, queerness, and the performative intimacies of death and dying.

Stephen Shaul has been living with Type 1 diabetes for over 30 years, and currently works as a system analyst for a multinational corporation. He served on Maryland's Advisory Council on Health and Wellness, helping in the development of the state's first diabetes action plan. You can find his work at the diabetes blog Happy Medium (http://happy-medium.net), as host of the podcast Diabetes By The Numbers, and anywhere the voice of the patient advocate is needed.

Valentina Sturiale is Chief Methodologist at Viralbeat as well as research associate in a number of research teams dealing with social media usage, the production of junk news and aging. She is T1 diabetic.

Samuel Thulin is a media artist and researcher holding a PhD in Communication from Concordia University, Montreal. Thulin is interested in sound, space and place, the datafication of everyday life, and relationships between chronic illness, disability, and art. Thulin's artwork can be found at: https://samuelthulin.com/.

Heather R. Walker is the Associate Director of Qualitative Research at the University of Utah Health and earned her PhD in Disability Studies at the University of Illinois at Chicago. Walker's research of diabetes has been featured in journals such as Qualitative Health Research, the Journal of Medical Internet Research Diabetes (JMIR Diabetes), Journal of Diabetes Science and Technology (JDST), The Diabetes Educator, and The Association of Diabetes Care and Education Specialists Perspectives in Practice Journal. You can find her on Twitter @Heather_RoseW.

G. William Zorn is a playwright and Ph.D. His research interests include the definition of "family" and the use of ghosts in contemporary American drama. You can find him at www.gwilliamzorn.com and his work in national booksellers.

Abbreviations

A1C+K27K41JJ1:K33	Hemoglobin A1C
AA	Alcoholics Anonmyous
AADE	American Association of Diabetes Educators
ACT UP	Aids Coalition to Unleash Power
ADA	Americans with Disabilities Act
ADA	American Diabetes Association
AUW	American Universalist Women
AZT	Azidothymidine
BIPOC	Black, Indigenous, and People of Color
CDC	Center for Disease Control and Prevention
CDC	Clara Barton Camp
CGM	Continuous glucose monitor
CHMK	Camp Ho Mita Koda
3D	3-Dimensional
DAT	Diabetes Association of Thailand
DDA	Diabetes Data Art
DKA	Diabetic ketoacidosis
dQ&A	Diabetes Question and Answer
FDA	Food and Drug Association
GMHC	Gay Men's Health Crisis
H/C	Hurt/Comfort
HHS	Health and Human Services
IDF	International Diabetes Federation
JDRF	(Formerly) Juvenile Diabetes Research Foundation
LADA	Latent Autoimmune Diabetes in adults
MD	Medical Doctor

MDA	Muscular Dystrophy Association
MODY	Maturity Onset Diabetes of the Young
NIDDK	National Institute of Diabetes and Digestive and Kidney Disease
NIH	National Institutes of Health
NYPD	New York Police Department
PhRMA	Pharmaceutical Research and Manufacturers of America
PSA	Public Service Announcement
SNL	Saturday Night Live
T1D	Type 1 Diabetes
T2D	Type 2 Diabetes
TF-IDF	Term's Frequency and Its Inverse Document Frequency
UPR	Unconditional Positive Regard
UK	United Kingdom
US	United States
YMCA	Young Men's Christen Assocaition

List of Figures

Introduction

Bianca C. Frazer and Heather R. Walker

On March 6th, 2020, a diabetic[1] podcaster shared a controversial image on Instagram with their then 6,697 followers. The post, which featured white text set against a black background, simply read: "The only disability is a bad attitude." This post relies on all-too-common beliefs about disability, including: (1) it is a feature of individual bodies, not a

The authors contributed equally to this work

[1] In this book, authors were given the flexibility to choose to use identity-first, person-first terminology, or a combination of the two. As editors, we prefer to use identity-first terminology because doing so honors diabetes as an integral part of identity and personhood. We also firmly believe in the way intentionally using this term works to reclaim it.

B. C. Frazer (✉)
Department of Disability and Human Development, University of Illinois Chicago, Chicago, IL, USA
e-mail: bfrazer@uic.edu

H. R. Walker
Medical Group Analytics, University of Utah Health, Salt Lake City, UT, USA
e-mail: heather.walker@hsc.utah.edu

B. C. Frazer, H. R. Walker (eds.), *(Un)doing Diabetes: Representation, Disability, Culture*, Palgrave Studies in Science and Popular Culture, https://doi.org/10.1007/978-3-030-83110-3_1

meaningful social category (2) it exists in one's mind and can be overcome by personal willpower and (3) choosing to identify as disabled constitutes an act of self-indulgence and self-loathing (Siebers 2010). On the post itself, followers' responses reflected support or criticism of these underlying ideas. Comments on the image ranged from agreement ("no 'able bodied' person has come to better understand this disease when I was sitting in a pool of self-pity") to disappointment ("Uhhhh. This is the wooooorst").

One follower added in the comments: "I usually love everything you put out. But this is so ableist." When the user identifies *ableism*, they are referring to the worldview that pathologizes those who might claim disability as a positive identity. Going beyond individual beliefs, community lawyer TL Lewis defines ableism as "*a system* [emphasis added] that places value on people's bodies and minds based on societally constructed ideas of normalcy, intelligence, excellence and productivity" (Lewis 2021). As exemplified by the follower's critique, diabetic people interact with varying degrees of awareness around the systemic nature of ableism. In this interaction, readers can witness diabetic communities debating their relationship to disability narratives and identity.

While this online conversation reveals the changing viewpoints in online communities, the public conception of diabetes remains firmly unchanged. Popular media representations continue to portray diabetes as a condition couched in lifestyle choices (i.e., caused by an individual's lack of self-control or overindulgence in junk food). In its most reductionist form, U.S. media depicts diabetes as a natural result of eating too much sugar.

We claim here that stereotypical depictions of all forms of diabetes focus on individual behaviors while excluding social-political factors. Therefore, in this volume, we pivot toward the larger systems and institutions that popular culture rarely examines. We ask, what do individualistic stereotypes *reveal* about the social conditions for the diabetic person? What do they *conceal*? How do these narratives perpetuate assumptions about a "normal" or "good" body? How might frameworks developed by disability activists and scholars help uncover ideas that often go unquestioned in representations of diabetes?

What This Book Offers

This volume, an assemblage of complementary critiques, introduces diabetes as a site of inquiry within the field of disability studies. For scholars familiar with disability studies, this book offers diabetes as a new case study to destabilize and complement historical and contemporary disability theories. For scholars entrenched in diabetes research, but unfamiliar with disability studies frameworks, this volume offers a set of analytical tools that can reveal how popularized representations of diabetes reveal and conceal the realities of living with diabetes in the United States today. Each of the 21 chapters in this book resist popular and seemingly commonsense ideas of diabetes, and many offer generative concepts and pathways to move forward. We collectively take on existing paradigms and offer new ones more focused on intersectional diabetes experiences and disability justice.

As such, this collection intervenes into the common ways that medical communities, political and public health campaigns, film, television, and even established diabetes community groups portray diabetes. In her analysis of Robbie McCauley's performance piece *Sugar*, Sheila Bock noted: "People's knowledge about diabetes is filtered through different modes of experience—individual, familial, community, cultural" (2015, 135). In this book, authors examine cultural artifacts (e.g. film, television, theater, literature, social media) that shape the public's understanding of diabetes. We believe that these depictions are so powerful, so subtle, and the underpinning assumptions so unquestioned, that many of the assertions in this book will be counterintuitive to readers.

We hope that this book primes readers to critique popular understandings of diabetes in public discourse, raise *disability consciousness* within diabetic communities, and further the goals of disability justice and activism. We hope chapters from this volume, empower, uplift, and invigorate individuals toward activism. We composed this collection of essays with the goal of generating shifts in inter- and intra-community discourses of diabetes. When dreaming about what this book could do, we envisioned a timely and rather unconventional academic text that featured perspectives from academics and community members alike. Considering nearly every author in this volume lives with some type of diabetes, our book holds to that promise as well. For diabetic scholars and diabetic people without academic training, this book offers openings to see yourself in these unfolding narratives, and the space to reflect and grow. For established and in-training scholars spanning the humanities, medicine, and the social sciences with only a faint interest in diabetes or disability studies, this book offers emancipatory takes on diabetes. From its inception, we imagined that this book would move readers, challenge, and change them.

As editors, we have over fifty years spent in confusion and discomfort as we've tried to navigate, challenge, and create shifts in public ideas about diabetes. Together, we bring humanities and social science training, as well as our own lived experience, to this project. Together, we bring specific levels of academic, racial, community, and class privilege to this project. We are keenly aware that diabetes experience is not monolithic, and there are many experiences within broad diabetes communities that we do not have. The authors within this collection bring their unique identities, histories, and/or positions in the diabetes community to their analysis. Additionally, since this is an interdisciplinary text, writers arrive from diverse fields with distinct training.

Bringing together scholars and diabetic activists spanning academic disciplines, fields, and experiences, authors in this collection *(un)do diabetes.*[2] *Undoing* diabetes means authors deconstruct assumptions the public commonly holds about diabetes, while *doing* diabetes seeks to understand the narratives community members create to represent themselves. Much like disability studies scholar Alison Kafer contends about the category of disability, we too assert that understandings of diabetes are political in nature. Reading diabetes as political situates it as "a category to be contested and debated" (2013, 3). In this spirit, we deconstruct and disrupt status quo representations of diabetes. By poking holes in the most insidious representations of diabetes, this books contests and debates even the most seemingly common-sense assumptions about the condition. Even disability studies scholars versed in the frameworks authors use here will hopefully be challenged to reconsider embedded and internalized stereotypical conceptions of diabetes. We believe discomfort invites the awareness and critique that is so necessary to shift public thinking about this ubiquitous condition.

[2] Here, we take pause to clarify that "undoing" diabetes does not refer to curing or putting diabetes into remission on a biophysical level. Rather, we chose this term as a playful pun and as yet another way to undo the unquestioned social and cultural conceptions of diabetes and diabetics. Bring playfulness into it our title lightens, lifts, and elevates the work.

Defining Diabetes: Contemporary Understandings

Messaging about diabetes emerges from sources with differing goals including the medical establishment, cultural representations, and social structures and institutions. With these areas in mind, the following sections definitions of diabetes expose a series of contradictions. In the following four definitions of diabetes, paradoxes and conundrums emerge that complicate how readers understand diabetes. The definitions we offer serve as analytical tools and guiding signposts for readers to understand how authors in this book have come to understand and evaluate representations of diabetes. As would likely occur in real life, we begin our exploration by defining diabetes from a medical perspective, *as disease*. From there, we look at how non-diabetic groups are using diabetes *as a metaphor*. After a dissection of diabetes-as-metaphor, we delve into social conditions of diabetes and describe *diabetes as disability*. By reimagining diabetes complexly, we then pivot to consider it as a *site of resistance*. At the conclusion of this section, we lodge an argument for using representation as a unit of analysis within this volume.

Diabetes as Disease

Diabetes, a non-apparent (often referred to as *invisible*) autoimmune and/or metabolic disease, expresses itself in multiple forms and is anything but uncommon. In the United States alone, 30.3 million people, about one out of every ten, have some form of diabetes (Centers for Disease Control and Prevention 2020). The National Institute of Diabetes and Digestive and Kidney Disease (NIDDK) defines diabetes as, "a disease that occurs when your blood glucose, also called blood sugar, is too high" (2021). This definition, published in a public online webpage addresses the reader as "you," which mimics the parlance of dichotomized clinical experiences between provider and patient. Not only is the provider-patient relationship hierarchical, but also often laden with medical paternalism (i.e. limiting the autonomy of a person or group of people under the assumption that such limitations are in their best interest).

The NIDDK definition and article, then, reinforce the power dynamics and assumed authority typical in such clinical relationships. The NIDDK elaborates by explaining that,

> Blood glucose is your main source of energy and comes from the food you eat. Insulin, a hormone made by the pancreas, helps glucose from food get into your cells to be used for energy. Sometimes your body doesn't make enough—or any—insulin or doesn't use insulin well. Glucose then stays in your blood and doesn't reach your cells.

Here, NIDDK uses the second-person pronouns, "you" and "your" to differentiate a diabetic body (presumably the reader) from the author through to the omission of first-person pronouns (i.e. "our" or "we"). Thus, while NIDDK's second-person definition describes the body's ability to produce or use insulin as characteristic of diabetes, it also instigates Othering by setting up the reader, the "you," as something identifiable and not species typical.

Characteristic of the groupings legitimized by the wider medical establishment in the United States, NIDDK then describes various sub-groups within the diabetic population. NIDDK's webpage goes on to explain the typography of diabetes, denoting bio-medical differences in the bodies of people with varying diabetes types (i.e. Type 1 diabetes, Type 2 diabetes, gestational, latent autoimmune diabetes in adults (LADA), prediabetes, maturity onset diabetes of the young (MODY), steroid-induced diabetes, and many more). NIDDK's sub-grouping differentiates diabetes types by diagnoses processes, called "onset," by required treatment varieties like oral medical and insulin, and by symptomology—a contrast to the monolithic portrait of diabetes just prior.

These subgroupings do not negate what people with all diabetes types share in common, but they do impose categorical identifiers based solely on the diagnosis. While bio-medical definitions like the one offered by the NIDDK are useful for laying out the nuts and bolts of *impairment* (a term disability scholars use to refer to bodily difference), they do not capture the lived experience of navigating the social world with a diabetic bodymind. The absence of social aspects within NIDDK's definition reveal a *medical model* view of diabetes. The *medical model of disability* in Western culture frames bodily difference as a problem that requires medical intervention and/or a cure. From the perspective of the medical model, the body has a problem producing or using insulin. Further, the medical model suggests the only solution to the problem is the individual who complies with the directives of Western medicine.

Diabetes as Metaphor

The public often uses the materiality of diabetes—that is, the physical symptomology occurring within the diabetic body—as a metaphor. In their exploration of metaphor, linguists George Lakoff and Mark Johnson found that people use metaphors as tools to take concrete experience and make abstract ideas more concrete (1980). Lakoff and Johnson warn readers that such borrowing often relies on assumptions about the concrete experience while shaping ideas about the abstract one (ex: saying you are "buying time" re-enforces capitalistic notions about the positive value of consumerism when metaphorically expressing that you need more time). Additionally, Lakoff and Johnson note that while metaphors reenforce the similarities between the more concrete ("buying") and the abstract ("time"), metaphors can conceal meaningful differences.

One place where groups rely on a set of beliefs about diabetes to shape a more abstract concept occurs when groups aim to legitimize the materiality of psychiatric disabilities. Relying on the notion that a reasonable person takes diabetes seriously and would never blame a diabetic person for the body's need for insulin, the 2018 Alcoholics Anonymous (AA) Message of Hope resource states:

> Fundamentally, alcoholism is a health problem—a physical and emotional disease—rather than a question of too little willpower or of moral weakness. Just as there is no point blaming the victim of diabetes for a lack of willpower in becoming ill, it is useless to charge the problem drinker with responsibility for the illness or to regard such drinking as a vice. (2021)

AA draws two parallels between diabetes and alcoholism. First, they draw a similarity in unfair stigma. That is, AA implies that outsiders unfairly blame both alcoholic and diabetic people for their health condition. Outsiders accuse both groups of lacking the moral character to maintain self-control and practice willpower. Secondly, to combat this blame, AA locates both diabetes and alcoholism as physical illnesses and as such, the person does not deserve scorn. The way AA positions alcoholism in relation to diabetes makes use of the cultural imagination. In other words, they play on a set of assumptions about diabetes to de-stigmatize alcoholism. Ironically, the use of this metaphor relying on one assumption does not acknowledge the immense stigma that diabetic people do experience.

Lawyers and rights-activists' groups also play on the cultural imagination arguing for the law to protect addiction as a disability under the Americans with Disabilities Act (ADA). The ADA National Network 2019 resource guide called, *The ADA, Addiction and Recovery*, uses vignettes and metaphorical thinking to make sense of evolving legislative policies. In one vignette, the fictitious character Tom takes a drug called Suboxone to aid in his recovery from an opioid addiction. When explaining why Tom would be protected under the ADA, the resource guide states, "Suboxone is a legally prescribed medication to help Tom function just like insulin is prescribed for the health and function of a person with diabetes. Tom's use of Suboxone cannot, by itself, justify a refusal to let Tom see his children on the weekend" (2019). Again, this guide references diabetes as an analogy for legitimizing addiction as a physical, material, illness caused by an imbalance within the body.

The problem with the AA and the ADA using diabetes as a metaphor lies not in the linkage between the two, but rather the set of assumptions that give the metaphors their meaning. The analogy assumes that doctors unreservedly prescribe insulin where needed without blame or shaming a patient, an idea that authors in this collection contest. The metaphor also hides the social realities of having diabetes in the United States. For example, as several authors will discuss in impending chapters, many diabetic people cannot access the insulin they need due to price gouging in the U.S. Also, as of 2017, judges are hearing cases from employers contesting the legitimacy of diabetes as a disability, despite historical inclusion under the ADA (Robertson 2017). Thus, tending to diabetes as a metaphor requires us to tease out the beliefs taken as concrete.

Diabetes as Disability

Legally in the United States, disability constitutes a protected class under the Americans with Disabilities Act (ADA), which passed into law in 1990. The ADA is an equal opportunity federal civil rights law that prohibits discrimination on the basis of disability and was modeled after similar legislation that passed in 1964 and 1973. Section 504 of the Rehabilitation Act of 1973 extended protections to those with diabetes using a medicalized narrative similar to NIDDK's definition. As advocates from the American Diabetes Association have argued in legislation, the Rehabilitation Act *implicitly* includes diabetes because diabetes impairs and substantially limits "the functioning of major bodily systems such as the endocrine system. Diabetes, by its very definition, limits the functioning of the endocrine system" (Association 2021). Perhaps because diabetes is not explicitly included in the ADA legislation, its legitimacy as a disability has been questioned in US courts. However, we also argue that the medical establishment and its pervasive influence over the cultural imagination also play a role.

Despite its implicit inclusion in the formidable ADA legislation, few in the medical profession consider diabetes a disability. Similarly, disability activism and scholarship have not often included diabetes, and thus have been left relatively untheorized. The broad lack of conceptualizing diabetes as disability partially stems from the episodic nature of diabetes—meaning that diabetes comes with fluctuations in health and medical institutions describe the impact of diabetes as reliant upon individual self-care and self-management (Boyd 2012). We argue, that by looking at diabetes as a disability, we generate entry points for theorizing diabetes experiences, identity, and embodiment.

As evidenced by the initial story in this introduction, we refer to the impulse for people to theorize diabetes as a disability as an increasing ***disability consciousness***. Disability studies and bioethics scholar Rosemarie Garland Thomson describes a "disability consciousness" as a growing awareness of the "history, culture, and politics of disability" (2019, 6). Garland-Thomson notes that in her own story her physical impairments had not changed, but her sense of community, identity, and activism ignited her disability consciousness. Investigating diabetes as a disability stems from community members and scholars resisting minimizing or medicalizing their lived experiences with diabetes, as well as from the increase in activism against unaffordable insulin and medical racism. We introduce disability consciousness here as an intervention and as an argument for using representation as a guiding unit of analysis for every chapter within this volume.

Looking at diabetes as disability calls for us to reimagine two main areas. First, theorizing diabetes as disability allows us to embrace disability notions of embodiment, care, and cure. For example, disability studies studies scholar Margaret Price popularized the term "bodymind" to describe how the mental, emotional, and physical are inextricably intertwined and never experienced in isolation (2015). Using Price's framework to formulate ***diabetic bodyminds*** de-medicalizes diabetes and resists the notion that diabetes constitutes a discrete, compartmentalized aspect of one's being.

Secondly, theorizing diabetes as disability calls us to critically situate the lived experiences of diabetes as an impairment against the disabling socio-political and cultural representations that sustain it as stigmatized and spoiled identity. Thinking through depictions of diabetes in and as disability invites readers to consider ableism as a dynamic in these representations. As authors in this collection analyze representations of diabetes in U.S. culture, politics, and society, they point to instruments of ableism and stigma at play in stereotypical ideas about diabetes. In so doing, our authors and this volume as a whole identifies ableism as a force of oppression operating at individual, social, cultural, and political levels.

Bringing together these two main areas of embodiment and social conditions, we can align with the language and tools from the disability justice movement to look back at this community. Queer, crip, BIPOC performance group Sins Invalid articulated ten principles of Disability Justice (Berne et al. 2018). Principles include intersectionality, leadership of the most impacted, anti-capitalist politic, commitment to cross-movement organizing, recognizing wholeness, sustainability, commitment to cross-disability solidarity, interdependence, collective access, and collective liberation. While the disability rights movement produced key legislation like the ADA, the disability justice movement brings forth essential tenets that benefit diabetes communities. For example, an anti-capitalist stance aligns with diabetes communities concerns with insulin price gouging, while intersectionality means a critical intervention in the over-representation of white diabetic people in major advocacy organizations.

Chapters in this volume use disability studies frameworks such as these to contend with ableism-based oppression in structures ranging from healthcare to internet algorithms, interpersonal microaggressions and relationship dynamics, and internalized shame and disgust by non-diabetics and diabetics alike. And by doing so, we debate how and where societal conditions and constructions create disablement for diabetic people. And we continue to question everything. How does the pressure to pass or cover diabetes as disability impact identification as a unified minority group? How do media, television, and film representations of diabetes perpetuate pervasive stereotypes of diabetes as a lifestyle disease? And what does complex embodiment, "which theorizes the body and its representations as mutually transformative," look like and require in the context of diabetes (Siebers 2010, 284)? When we look at diabetes as a complexly embodied disability, we gain the tools used by disability studies scholars to analyze both apparent and non-apparent disabilities. By deploying disability studies frameworks and principals from disability justice and analytical tools against stereotypical representations of diabetes, we poke holes and call out the racist, ableist, and ageist assumptions built into them. In other words, we weaken stereotypes by challenging their stigmatizing oppressive roots.

Diabetes as a Site of Resistance

Defining diabetes as a *site of resistance* requires that we highlight the narratives diabetic people use to describe themselves. Often, these narratives work to counter diabetes stigma and stereotypes. Diabetes as a site of resistance encapsulates the socio-political conditions of diabetes that medical definitions miss while elevating the way diabetic people portray themselves. It includes the representational strategies individuals use to protest the way diabetes is talked about by their friends and family. It includes the counternarratives diabetic people deploy, whether directed toward the public or within diabetes communities.

And notably, defining diabetes as a site of resistance includes community and scholarly efforts to transform the structural inequalities and discrimination that maintain stereotypical formulations of diabetes. For example, in 2006, writer and medical ethicist Harriet Washington coined the term *medical apartheid* to contextualize racialized interpretations of data, such as higher incidence of diabetes in marginalized communities (2006). Washington demonstrates how these rates are not evidence of recklessness or laziness on the part of marginalized groups, but rather of centuries of racism and inequity in medicine, healthcare, housing, food access, and situational stress. Washington's terminology resists and disrupts stereotypical formulations of diabetes and effectively positions that resistance as a political act. That is, by linking to areas of structural inequality reproducing the incidence of diabetes in certain minority groups, Washington pivots away from the conception of diabetes as an individual problem and toward it as a social one.

Similar to scholarship exploring disability identity in autistic and D/deaf communities, the acts of resistance described by authors in this book sometimes point in opposing directions. Most notably, representational strategies can be counter-productive for the wider diabetic population and can cause splintering into sub-groups based on diagnosis. For example, many with Type 1 diabetes urgently push against stigmatizing representations of diabetes in media and entertainment; however, they employ the strategy of defensive othering. Sociologist Matthew B. Ezzell defines defensive othering as, "subordinates distancing themselves from other subordinates and reinforcing the legitimacy of a devalued identity in the process" (2009). For the Type 1 diabetes community, this often looks like telling others how incorrect and unfair representations of diabetes are that depict diabetes as the result of eating too much sugar. They claim these stereotypes are not true for *them*, insinuating that they are true for *those other* diabetics, referring to those with Type 2. As many will argue in this book, defensive othering is a highly problematic representational strategy. Considering how frequently it is deployed, however, we must invest time and space to interrogate the motivations behind its use. In so doing, authors identify opposing or alternative strategies with less problematic effects.

Examining diabetes as a site of resistance takes on terrifying urgency during the COVID-19 pandemic. The COVID-19 pandemic confirmed that the public conceives of the broad category of diabetic people as altogether undeserving of resources regardless of type. In online contexts, diabetic people noted a lack of empathy for those infected with COVID. Tracey Berg-Fulton (@BergFulton, 2020), an engineer with diabetes, shared on Twitter:

> If I die from COVID, you'll blame it on my T1 diabetes. You'll wave me off because 'underlying conditions' make my death palatable, expected, predictable. I should have been 'healthier' 'tried harder.' Will you even feel for my family? Or am I an acceptable loss b/c I'm 'sick.'

As the conversation moved from COVID infections to vaccine distribution, members of the Type 1 community advocated for Type 1 to be prioritized alongside Type 2 diabetics for vaccination. Their representational strategy, here, suggests that when the urgency is there, Type 1 groups will advocate to be recognized as a part of the wider diabetic population, forgoing a strategy of defensive othering.

Authors cover a range of perspectives here: from writing about specific types of diabetes to focusing on the shared struggle of being judged for every micro-decision involved in diabetic life. Resistance brings together people with different types of diabetes and looking at resistance illuminates responses to oppressive forces. According to disability studies scholars Susan Gabel and Susan Peters, "Resistance is inherently political but because it accommodates diverse stakeholders in fluid coalitions and assumes that they can co-resist oppression, its processes can inclusively unite across paradigmatic boundaries. Furthermore, resistance theory acknowledges the social forces opposing disabled people (also resistant processes) and illuminates responses to these forces." Defining diabetes as a site of resistance, then, necessitates we move beyond identifying stereotypes and toward what various stakeholders do to dismantle them. Several essays within the collection discuss how particular acts of resistance, activism, and advocacy have changed the social landscape of diabetes.

Representations of Diabetes

In his counsel to a group of actors, Hamlet declares the purpose of "playing" is to "mirror up to nature," meaning to accurately represent a story so the audience might see themselves in it (and their guilty actions). German playwright, director, and theater theorist Bertolt Brecht pushed back on Hamlet's belief about the role of art in society, writing: "Art is not a mirror to reflect reality, but a hammer with which to shape it." According to Brecht then, representations have the power to reflect and shape reality, and to help audiences see themselves and the world in new ways. Art, in this way, is generative. Disability activists and scholars use a similarly generative approach when they identify as *crip* (abbreviated from cripple) and utilize *crip theory*. By claiming these identities, they complicate any efforts to be normal and be ruled by dominant ideas about how bodies be and exist in the social world. In resisting the normative, taking a hammer and smashing the oppression that comes with ableism and its bias against diabetes, Gloria Anzadúa tells readers the new consciousness that must emerge: "Nothing happens in the 'real world' unless it first happens in the images in our heads" (1987, 87). While some representations reflect the status quo and the past, others explored in this volume may open readers to a disability consciousness and new visions for living in and reading the diabetic bodymind.

In this volume, multi-disciplinary contributors use disability studies as their lens to analyze representations of diabetes. Disciplines throughout wider fields like the humanities and social sciences contain multiple theories, processes of analysis, and methods of engaging with representation. Thus, this book collectively offers a broad range of representations as objects of study. With that said, for the collection as a whole, we theorize *representations* as objects in public view, marked as relating to diabetes in some way, and imbued with assumptions so much that it does not fully explain itself. Representation relies on the viewer to already have some idea and meaning tied to the object. This means that when describing and analyzing representation in their respective chapters, authors draw out the unspoken assumptions and pull apart the pieces of a given representation and its messaging.

When identifying various representations, our goal is not to point at some representations and identify them as good, and others as bad. In her work on disability and representation, Carrie Sandahl advocates for analyzing disability representations as "representational conundrums." By aiming our analysis toward conundrum, we can open ourselves up to wrestle with the "challenging, puzzling, or paradoxical issues that are unique to or complicated by disability's presence" (2018, 130–131). Using Sandahl's approach as a guiding principle, our authors attend to the complexities of diabetes representations, rather than naming a list of do's and don'ts. Take, for example, hypoglycemia. Film scholars and community members have critiqued scenes showing hypoglycemia as being melodramatic and sensationalized for the sake of the nondisabled viewer. However, writers in this volume complicate scenes of hypoglycemia in film by looking at them within real-life contexts. For example, one author describes using a scene of hypoglycemia in film as a complex way to "come out" to their friends or family, while another appreciates the suspense of their lived experience, and a third investigates interdependence. Authors are not unified in their critiques of their objects of study, but they consistently reject common tropes of pity, charity, patronizing, or overcoming narratives. Such refusals are hallmarks of disability studies frameworks.

Situating this Volume in Disability Studies

(Un)doing Diabetes is the first collection of essays using disability studies theories and frameworks to explore representations of diabetes across a wide range of mediums- from Twitter to TV and film, to theater, fiction, fanfiction, fashion and more. How might people understand representations of diabetes when they encounter them in culture, politics, and society, if they did so with disability consciousness? A disability studies approach to diabetes locates an individual's experiences of diabetes within historical and contemporary social conditions. Using disability studies also requires greater care and attention of the diabetic bodymind. Readers are invited to begin understanding representations of diabetes as a disability, tending to the diabetic bodymind as an embodied physical, mental, and

emotional social identity with interpersonal and socio-political consequences.

Within disability studies literature, this collection engages crip theory by "cripping" diabetes. *Cripping*, according to disability and performance scholar, Carrie Sandahl, is a kind of critique used by academics and activists to "spin mainstream representations or practices to reveal able-bodied assumptions and exclusionary effects" (2003, 37). Sandahl advocates for reclaiming "crip" from the historically derogatory "cripple" similar to queer studies and activism. Sandahl articulated "cripdom" as a "radical stance toward concepts of normalcy" (2003). Robert McRuer further developed this framework into *crip theory*, encouraging disability scholars and activists to resist compulsory normalcy and instead to experiment with the potential to offend, to politicize, and to generate pride (2006). This volume *crips* diabetes by exposing traditional and unquestioned conceptions of diabetes permeating the medical and social science literature to theories that liberate the body, complicate meanings, and deconstruct ideologies that maintain the status quo of diabetes perceptions, care, politics, and practice. Thus, *cripping diabetes* allows us to shift the landscape of diabetes scholarship to reflect more radical, political, and empowered views.

This book also brings diabetes into conversation with the burgeoning area of research around chronic illness and non-apparent disabilities—effectively filling a gap noticed by scholars in the field. Alison Kafer confirmed in her text *Feminist, Queer, Crip* (2013) that while several writers, including Susan Wendell, Ellen Samuels, and Margaret Price, have examined chronic illnesses such as chronic fatigue syndrome and psychiatric disability, conditions like diabetes remain unexamined. While Kafer highlights the lack of literature about diabetes in disability studies, critical diabetes research has emerged from other fields such as Medical Anthropology, Communication, and English.

This collection of interdisciplinary essays features scholarship commissioned exclusively for this volume from both leading scholars and emerging voices in the study of social, political, and cultural conditions of diabetes. Our authors use principles of disability justice, feminist critiques, and critical race theories in a way that benefit the study of diabetes and also the theories themselves. Perspectives from fat studies also inform discussions of food justice, medical racism, and embodiment. As it stands now, diabetes scholarship remains medicalized and hyper-focused on individual willpower and symptom management. By including current and historical accounts of community efforts to create change to those representations, this book will enter diabetes activism into the historiographical record as a part of disability rights activism and disability justice in a moment of critical change for diabetes communities. As a collection, this volume will take on existing paradigms and offer new ones more focused on intersectional diabetes experiences and disability justice.

To that end, our collection adds to the growing literature exploring the racialized history of diabetes (Hatch 2016; Tuchman 2020; Washington 2006). We extend this work unpacking the problematic history of diabetes and white supremacy in the U.S. through the lens of ableism. The field of disability studies has made efforts to de-center the white, disabled experience with critical works such as Christopher M. Bell's pivotal anthology, *Blackness and Disability: Critical Examinations and Cultural Interventions.* Bell's work challenged historical segmentation in disability studies scholarship bringing to light issues of marginalization based on race and ethnicity (2011). *(Un)doing Diabetes* furthers Bell and others' important expansions by addressing the role of race and representations of diabetes. Another consideration in the field is the move beyond disability rights toward disability justice, which holds intersectionality as a primary value; our collection applies that lens to diabetes.

This volume arrives at a moment when crip identity and disability consciousness are rising and thanks in large part to the dissemination of information and resources online, there is now an upswell of understanding of how ableism and racism shape diabetic bodyminds. Now, more than ever, diabetic people are linking their experiences with diabetes to mental health (Fergie et al. 2016). Furthermore, the insulin crisis has created cross-disability solidarity within diabetes communities while increasing the political and historical conversations about causes of disability and access to resources. We offer this book up now as diabetics in the United States are dying due to insulin unaffordability, as politicians villainize people with diabetes under the pretense of rising health care costs, and as television and film continue to riff off of stigmatized representations of diabetes as a lifestyle disease. Each essay within this book calls attention to the devastating consequences of unchecked diabetes stigma and stereotypes in real-life situations.

Part 1, "Social Media, Social Worlds & Activism," includes authors that evaluate representations of diabetes activism in online spaces. In part 2, "Film, Television, Visual Art, and Performance," essays interrogate examples of art and entertainment in order to challenge common representations of diabetes. The contributors to part 3, "Staring, Coding, and

Reading the Diabetic Body," take up questions of race, gender, and class and how disability troubles these boundaries. Part 4, "Re-Scripting and Resisting Spoiled Identities," features writers who contest representations of diabetes that use stigma and shame as strategies to impose normalcy on diabetic bodies. And finally, part 5, "Disability Identity, Crip Futures and Liberation," explores the role of disability identity for diabetic people across a variety of contexts including online, diabetes camp, and advocacy work. At the start of each section, we provide an overview of the chapters within it, overlapping themes, and guiding questions.

References

Anonymous, Alcoholics. 2021. Is There an Alcoholic in Your Life? A.A.'s Message of Hope. https://www.aa.org/assets/en_US/p-30_isthereanalcoinyourlife.pdf.

Anzaldúa, Gloria. 1987. *Borderlands/La Frontera: The New Mestiza*. 1st ed. San Francisco: Spinsters/Aunt Lute.

Association, American Diabetes. 2021. Section 504 of the Rehabilitation Act of 1973. https://www.diabetes.org/resources/know-your-rights/section-504-rehabilitation-act-1973.

Bell, Christopher M. 2011. *Blackness and Disability: Critical Examinations and Cultural Interventions*. Vol. 21 *Forecaast*. East Lansing: Michigan State University Press.

Berg-Fulton, Tracey (@BergFulton). 2020. If I die from COVID.... Tweet, 8/16/20.

Berne, Patricia, Aurora Levins Morales, and David Langstaff. 2018. Ten Principles of Disability Justice. *WSQ: Women's Studies Quarterly* 46 (1): 227–230. https://muse.jhu.edu/article/690824.

Bock, Sheila. 2015. "Grappling to Think Clearly": Vernacular Theorizing in Robbie McCauley's Sugar. *Journal of Medical Humanities* 36 (2): 127–139. https://doi.org/10.1007/s10912-015-9326-8. https://www.ncbi.nlm.nih.gov/pubmed/25605651.

Boyd, Vic. 2012. Are Some Disabilities More Equal Than Others? Conceptualising Fluctuating or Recurring Impairments Within Contemporary Legislation and Practice. *Disability & Society* 27 (4): 459–469. https://doi.org/10.1080/09687599.2012.662828. https://www.tandfonline.com/doi/abs/10.1080/09687599.2012.662828.

Centers for Disease Control and Prevention, CDC. 2020. *National Diabetes Statistics Report, 2020: Estimates of Diabetes and Its Burden in the United States*. https://www.cdc.gov/diabetes/data/statistics-report/index.html.

Ezzell, Matthew B. 2009. "Barbie Dolls" on the Pitch: Identity Work, Defensive Othering, and Inequality in Women's Rugby—University of Illinois at Chicago Library. *Social Problems* 56 (1): 111–131. https://i-share-uic.primo.exlibrisgroup.com.

Fergie, G., K. Hunt, and S. Hilton. 2016. Social Media as a Space for Support: Young Adults' Perspectives on Producing and Consuming User-generated Content about Diabetes and Mental Health. *Soc Sci Med* 170: 46–54. https://doi.org/10.1016/j.socscimed.2016.10.006.

Garland-Thomson, Rosemarie. 2019. Becoming Disabled. In *About Us: Essays from the Disability Series of the New York times*, ed. Peter Catapano, Rosemarie Garland-Thomson, and Andrew Solomon, 1st ed. New York, NY: Liveright Publishing Corporation, a division of W.W. Norton & Company.

Hatch, Anthony Ryan. 2016. *Blood Sugar: Racial Pharmacology and Food Justice in Black America*. Minneapolis: University of Minnesota Press.

Kafer, Alison. 2013. *Feminist, Queer, Crip*. Bloomington, Indiana: Indiana University Press.

Lakoff, George, and Mark Johnson. 1980. *Metaphors We Live By*. Chicago: University of Chicago Press.

Lewis, Talila A. 2021. Ableism 2020: An Updated Definition. http://www.talila-lewis.com/1/post/2020/01/ableism-2020-an-updated-definition.html.

McRuer, Robert. 2006. *Crip Theory: Cultural Signs of Queerness and Disability. Cultural Front*. New York: New York University Press.

Network, A. D. A. National. 2019. The ADA, Addiction and Recovery. https://adata.org/factsheet/ada-addiction-and-recovery.

NIDDK. 2021. Diabetes. https://www.ncbi.nlm.nih.gov/pubmed/.

Price, Margaret. 2015. The Bodymind Problem and the Possibilities of Pain. *Hypatia* 30 (1): 268–284.

Robertson, Marjory D. 2017. Diabetes Not a Disability under the ADA?. Sun Life Financial Inc. https://www.lexology.com/library/detail.aspx?g=a4c7ab08-ba0f-45e4-9643-a2fe247ecf34.

Sandahl, Carrie. 2003. Queering the Crip or Cripping the Queer?: Intersections of Queer and Crip Identities in Solo Autobiographical Performance. *GLQ: A Journal of Lesbian and Gay Studies* 9 (1–2): 25–56. https://muse.jhu.edu/article/40804.

———. 2018. Using Our Words: Exploring Representational Conundrums in Disability Drama and Performance. *Journal of Literary & Cultural Disability Studies* 12 (2): 129–144. https://muse.jhu.edu/article/694071.

Siebers, Tobin. 2010. Disability and the Theory of Complex Embodiment—For Identity Politics in a New Register. In *The Disability Studies Reader*, ed. Lennard J. Davis, vol. xiii, 653. New York: Routledge.

Tuchman, Arleen Marcia. 2020. *Diabetes: A History of Race and Disease*. New Haven: Yale University Press.

Washington, Harriet A. 2006. *Medical Apartheid: The Dark History of Medical Experimentation on Black Americans from Colonial Times to the Present*. 1st ed. New York: Doubleday.

PART I

Social Media, Social Worlds & Activism

This book, in its entirety, serves as a counter theory to challenge dominant ideas and theoretical considerations of diabetes in the cultural imagination. Thus, to open the book, Part I: Social Media, Social Worlds, and Activism focuses on the representational strategies diabetic people use to change the social, political, and cultural landscape of diabetes. In these four chapters, Jeffrey Bennet, Lora Arduser, Valentina Sturiale, Guido Anselmi, and Clair Irwin describe the shifting tone and performance of activism in online diabetes groups. From a first-hand account to an empirical study of Twitter data, these chapters delve into the efforts, motivations, and impacts of diabetes activists. They describe the lived experience of diabetes as inherently political. Collectively, these chapters articulate the urgency for change, most notably evidenced by the insulin crisis in the United States.

In the first chapter, "Diabetes Twitter: A Communal Retort to Capitalism," author Jeffrey Bennet describes the rhetorical dynamics diabetes activists use on Diabetes Twitter to shift public thinking. Bennet argues that activists on Diabetes Twitter use the platform to center capitalism and oppressive capitalist structures as the generators of harm to diabetic people. Bennett describes and questions how generative this approach might be, ultimately arguing that their activism "will remain a source of anger and moral righteousness in the face of a system that has little regard for the lives of people living with this most precarious of diseases." Where Bennett's chapter presents a focused and relatively unified activist message, the next chapter details an intra-community conflict in these online advocacy spaces.

Lora Arduser in "What's in a Name? The Diabetes Civil War," explores the narrative conflict between Type 1 and Type 2 diabetics evident in online fora, online newspaper comments, and a Change.org petition. Arduser's chapter dissects classifications of diabetes and how diabetic people (particularly Type 1) have utilized knowledges of typography to convey expertise of medical knowledge. In other words, Arduser illuminates the representational strategy of using scientific and medical knowledge to demonstrate credibility and identify as an *expert patient*. After establishing use of medical knowledge as a representational strategy, she problematizes it when deployed as an act of defensive othering. As Bennett and Arduser's chapters talk about rhetorics and social dynamics of diabetes online communities more broadly, Clair Irwin and Valentina Sturiale and Guido Anselmi's chapters directly explore the #insulin4all social movement unfolding since early 2014.

In the chapter, "The #insulin4all Movement: A Few Committed Individuals Isn't Enough," activist scholar Clair Irwin details a first-hand auto-historiographical account of the movement from within. As a #insulin4all chapter leader, Irwin breaks down how diabetes activists borrowed representational strategies from AIDS activists of ACT UP. Irwin complicates the story of #insulin4all and their approach to activism by outlining how the supercrip narrative of disability underlays internal group dynamics. To conclude her chapter, Irwin offers suggestions for how #insulin4all as a movement might shift and re-tool group dynamics.

In the final chapter in this section, Valentina Sturiale and Guido Anselmi's piece entitled "One or Many Voices, Narratives from #insulin4all" takes an empirical turn toward existing activist strategies. They analyze longitudinal Twitter content and news media coverage of the insulin crisis to argue that diabetic activists use personal story as a representational strategy to shift the blame for diabetes burden onto systems rather than individuals.

Together, four central questions guide the works in part one. Readers can expect chapters in this section to draw out tensions and frictions in their answers.

- How are activists and activist groups using representational strategies to shift public thinking and discourse around diabetes?
- How does *empowered consciousness* operate in diabetic activist groups?

- What can relocating the problem of diabetes from individual bodyminds to structural apparatuses do to the cultural imagination of diabetes?
- What does it mean to be diabetic in an unchanging ecosystem perpetuating diabetes as a simple, blameworthy, lifestyle disease?

Diabetes Twitter: A Communal Retort to Capitalism

Jeffrey A. Bennett

Laura Marston is perhaps the most vocal and prominent advocate for people living with Type 1 diabetes on Twitter. Marston was diagnosed with the disease when she was a teenager in 1996. She routinely tells her social media followers that the insulin she first used to manage the condition—Humulin—cost a mere $10 a month. Like many people with diabetes in the United States, Marston was later switched to the fast-acting insulin Humalog, which was more expensive ($21) but still affordable so long as she had health insurance. But in 2012 Marston lost her job, leaving her to pay for an expensive insurance plan out of pocket that still required her to doll out hundreds of dollars a month for insulin.[1] By that time the price of

[1] Carolyn Johnson, "Why Treating Diabetes Keeps Getting More Expensive," *Washington Post*, October 31, 2016.

J. A. Bennett (✉)
Department of Communication Studies, Vanderbilt University,
Nashville, TN, USA
e-mail: jeff.bennett@vanderbilt.edu

B. C. Frazer, H. R. Walker (eds.), *(Un)doing Diabetes: Representation, Disability, Culture*, Palgrave Studies in Science and Popular Culture, https://doi.org/10.1007/978-3-030-83110-3_2

the medicine had skyrocketed even though no significant change to its formula had been developed by the industry. This specious pharmaceutical malpractice that creates a zero-sum choice between life and death for people with diabetes weighed heavily on Marston's well-being. She has sold all of her possessions at least twice and at one point even had to give away her dog, Nicky, to make ends meet.[2] For all these reasons and more, Marston has said that "The price of insulin radicalized me."[3] Her story is all too familiar to people living with diabetes who are left at the mercy of opportunistic corporations that privilege profits and stock holders over patients and access to care.

Marston's social media feed reveals a deep-seeded devotion to making the world a more equitable place for people living with diabetes. As I write this in fall 2020, a year that has been as volatile as it has been long, it is hard not to note the intense focus Marston gives to the price of insulin in the face of so many pressing social issues. While making some reference to world events, and a few welcome appearances by her cat Bear, Marston's Twitter presence is dedicated almost entirely to raising awareness about pharmaceutical price gouging and the complications that stem from diabetes in a capitalist system. Any discussion of diabetes in the United States inevitably circles back to the exorbitant and immoral price of insulin, which can sometimes cost over a $1000 a month. This fact is especially noxious when we consider that the patent for the medicine was sold to Eli Lilly for only $3 so that patients could purchase it.[4] The urgency provoked by this disaster capitalism has even led Marston and others to help facilitate the distribution of donated insulin to people in need, as was the case after the massive fires that swept the U.S.'s West Coast in 2020. Like many on Twitter eager to raise awareness of diabetes risks, Marston retweets posts that shed light on the dangers posed to people with diabetes when they are hospitalized and staff are uneducated about insulin dosing. She relays the threats posed by police who mistake hypoglycemia for intoxication and points out the complications that often arise from the shortcomings of diabetes technologies. But it is Marston's intense focus on prices, capitalism, and the mendacity of the drug industry that dominates her timeline.

[2] Ritu Prasad, "The Human Cost of Insulin in America," *BBC News*, March 14, 2019.

[3] Laura Marston, May 17, 2020, https://twitter.com/Kidfears99.

[4] Michael Bliss, *The Discovery of Insulin* (Chicago: University of Chicago Press, 2013), p. 178.

In this chapter I engage the rhetorical dynamics of the collective colloquially known as "Diabetes Twitter" to ascertain the ways they use the platform to intervene in, and reshape, conversations about the disease. In particular, I focus on how these communities perform a vernacular intervention into exchanges about capitalism that have grown more intense and visible as the cost of insulin has continued to soar. Pharmaceutical companies have raised the price of insulin for decades without fear of reappraisal. All the while, people with diabetes have continually attempted to intercede in these duplicitous practices to combat the mystification perpetuated by a system that constantly works against them. Social media users spotlight and rebuff the tight associations among lobbyists, nonprofits, and politicians, arguing that the conventional ways of doing business actively endanger their lives. Rather than be trapped by a discourse that reiterates the familiar refrain that prices are going up and lives are being lost, those living with the condition, and their loved ones, give prominence to the matrix of capitalist forces destroying their longevity. In doing so, diabetes advocates incrementally move the language of management away from individual scripts of self-care and reliance and toward systemic critiques that highlight the precariousness of living with the disease. Rather than be gaslighted into believing that high prices will produce newer and better innovations, these critics emphatically implore industry executives and political operatives to remedy the manufactured crisis wreaking havoc on their community.

Media outlets such as *The New Republic* contend that insulin has become a metonym for the necessity of universal healthcare programs such as Medicare for All. Diabetes advocates have acted as a catalyst for this discourse by incessantly repeating arguments about cost, disseminating information about suspicious industry practices, and retorting loaded data put forth by pharmaceutical lobbyists.[5] Using their everyday experiences to craft an ethos of expertise underscored by outrage, these self-appointed authorities have propagated the mantra that insulin prices, much more than individual management, are a death sentence for those living with the condition. They marshal their experiences with diabetes to forward an array of solutions to the crisis, which range from insulin price caps to making the medication available over the counter. Here, I look to the controversies that have underlined the ascendancy of "Diabetes Twitter" to think

[5] See, for example, Natalie Shure, "How Insulin Became the Poster Child for Medicare for All," *The New Republic*, February 27, 2020.

through the possibilities and constraints of this labor in the face of industry malfeasance.

A quick caveat: I am not interested in the veracity of truth claims being made by diabetes advocates at all times. With millions of users, including thousands making arguments about the cost of insulin, there is invariably some discrepancy in the metrics being used to advance their cause (including statistical evidence about price increases). But this contestation of facts is also true when we look to the data presented by corporations eager to protect their profits. Rather, I am compelled by the form of the arguments that tend to resonate on Twitter. Subscribers to the platform fabricate a Manichean dichotomy between good and evil to enliven their cause. This narrative, when collectively assessed, ultimately calls for a complete shift in capitalistic practices that are facilitating the slow death of the population. In this way, these forumites follow the trajectory of disability movements that spotlight the political and relational forces that produce and reiterate reductive medicalized scripts about the body.[6] This analysis unfolds by looking to critiques made against pharmaceutical companies, diabetes advocacy groups, and politicians. Although any of these could merit a book-length study about the interrelationship between diabetes and capitalism, I argue that these three are central to understanding the impulses of Diabetes Twitter and the changes that collective aspires to instigate.[7]

Social Media and the Crafting of a Collective Diabetes Persona

Social media activism has been a centerpiece of debate about the role of advocacy in the public sphere for well over a decade. Academics and public intellectuals alike have pondered the degree to which participating in on-line persuasive efforts is similar to face to face or "in-the-street" activity, as well as the limits of these analogic frames. Thinkers such as Malcolm Gladwell, for example, have dismissed the potential of on-line activism, arguing that it tends to foster "weak ties" in movement organizing, rather

[6] Alison Kafrer, *Feminist, Queer, Crip* (Bloomington, IN: Indiana University Press, 2013), 4–10.

[7] I have made the choice to reproduce the tweets as they appear in their original form on Twitter. The rhetorical choices advocates make highlight variations in voice, reflect emotions otherwise lost on the medium, and sometimes signal their variable uses of the technology as a means of identification.

than "strong ties," that catalyze citizens to action. He points to the 1960s lunch counter protests as an example of these "strong ties" while remaining skeptical of home-bound participation in a cause.[8] Others, such as Henry Jenkins, have suggested that internet activism is an extension of practices that have long existed among groups of people with shared interests. He insists that we only need look to the history of resource sharing and collective intelligence among internet enclaves to find noteworthy parallels to traditional movements.[9] In my own classroom, students eagerly embrace inquiries about the degree to which expressing support from their screens is a form of "slacktivism" or an extension of moral commitments to be celebrated.

The choice between "slacktivism" and "real" activism is, to my mind, a false dichotomy that reduces complex and conflicting behaviors for purposes that occlude the varying functions of social media and the complicated identities of actors using such sites. Nonetheless, critics continue to be captivated by the implications that people might be retweeting or posting content to social media sites out of self-directed affirmation and not necessarily the public good. Social media scholar danah boyd, for example, recently asked, "What constitutes the public when we're each living in our personalized world? How do we engender public-good outcomes when our tools steer us toward individualism?"[10] boyd was engaging in dialogue with her co-authors (Mizuko Ito and Jenkins) when she posed this question. Each of them agree, to different extents, that mediums such as Twitter can be used for both egocentric purposes, as well as collective action.[11] Their consensus on this point might suggest that the idea of "public" should be pluralized, constituting not simply *a* public but *multiple* publics and variable ways of being public, sometimes simultaneously. This seems particularly true when people living with chronic conditions and disabilities utilize the internet as a space of resistance. As Heather Walker observes, being on-line has changed the fundamentals of protest by allowing greater flexibility in the construction of

[8] Malcolm Gladwell, "Small Change: Why the Revolution will not be Tweeted," *The New Yorker*, October 4, 2010.

[9] Henry Jenkins, Joshua Green, and Sam Ford *Spreadable Media: Creating Value and Meaning in a Networked Culture* (New York: NYU Press, 2013), 30.

[10] In Henry Jenkins, Mizuko Ito, and dana boyd, *Participatory Culture in a Networked Era* (Cambridge: Polity Press, 2016), 28.

[11] Ibid., 28–30.

identities but also decreasing the risks typically associated with conventional demonstrations.[12]

Jenkins contends that the medium demarcating political communities is less important than mutual practices of identity formation, such as the collective ownership of stories and the development of sharing economies.[13] The narratives embraced to constitute communal identities, for example, are not exclusive to face-to-face communicators and illustrate both the strategic uptake of identification by on-line cohorts and the tactical use of these assemblages in situ. Diabetes Twitter has adopted many of these precepts to forge a social media presence. The story about the sale of insulin's patent, for instance, is a staple of on-line storytelling and one that has not been easily manipulated by pharmaceutical companies. The commonalities expressed among people with Type 1 diabetes on the social media platform, be it with their origin stories, their experiences with the high cost of insulin, or their cantankerous relationship with big pharma, help to cement a collective identity.

These community collaborations echo the ways people with disabilities have seized opportunities brought by technological shifts to intervene in the social world. Such developments have often been accompanied by political, legal, and social challenges but have also illustrated the variable identities assembled under the broad rubric of "disability" and the divergent ways access might be understood.[14] Katie Ellis and Mike Kent argue that technological engagement has redefined concepts such as the "social model of disability," which casts disability as a product of the environment and not simply a medicalized projection of the body. "The production of disability," they assert, "is a dynamic process that is shaped by technology, culture, and the underpinning moral order" and these practices and ideas are not easily captured by a singular theoretical heuristic.[15] Alison Kafer likewise contends that, "What we understand as impairing conditions—socially, physically, mentally, or otherwise—shifts across time and place,

[12] Heather Walker, "#CripTheVote: How Disabled Activists Used Twitter for Political Engagement During the 2016 Presidential Election," *Participations: Journal of Audience and Perception Studies* 17 (2020): 147–171.

[13] Ibid., 28.

[14] Katie Ellis and Mike Kent, *Disability and New Media* (New York. Routledge, 2011), 16, 94; Sarah Parsloe and Avery Holton, "#Boycottautismspeaks: Communicating a Counternarrative Through Cyberactivism and Connective Action," *Information, Communication, and Society* 21 (2018): 1116–1133.

[15] Ellis and Kent, 97.

and presenting impairment as purely physical obscures the effects of such shifts."[16] Whereas Kafer notes that more work needs to be done in the humanities to understand diseases such as diabetes as a disability, users to platforms such as Twitter use the medium to energize such identities and thereby reposition a slew of political, medical, and communal relationships.[17] They spotlight the creation and maintenance of debility as a central component of the capitalist enterprise.[18]

Twitter, in particular, lends itself to the constitution of a specific style of address and identity formation, even as it serves multiple functions not reducible to simplistic classificatory schemas. Jean Burgess and Nancy Baym observe that "Twitter remains a site of uncertainty and contestation not only over what kind of communication it should be used for, but over the purpose and value of different kinds of human communication in general."[19] The social network tends to have fewer adherents than Facebook or Instagram, though it still draws about 145 million users daily. Despite these impressive numbers, social media critics warn that the information circulating on Twitter, including its affective political attitudes and popular policy posts, do not necessarily reflect the disposition of the larger polity.[20] In some ways, Twitter might actually reflect the tendencies of older forms of organizing documented in social influence studies, wherein opinion leaders steer the direction and tenure of public conversation. In such models users in a network influence one another even when an opinion leader is not present by seeking out and distributing information that reinforces beliefs about themselves and the world they live in.

Additionally, the rhetorical stylistics of Twitter represent a defining component of its public disposition because it is enlivened by particular modes of address and interactive dynamics. These constraints, which facilitate the possibilities and limitations of user creativity, include the medium's character limit and the fabrication of resonant hashtags. In their study of Donald Trump's Twitter habits, Brian Ott and Greg Dickinson argue that the former president's obsessive use of the medium is best understood as a mechanism for developing a curated persona. Twitter enables figures such as Trump to craft a rhetorical style that privileges an

[16] Kafer, 7.

[17] Kafer, 12.

[18] Jasbir Puar, *The Right to Maim: Debility, Capacity, and Disability* (Durham: Duke University Press, 2017).

[19] Jean Burgess and Nancy Baym, *Twitter: A Biography* (New York: NYU Press, 2020), 13.

[20] Alexis Madrigal, "Twitter is not America," *The Atlantic*, April 24, 2019.

aesthetic character over a conceptual one and allows him to stress affective rather than rationally plotted thoughts.[21] It perhaps goes without saying that Trump's rhetorical style reflects some of the worst tendencies of white rage grievance politics, which has helped him amass followers and garner a constant drip of attention from U.S. media outlets. Twitter's format, demanding simplistic messages, but underscored by an impulsivity and incivility in its users, has depersonalized interactions and enabled exchanges that are not always productive, especially for the purposes of democratic deliberation and the civic good.

Whereas Ott and Dickinson study the rhetorically-crafted persona of a notorious politician to note the drawbacks of the medium, I ponder the extent to which a collective persona can be cultivated among a multitude of users to redirect conversations about a social issue such as healthcare. Does the simplicity of message construction that is so harmful to some portions of our democratic culture serve an important function when contemplating the bureaucratic red tape erected around pharmaceutical corporations that engage in price gouging? Advocates on Twitter turn to the platform for a variety of reasons but I will contain my analysis to three topics that appear frequently in their rhetoric: First, these social media monitors openly retort the pharmaceutical industry for the high price of insulin and the outlandish cost of diabetes technology. Second, they lobby politicians on the state and national level to make insulin more affordable. Third, they critique diabetes organizations such as the American Diabetes Association (ADA) and the JDRF (formerly the Juvenile Diabetes Research Foundation) for being too closely aligned with insulin manufacturers. After examining each of these subjects, I illustrate the extent to which Diabetes Twitter offers broad critiques of capitalism to advocate for changes to healthcare policy. Each of these foci attempts to move the language of management from the individual mechanisms of discipline to one that emphasizes the complications of treatment in a system that views them as profit-generating consumers, not citizens worthy of care.

[21] Brian Ott and Greg Dickinson, *The Twitter Presidency: Donald J. Trump and the Politics of White Rage* (New York: Routledge, 2019).

Retorting Pharmaceutical Corporations

Three pharmaceutical companies, Eli Lilly, Novo Nordisk, and Sanofi, control over 90% of the global insulin market. Healthcare advocates such as Marston are quick to note that these businesses gross billions of dollars in profits annually from the medication.[22] For years, people with diabetes have pushed the leaders of these entities to reduce the list price of insulin and bring biosimilars, which are essentially generic insulins, to the market. Time and again, however, these multi-national corporations have raised insulin prices, often simultaneously, and forced people with diabetes to ration the substance to make ends meet. To be more specific, roughly a quarter of all people with diabetes have resorted to rationing insulin, putting themselves at risk of diabetic ketoacidosis (DKA), hospitalization, and death.[23] It is little wonder these entities are not often regarded as partners in diabetes care but enemies to the cause.

The sharp contrast between financial ruin and debilitating complications for people with diabetes and the bottomless well of corporate greed exhibited by pharmaceutical executives has established a dramatic us/them dichotomy that resonates on a medium like Twitter. Contributors with diabetes provide a profusion of testimonials about the suffering derived from corporate exploitation and those stories carry tremendous weight on a medium that thrives on short, easily digestible anecdotes. Critics on Twitter literally provide the receipts that illustrate they are dying from the effects of unchecked capitalism rather than contrived notions about individual management. For example, on August 1, 2020, Twitter user Michelle Fenner pointed out that promises to reduce insulin prices during the COVID-19 pandemic had been retracted. She tweeted a picture of a pharmacy receipt, commenting, "Remember the $35.00 insulin by @LillyDiabetes for the pandemic. Yeah they raised the price again. It's 1102.30 for 4 vials so if you were on the special due to COVID or assistance it's over. So far 4 people have had it increased from 35.00 to 275.00

[22] Marston noted on October 15, 2019 that Eli Lily made "24.5 BILLION (with a B) in revenue in 2018 and got a $186.2 million dollar TAX REFUND along with paying 0% federal income tax. While diabetics die bc we can't afford basic insulin." Marston, October 15, 2019.

[23] Darby Herkert, Pavithra Vijayakumar, Jing Luo, Jeremy I. Schwartz, Tracy L. Rabin, Eunice DeFilippo, Kasia J. Lipska, "Cost-Related Insulin Underuse Among Patients With Diabetes," *JAMA Internal Medicine* 179.1 (2019): 112–113.

a vial #T1D #Insulin4all."[24] A Lilly representative replied to the tweet and claimed that the co-pay cap had not ended: "Many factors affect pharmacy experiences, like changing from employed to unemployed or new insurance." The company faced immediate push back from patients who supported Fenner's observation and testified that they shared similar experiences. One forumite pointed to the disclaimer at the bottom of a Lilly press release that stated: "There is no guarantee that we will be able to continue uninterrupted insulin supply or that our insulin and/or glucagon affordability programs will significantly lower or cap monthly out-of-pocket costs for people."[25] The company, unable to defend its practices in the face of this collective intelligence, offered a canned response to the complaints. "We want to Help. Please call the Lilly Diabetes Solution Center…to learn about our cost-saving solution."[26] But for people living with the disease, refrains about aid or faux solutions to the insulin crisis have never materialized as long-term fixes to complications that accompany capitalism.

Interestingly, the cost of insulin is never sidelined in such exchanges. Price remains the focal point of the conversation for each interlocutor, offering presence to the issue and cementing the interpretive lenses employed by those on social media. Lilly itself raises the issue of affordability in each of its tweets, thereby reinforcing the framework drafted by the advocates about personal expenditures. Lilly never has the appearance of holding the moral high ground in these disputes. In another instance, a company spokesperson posted: "Whether you're uninsured or have commercial insurance, the Lilly Insulin Value Program could reduce your out-of-pocket costs for Lilly insulin. Download the co-pay card at [their web site] to access these savings."[27] The tweet received few responses, but those who engaged it were highly critical of the sentiment. Molly King, for example, replied, "Or you could quit charging people over $3K for insulin that costs less than $20 to make. I get needing to make a profit but that profit margin is ABSURD and criminal."[28] Another monitor responded, "Instead of devoting this time and money to pay someone to help you brand yourselves as a company that 'cares,' why not just ACTUALLY

[24] Michelle Fenner, August 1, 2020, https://twitter.com/FennerMichelle.
[25] Elizabeth Snouffer, August 2, 2020, https://twitter.com/ElizabethType1.
[26] Eli Lilly and Company, August 2, 2020, https://twitter.com/LillyPad.
[27] Eli Lilly, August 3, 2020, https://twitter.com/LillyPad.
[28] Molly King, August 31, 2020, https://twitter.com/yesthisismolly.

make insulin accessible for people who need it to live? Your CEO is worth $22mil and my dead friend's blood is on his hands."[29] In yet another lengthy exchange, Curly Andr0id, wrote:

> I applied for this program since I am type 1 & uninsured. I received two discount cards to purchase both my long-acting, & fast-acting insulins via email. When I went to pick up both my insulins at the pharmacy…the pharmacist explained I am only allowed to use the $35 copay card on one of my insulin prescriptions at a time. The pharmacist even called your customer service line because she couldn't understand why you would give me 2 different discount cards but I can't even use them? I would assume you realize most type 1 diabetics need BOTH insulins to survive. so I'm put in a situation where I have to choose between which insulin I can pick up under you 'assistance' program.[30]

Lilly extended a perfunctory expression of thanks to the user, insisted that she was mistaken, and claimed to be looking into the problem. For people with diabetes, their dismissive response exacerbates the long and arduous process of attempting to access insulin and the unnecessary barriers erected to prevent them from doing so. A medication that is affordable and readily available over the counter in other countries is weighed down by a complicated and costly process that puts this person's life at risk.

In one of the more baneful developments I encountered during this study, the Pharmaceutical Research and Manufacturers of America (PhRMA), the lobbying organization that represents the nation's largest pharmaceutical companies, attempted to block a Minnesota law aimed at bringing down the price of insulin. The influence group claimed that the state's new emergency insulin program constituted "an unlawful taking of private property without compensation" because it requires corporations to reimburse retailers that provide emergency supplies of insulin to people with diabetes and "to offer insulin to low-income patients through companies' charitable patient assistance programs."[31] The law was named after Alec Smith, who died at the age of 26 after having to ration his insulin due to cost. His mother, Nicole Holt-Smith, has become a tireless advocate for insulin affordability. She responded to the suit by noting that insulin man-

[29] Molly King, August 16, 2020, https://twitter.com/yesthisismolly.

[30] @Curly Andr0id, August 3, 2020, https://twitter.com/Andr0idCurly.

[31] Peter Callaghan, "State says PhRMA doesn't have standing to challenge constitutionality of Minnesota's emergency insulin program," *MinnPost*, September 1, 2020.

ufacturers and their lobby have persistently refused to participate in talks that would lower the cost of the medication. She wrote, "we have tried speaking with the pharmacies but without direction from the board of pharmacy they are reluctant to participate, its frustrating because they have all been sent the information and were invited to participate in a zoom call, i think its more about the law suit."[32] Time and again pharmaceutical companies attempt to deflect attention away from their profit-generating machine and Diabetes Twitter points to their malfeasance in equal step.

Correcting and Educating Politicians

Social media users fighting for a more equitable and transformative approach to healthcare have repeatedly been daunted by the institutional gradualism that prohibits the success of forward-looking policies. Despite wide-spread public support for access to affordable care, attempts to alter entrenched cultural practices can prove overwhelming for proponents of change, especially when engaging politicians who are seemingly unmoved by the effects of deleterious policy decisions. Ellis and Kent contend that people with disabilities are frequently marginalized in policy discussions due to ableist scripts of productivity.[33] Diabetes Twitter highlights the burdensome work that advocates must perform in order to intervene in conversations about their lives and mitigate the risks posed by uninformed public servants. Politicians are often ignorant about the kinds of insulin on the market, its variable uses, or its centrality to the everyday lives of people with diabetes. Donald Trump, who has frequently contended that his policies would solve the insulin crisis (they have not), offers one of the more egregious examples of this obtuseness. He said during a press conference, "I don't use insulin. Should I be? Huh? I never thought about it."[34] Further, in the first presidential debate against Joe Biden, he remarked that insulin is "so cheap, it's like water" (it is not). Such attitudes illustrate why Twitter users often provoked exchanges with politicians who were at best blissfully ignorant and at worst purposefully dense. This included representatives on the state level in places such as Colorado and Minnesota, where lawmakers had drafted legislation to reign in the price of insulin.

[32] Nicole Holt-Smith, July 8, 2020, https://twitter.com/NSmithholt12.

[33] Ellis and Kent, 94.

[34] Daniel Dale, May 26, 2020, https://twitter.com/ddale8.

Healthcare reformers often worried that bills being introduced into session were not expansive enough to cover all people with diabetes, even when press coverage made it appear otherwise. Following the passage of Colorado's insulin price capping legislation, for example, several influencers argued that the law did not go far enough to protect patients because it was explicitly tied to insurance. Colorado's bill dealt with co-pay caps and not list prices, meaning only a fraction of citizens would be covered. Marston noted, "This is why copay caps are BAD POLICY. They help less than 20% of citizens, leave the uninsured paying the most, and lawmakers deem them as a panacea for the insulin price crisis. WE MUST STOP LETTING ADA RUN THE SHOW WHEN OUR LIVES ARE AT RISK."[35] I'll return to advocacy groups such as the ADA in the next section. For now, I want to draw attention to the policy decisions being made at the state level and how those maneuvers were not extensive enough to satiate advocates. If one looked only to the national media or to the press releases of state lawmakers, they might believe that a major social problem had been solved when, in fact, it had not. If anything, the Twitterverse highlighted that the law actually contributed to income inequality rather than leveling the playing field.

In a separate but highly publicized controversy, Diabetes Twitter was quick to correct a Minnesota state representative who was spreading misleading information about the accessibility of affordable insulin. In September 2019 Republican Jeremy Munson posted a video to social media and claimed that people with diabetes need not ration their insulin because, he insisted, they can simply go to Walmart and buy an older form of the medicine for less than $25. This is a common, though false, argumentative trope well-known to people with diabetes who champion price caps on insulin. The substance that Munson was peddling is an outdated insulin that has not been in wide use since the early 1990s. "Walmart insulin" gives people with diabetes substantially less flexibility than newer forms of the substance. As a result, it puts people at high risk of death when changing medications without the strict supervision of a physician (which many patients cannot afford if they are switching to such insulins). I have written elsewhere about the dangers of so-called Walmart insulin and its propensity for harm.[36] Social media users pointed out the

[35] Laura Marston, February 17, 2020, https://twitter.com/Kidfears99.

[36] Jeffrey Bennett, "Why Telling People with Diabetes to Use Walmart Insulin can be Dangerous Advice," *The Conversation*, November 14, 2019, https://theconversation.com/why-telling-people-with-diabetes-to-use-walmart-insulin-can-be-dangerous-advice-125528.

recklessness of Munson's arguments, including his repeated use of testimony from a disreputable physician to back his unscientifically supported claims.

Lija Greenseid, a self-described "passionate healthcare advocate," and whose daughter lives with Type 1 diabetes, was among those who publicly retorted Munson. She was especially critical of the lawmaker's embrace of the aforementioned doctor who had routinely profited off the pharmaceutical industry's fleecing of people living with Type 1 diabetes. She wrote, "Let me say this more clearly. Rep Jeremy Munson frequently cites testimony from a Dr Richard Dolinar to argue against the Alec Smith Emergency Insulin Act. Since 2013, Dr. Dolinar has been paid $700K from pharma, including about $120k from Lilly and Novo Nordisc in 2018 alone."[37] Greenseid posted testimony that Dolinar had delivered to the Minnesota legislature, in which he called Walmart insulin a "viable option" for people with diabetes experiencing an emergency. She contrasted that with an opinion piece Munson had published in the *Star Tribune* that leans heavily on Dolinar's words, and linked to a site that highlighted how much money the endocrinologist had scored from insulin manufacturers.[38] Munson's remarks eventually drew the ire of numerous legislators, including one who actually lived with Type 1 diabetes.[39] Ultimately, Munson's declarations were rejected when the Alec Smith insulin bill was passed into law in April 2020.

Holding Diabetes Nonprofits Accountable

Diabetes non-profits such as the JDRF and the ADA have long pushed for increased federal funding for research, lobbied Congress to support the Special Diabetes Program, and brought together public figures that are invested in finding a cure. The ADA has traditionally been identified as a physician's lobbying group while the JDRF is composed of children living with diabetes and their families. In more recent years organizations such

[37] Lija Greenseid, October 4, 2019, https://twitter.com/Lija27.

[38] Jeremy Munson, "Counterpoint: Over-the-counter insulin is a viable option," *Star Tribune*, October 3, 2019, https://www.startribune.com/counterpoint-over-the-counter-insulin-is-a-viable-option/562115132/

[39] Adam Uren, "GOP lawmaker's Walmart insulin video criticized as 'irresponsible,'" *Bring Me the News*, September 24, 2019, https://bringmethenews.com/minnesota-news/gop-lawmakers-walmart-insulin-video-criticized-as-irresponsible

Beyond Type 1 (founded by Nick Jonas of the Jonas Brothers) and T1 International have appeared as noteworthy players in diabetes advocacy, though with discrepant messages and varied methods for reaching their audiences. T1 International, in particular, has become an essential voice in the fight for accessible insulin, including its widely used Twitter hashtag #insulin4all.

Those active on the platform have increasingly criticized the ADA and JDRF for their close ties to pharmaceutical companies and the compromising position such affiliations may engender. Rather than agitate on behalf of people with diabetes, there is a persistent worry that such sponsorship will, at the very least, mute necessary critiques of multi-national corporations that have facilitated immeasurable harms. Importantly, these corporate associations are well known in diabetes communities and are generally made public by the nonprofits. On their web site, the JDRF notes that they have been partners with Eli Lilly since 1997 and have collected contributions from the manufacturer that soar above $13 million. They have likewise collaborated with Novo Nordisk since 2000, generating roughly the same amount of cash. Other frequent partners include diabetes conglomerates Medtronic, Dexcom, and Sanofi.

Social media advocates frequently spotlight how these non-profits appropriate the struggles of people with diabetes without necessarily putting pressure on drug manufacturers and lawmakers to make insulin more affordable. For example, Smith-Holt took to Twitter in June 2020 to relay a negative encounter she had with the JDRF. The organization wanted to highlight her son Alec's story and the legislation that was passed in his name. But Smith-Holt decided to include in her narrative the JDRF's and ADA's silence about the high cost of insulin.[40] The group attempted to rewrite a 250 word story that she submitted and asked her to be in a video using a script they composed instead. Smith-Holt rejected the offer and aired her grievances on Twitter. She remarked that she was disappointed in the nonprofit for not more vocally supporting efforts that would make insulin accessible for all. She insisted that the JDRF never lobbied the Minnesota legislature to get the bill passed and said resolutely that she would not "support an organization who is in bed with PHARMA."[41]

Sharp critiques like the one Holt-Smith made of the JDRF have also been directed at newer groups such as Beyond Type 1. In summer 2020,

[40] Nicole Holt-Smith, June 23, 2020, https://twitter.com/NSmithholt12.
[41] Ibid.

the non-profit's Twitter account posed the following question: "What is the main reason you're NOT using a Continuous Glucose Monitor? Tell us in the Comments!" Following the query, there was an additional tag that noted, "Posted in partnership with Abbott FreeStyle."[42] Immediately, a self-described parent of a person living with Type 1 replied with a screen-shot of the tweet. "Amammamous" retorted, "You cannot convince me that they do not expect the replies to be overwhelmingly about cost…and that the 'low-priced' Libre 2 is going to be an answer in a future post."[43] The casual dismissal of the tweet exacerbates what many people with diabetes have come to see as a problematic coupling of organizations claiming to lobby in their name but with the intent of pushing products and not productively transforming the politics that dictate their lives. Rather than being hailed as passive consumers in a seemingly corporate shell game, this social media advocate anticipated the absurdity of the tweet and discarded its market logic. The capitalistic enterprise underlying the message does little to make life more livable for people with diabetes—it simply positions them as customers in a marketing-scheme.

This is not the first time Beyond Type 1 ran into problems on Twitter in 2020. In May the organization's front man, Jonas, himself a person with Type 1 diabetes, tweeted, "Are you or someone close to you impacted by diabetes? The @JDRF and @BeyondType1 Alliance has brought over 100 partners together to protect those most vulnerable to COVID-19. Guidance + important info at: coronavirusdiabetes.org #BigLittleChanges."[44] Marston, unimpressed with the outreach, replied: "Literally FUCK YOU @ nickjonas. Your fellow diabetics are dying from insulin rationing and you're pushing a website sponsored by every insulin company and every Phrma shill group ever? Is money more important than your life? Or is it just more important than ours? #PhrmaShill."[45] Another user wrote that Beyond Type 1, "has brought over 100 partners together to take the money of people with diabetes until they die.*"[46] And yet another person with the Twitter handle "the moody diabetic" wrote: "Are you or someone close to you impacted by diabetes? The @JDRF @BeyondType1 Alliance has continued to ignore the fact that price gouging insulin kills several people a year.

[42] Beyond Type 1, June 28, 2020, https://twitter.com/BeyondType1.
[43] Amammamous, June 28, 2020, https://twitter.com/Amammamous.
[44] Nick Jonas, May 12, 2020, https://twitter.com/nickjonas.
[45] Laura Marston, May 12, 2020, https://twitter.com/Kidfears99.
[46] @autoimmuneallie, May 12, 2020, https://twitter.com/autoimmuneallie.

if you want to actually make a difference, please join your state's #insulin4all chapter:)."[47] Although some applauded the coalition, the majority of posts displayed little sympathy for the tweet. At every turn, it would seem that people with diabetes have become averse to the capitalist tendencies that continually put their lives at risk.

Capitalism and Diabetes Twitter's Discontents

This chapter has explored the ways that people with diabetes navigate and retort a matrix of capitalist forces that put lifesaving medications such as insulin out of reach. Although capitalism is not always explicitly mentioned by Diabetes Twitter, it is unquestionably implied in daily threads that appear on the platform. Advocates point to the vacuous nature of claims about insulin prices leading to further innovation, they call out CEOs like David Ricks of Lilly or Steven Ubl of PhRMA (who has a child with T1D) for the lifestyles they are subsidizing, and they breathlessly demand an end to exorbitant prices. At every turn, a system underwritten by capitalism is heckled for its murderous effects. On January 11th, 2020, a user by the name of Jerry Coyne noted that it was the 98-year anniversary of then 14 year-old Leonard Thompson being given the first injection of insulin. Marston retweeted the post and noted, "98 years later, many insulin-dependent diabetics in the United States can't afford the insulin we need to survive. Could you come up with $1,000 a month every month for the rest of your life to save yourself from certain death?" The question is not merely rhetorical. For many living in the United States this answer is abundantly clear: absolutely not.

Proponents of change, such as Marston, highlight the capitalist exploitation of people living with diabetes to show that no amount of individual management can account for the structural impediments foisted upon them. In February 2018 the American Enterprise Institute posted a "chart of the day" listing the long-term consumer price change to numerous U.S. goods and services. Among the most expensive changes were the costs of hospital services, college textbooks, and tuition. Twitter user Hannah Crabtree modified that chart to include the price of insulin and has since circulated the graphic several times because it so quickly goes viral. Whereas hospital services went up by well over 200%, Crabtree

[47] @whatsarave, May 12, 20020, https://twitter.com/whatsarave.

illustrated that the price of insulin has risen by almost 1200%.[48] In another vein, a Twitter user with the handle "Miss InsulinDependent MD" relayed that she had saved $6,000 by switching to her "insurance preferred insulin." But this was not a happy tweet. She wrote: "You too can significantly increase your A1C and decrease your quality of life when you live in a country with private-for-profit healthcare."[49] Users to the medium incessantly and insistently communicated that capitalism was destroying them, enlivening public claims about the inaccessibility of insulin and the ravenous effects of consumerism on the diabetic body.

From a communication perspective, the intense focus on disseminating a particularly narrow message about insulin prices, rather than adapting those claims to potential audiences, raises questions about the effectiveness and influence of actors on Diabetes Twitter. Eschewing organizations that have any ties to pharmaceutical companies, for example, is challenging in the U.S.'s capitalistic-driven system, even if the motivation for these concentrated directives is both laudable and understandable. People with diabetes have repeatedly witnessed multiple members of their community die without cause and efforts to persuade representatives on any other terms must feel like an exercise in cultural charades. Still, just as there is no denying that the political sentiments expressed on Twitter are not always reflected in the larger public sphere (few people on Twitter were arguing for Joe Biden to be president during the 2020 primaries), the work of these forumites might foresee something yet unrealized. Diabetes Twitter is a necessary and welcome voice but one whose effects may be limited in a system built on gradualism and capitalist exploitation. Unlike the saccharine glow of Diabetes Instagram, these advocates do not picture the disease and its technological accompaniment as aesthetically productive—they imagine the condition and insulin's outrageous list price as resolutely fatal. And while fatalism can be potentially generative in the political sphere when confronting the realities of diabetes, it is yet to be seen how effective this collective effort will be.[50]

The coming years might prove to be exceedingly difficult for people living with diabetes. The Affordable Care Act, which has offered legal

[48] Hannah Crabtree, "The Price of Insulin vs. the Price of Other Goods," *Data for Insulin*, June 18, 2019, https://insulin.substack.com/p/the-price-of-insulin-vs-the-price

[49] @msinsulindpndnt, July 7, 2020, https://twitter.com/msinsulindpndnt.

[50] See, Jeffrey Bennett, *Managing Diabetes: The Cultural Politics of Disease* (New York. New York University Press, 2019), 77–111.

protections to those with pre-existing conditions, may be dismantled by the Supreme Court, thereby facilitating the slaughter of people living with the disease. Even with the law intact, the high cost of insulin in the U.S. has continued to escort people to an early grave. The public advocacy performed by lay experts on Twitter may not be able to prevent the slow death of their community. Yet it will remain a source of anger and moral righteousness in the face of a system that has little regard for the lives of people living with this most precarious of diseases.

What's in a Name? The Diabetes Civil War

Lora Arduser

Introduction

As the incidence of diabetes climbs, diabetes online communities periodically erupt into an ongoing "civil war." This phrase, picked up in a November 22, 2010, article by Julie Deardorff in the *Chicago Tribune*, highlights a community rift. Deardorff writes, "As rates of Type 2 diabetes soar, tempers are flaring in the diabetes blogosphere, where many people with Type 1 diabetes are lobbying for a new, distinct name for their condition in hopes of clearing up misconceptions and securing more resources to put toward a cure" (para 4). I find this notion of a civil war, a war between citizens of the same country, to be an apt metaphor for what I have observed in this project for two reasons. First, because it mirrors the way in which the American Civil War (fought from 1861 to 1865) often pitted family members against each other. In hundreds of families, brothers fought one and other or sons fought on the opposite side of their fathers. This familial division was symbolic of the divided nation, a division

L. Arduser (✉)
University of Cincinnati, Cincinnati, OH, USA
e-mail: Lora.arduser@uc.edu

B. C. Frazer, H. R. Walker (eds.), *(Un)doing Diabetes: Representation, Disability, Culture*, Palgrave Studies in Science and Popular Culture, https://doi.org/10.1007/978-3-030-83110-3_3

that remains a cultural phenomenon today. The second reason is related to how bodies were related to a hierarchy through the Enrollment Act (1863) (The Conscription Act). The Enrollment Act, the first military draft in American history, gave any draftee who was not excused the ability to hire a substitute, or to pay a fee of $300. The $300 fee soon became the most controversial part of the act, leading to the perception of the war as "a rich man's war and a poor man's fight" (McPherson 1989). In other words, by separating or categorizing the bodies of potential draftees, the Act created an economical hierarchy of these individuals.

The civil war between people with diabetes also reflects a hierarchal structure of particular bodies—bodies with Type 1 or Type 2 diabetes—and their cultural representations (an identity that stands for or denotes another symbolically). To address assumptions made about this identity, this chapter examines the online discourse generated about a petition on Change.org started by two mothers of children with Type 1 diabetes. The petition urges decision-makers at the American Diabetes Association (ADA), the National Institutes of Health (NIH), and the International Diabetes Federation (IDF) to revise the names of both Type 1 and Type 2 diabetes to more clearly differentiate the nature of each disease.[1] In the petition the writers state: "Our sons face this life-threatening disease with strength, courage and perseverance despite being subjected on a daily basis to ignorance and misconceptions. It is with their future in mind that we file this petition to bring clarity to two very different diseases—Type 1 and Type 2 Diabetes" (Perez 2013). The petitioners' argument for a name change largely revolves around a perceived need to educate the public about the kind of disease their children have. In the petition writers' efforts to re-label Type 1 and Type 2 diabetes, however, a rift within what is often characterized as a monolithic community is exposed.

To address the implications of the representations of "categories" of diabetes *within* the community of people living with the illness, I draw on the concept of counterpublics in public sphere theory and the identity of "expert patient"—a term coined by the UK's Department of Health following an observation often made by doctors, nurses, and other health professionals that people with particular chronic diseases, including diabetes, understand their disease better than medical professionals do. And while this knowledge is often referred to as "lived experience," it is more

[1]As of 2020, there has been no indication that decision makers have responded to this petition.

complex than that and thus deserves more consideration. As I pointed out in my book *Living Chronic: Agency and Expertise in the Rhetoric of Diabetes* (2017), chronic patients often work in partnership with their health care providers: the physician informs the patient of all the data relevant to making the decision about treatment and the patient provides information such as her values, preferences, lifestyle, and beliefs. However, because the patient is making daily, if not hourly, decisions about her care in between these brief encounters with medical professionals, she acquires a level of expertise medical providers are not able to achieve. Therefore, expert patients' identity status lies categorically beyond the boundaries of both "medical expert" and "patient." As I argue in this chapter, the expert patient identity is based on an ethos drawing from both lived experience in the form of expert testimony and scientific/medical claims of knowledge.

In the critical discourse analysis that follows, I trace the sources of evidence the petitioners and others use, specifically acts of classification and scientific ethos building, to make their arguments for or against a name change. This tracing reveals that the discourse related to the petition reinforces cultural stereotypes in ways that are detrimental to an expert patient identity and exposes efforts to stigmatize those with Type 2 diabetes in particular. This form of stigmatization, referred to as defensive othering, occurs when marginalized persons "[accept] the legitimacy of a devalued identity imposed by the dominant group, but then [say], in effect, 'There are indeed Others to whom this applies, but it does not apply to me'" (Schwalbe et al. 2000, 425). Schwalbe et al. further define defensive othering as "identity work done by those seeking membership in a dominant group, or by those seeking to deflect the stigma they experience as members of a subordinate group" (p. 425). Schwalbe et al. offer examples of a study of homeless men calling other homeless men "lazy bums" (Snow and Anderson 1987) and Irish immigrants distancing themselves from other immigrants who encourage a stereotype of the Irish as loud drunks (Field 1994). By stepping just outside the stereotype, these individuals are declaring themselves an exception to the rule while reinforcing the legitimacy of the stereotype. In sum, actions of defensive othering result in the reproduction of inequality.

Here I am interested in understanding how the defensive othering of people with Type 2 diabetes by other people with diabetes in the public sphere impacts the empowering identity of expert patient. Along with implications about identities, such hierarchal divisions of bodies can be used to "legimat[e] an unequal distribution of resources, status, and power within a biased social and architectural environment" (Garland-Thomson 2002, 5). In this case, these resources are often seen as access to research funding for a cure for Type 1.

I come to this project as a researcher interested in diabetes communication, but I am also a person with diabetes. I tend to struggle with my own positionality with my research about rhetoric and diabetes. As a person with latent autoimmune diabetes in adults (LADA) I've often thought of myself as privileged to have insider status. Quite frankly, it has been a useful status in terms of gaining the trust of my research participants. As I noted in my 2011 article about a diabetes online community, people with diabetes tend to trust others with knowledge of the disease (Arduser 2011). But over the years, and in part because of my work on this project, I've grown to realize that I had been viewing the expert patient as its own "monolithic totality" (Keränen 2014, 104). I think this is largely due to the ideas that attach themselves to chronicity—ideas that prioritize the divide between medical practitioner and people doing the daily work of chronic illness. This divide between chronic patients and medical professionals can hide other divisions including the one under discussion here.

Diabetes in the Public Sphere

In the last decades disability studies scholars have prioritized the social model of disability over the medical model of disability. According to Michael Oliver, the social model was developed by disabled people in an effort to reject the fundamentals of the individual/medical model of disability—which locates the problem of disability within individual bodies and as originating from physical or mental limitations (Oliver 1990). A major focus of the social model is what Alison Kafer (2013) calls the built environment, stairs and sidewalks and other material elements with which our bodies interact. As Kafer points out, however, our built environment also consists of the relational, political, and virtual spaces in which people with disabilities interact. Scholars in disability studies as well as scholars of the rhetoric of health and medicine have long discussed the use of online forums for people with various ailments, chronic disease, and disabilities (see Atwood et al. 2018; Bakke 2019; and Ghiaciuc 2011 for examples). In some of my own work, I have looked at one such online community for people with diabetes—a community I joined soon after being diagnosed with LADA at the age of 33. Like many researchers of other forums created for and inhabited by people with similar issues, my analysis of the communicative purposes of this space concluded that people come to the forum for support and information (Arduser 2011). But our virtual worlds do not encompass only these types of communal supportive spaces, as the Change.org website illustrates. Rather than being a community, this site functions as a sphere of public discourse in which "forms of social activism and resistance" can produce "notable effects on society" (Warnick 2007, 3).

Traditional public sphere scholarship, grounded in Jürgen Habermas's (1974) concept, defines the public sphere as an assemblage of individuals who gather to discuss matters of public concern or of common interest. It is, "a realm of our social life, in which something approaching public opinion can be formed" (49) and is characterized as facilitating rational discourse of public affairs directed toward the common good. Other scholars have expanded, revised, and criticized what has been described as an idealized version of the public sphere. Most notably, Goodnight's (1982, 1987) landmark work with technical, public, and personal spheres has updated what was once seen as a singular entity, or what Lisa Keränen (2014) has described as a "homogenous mass" (104). As Keränen explains, a rhetorical lens on publics "replaces the vision of the public as a monolithic totality with a view of multiple, overlapping, and interrelated groups whose members engage one another in dialogue about matters of mutual interest" (104). These less bounded groups can organize around a topic in ways that highlight these topics as being important in various spheres, including public, private, and technical.

And while "personal exchange, through dialogue, achieves genuine power to displace long-established outlooks, expectations, and experiences" (Goodnight 2012, 265), such as stereotyped cultural identities, deliberations between experts like people with chronic diseases in public argument spheres, can also result in acrimony that fragments collective social action. It is within such a public sphere that stigma becomes revealed in new ways. As Goffman stated:

> When normal and stigmatized do in fact enter one's immediate presence, especially when they there attempt to sustain a joint conversational encounter, there occurs one of the primal scenes of sociology; for, in many cases, these moments will be the ones when the causes and effects of stigma must be directly confronted on both sides. (2017, 139).

In the case at hand, this confrontation results in a split into counterpublics—what Nancy Fraser defined as "parallel discursive arenas where members of subordinated social groups invent and circulate counter discourses to formulate oppositional interpretations of their identities, interests, and needs" (1990, 67). As Fraser argued, when the public is understood as a single concept, there are no places for members of "subordinated groups" (64). Fraser defines such groups as women, workers, peoples of color, and gays and lesbians, who gather to deliberate. Here, I argue that people with diabetes are included within another subordinated group: those with disability. I argue that as one such group, they function as a network of "*partially* [emphasis mine] intersecting and overlapping, directly and indirectly connected, sites of discourse" (Asen 2000, 270).

In the case of expert patients, this partial intersection is an artifact of the counterpublic in relation to other publics—the general public and the medical public. When set up in opposition to these two publics, the expert patient can easily be viewed as its own "monolithic totality"—a phrase Keränen also uses to describe what a nonrhetorical view of publics can produce (2014, 104)—with entirely overlapping and interrelated views and interests. The rhetorical tactics, such as using numbers to make arguments, used in the public sphere in which these arguments occur clearly show that people with (and related to people with) Type 1 diabetes and people with Type 2 diabetes are members of a subordinated group who join together in private settings to discuss issues related to their multiple identities, needs, and interests. As Bill Hughes (2009) notes in his analysis of the wounded, monstrous, and abject tropes of the disabled body, the concept of the subaltern has not had much influence in disability studies. He does, however, also note that two aspects of the concept might be useful. First, "It refers to a minor that is in a position to subvert the hegemonic group." Additionally, "it recognises that the presence of the subaltern is central to the self-definition of the majority." In lodging these arguments, Hughes reasons that agency is bestowed to the subaltern as "other."

I argue that in the particular incident under investigation here, the discussions taking place lead some members of this particular counterpublic to purposefully stigmatize others. Interestingly, in doing so, they also stigmatize themselves and/or their children. In these texts the writers divide wounded and monstrous identities often associated with disabled people (Hughes 2009). Doing so can lead to the identity of expert patient not emerging and the sides battling each other in ways that undermine the arguments they try to build on expert identity.

Investigating Language Used in a Virtual Public Sphere

Discourse analysis looks at language-in-use: "People use language to communicate, co-operate, help others, and build things like marriages, reputations, and institutions. They also use it to lie, advantage themselves, harm people, and destroy things like marriages, reputations, and institutions" (Gee 2011, iv). And while there is no one way to approach discourse analysis, this method emphasizes the contextual meaning of language, focusing on the ways people use language to achieve specific effects (e.g,. to build trust, evoke emotions, or manage conflict).

Barbara Johnstone and Christopher Eisenhart concur in the introduction to their edited collection (2008) that researchers using discourse analysis are interested in the structure and function of a piece of text, but the approaches taken to discourse course analysis are diverse, including studies of spaces such as the chapter in the collection called "Ethos and Narrative in Online Educational Chat" by Martha Sylvia Cheng. Teun A. Van Dijk (2018) also notes that in a critical discourse analysis a cohesive method is less important than the cohesive interest in the topic examining important social problems, including projects that focus on stigma and identity production, like this one. Here I follow the general steps involved in discourse analysis: (1) defining the research question and selecting the data for analysis (2) analyzing the content for themes and patterns, and (3) reviewing results and drawing conclusions.

Ethical Concerns of Internet Research

The ethical concerns of using textual data from internet groups such as online communities are multiple. In earlier work (Arduser 2011, 2017) with the online TuDiabetes community my experience was that the site moderators were more concerned with this privacy than members of the community were. When I began my research projects with this group is was an informal process: I contacted the site founder, described my project, and asked for his blessing. Once I received that, community members were not only willing but expressed excitement to talk with me.[2]

Institutional Review Boards (IRBs) often handle these projects in various ways. In my case, the data collected for this project was part of a larger IRB protocol that included interviews. The IRB was not concerned with nor offered any guidance on the textual data I was collecting; they were specifically concerned with my work with "human subjects" (i.e., the interviewees). As Heidi McKee and James Porter (2009) point out, however, members of online communities often view their postings as private despite the fact that many of these may be publicly available to anyone browsing the Internet. Because of these concerns McKee and Porter (2009) suggest that researchers consider the following when conducting writing research online: (1) public vs private, (2) data identification, (3) degree of interaction, (4) topic sensitivity, and (5) subject vulnerability. These factors, they argue, help researchers make decisions on consent.

For this project, therefore, I focused exclusively on digital posts that were expressly public. This included online blogs and comments, online news stories and comments, and the Change.org petition and comments. These genres are all designed to be public and reach the broadest audience possible. None of these data sources required a password or membership to access. Because of this, the data are easily searchable and identifiable online. In collecting the data, I did not interact with any of the individuals posting original entries or comments on those entries.

War of Words

Employing a critical discourse analysis strategy for analyzing and conceiving of discourse, the following inquiry looks at texts concerning the Change.org petitions. The material for this chapter specifically comes from the petition and comments on it as well as the *Chicago Tribune* article and online comments and three blog posts and comments. With regard to changing the names of Type 1 and Type 2 diabetes, I examine the way these texts are produced, circulated, distributed, and consumed in this public sphere and the ideology surrounding the examined discursive practices. The results show that the rhetors in this public sphere rely on the

[2] Over the years, as more researchers become interested in working with this community; however, the site administrators set up a formal process to vet and approve research projects occurring within their space.

scientific concept of classification and a scientific ethos to bolster an expert identity. More specifically, they rely on the concept of classification, reliance on a certainty of numbers, medical knowledge of the disease, and expert testimony as ways to build and exercise an expert patient ethos. By inhabiting this particular identity in this particular space, however, this disease community fractures in ways that result in different stigmatized identities for people with diabetes.

Classification

Ever shifting scientific classification exercises have a long-established history as a tool for medicine in terms of both treatment and diagnosis. In an age when scientific reason and objectivity are given so much credence, it is easy to forget that the act of classification is a process based on mental constructs that provide "a spatial, temporal, or spatio-temporal segmentation of the world" (Bowker and Star 1999, 6). As such, classification systems generate hierarchies that imply priorities. In other words, scientific and biomedical naming and classification are not neutral processes. Rather, "On the contrary, names can constitute powerful instruments of persuasion and manipulation" (Macagno and Walton 2009, 83). In other words, "to choose a definition is to plead a cause" (Zarefsky et al. 1984, 113). The cause the petitioners' plead is to "correctly" name Type 1 and Type 2. The petition asks decision-makers to revise the names of both Type 1 and Type 2 diabetes to more discursively reflect the nature of each disease (i.e. the unique nature of Type 1 would be reflected in a name such as Autoimmune Beta Cell Apoptosis Diabetes and the unique nature of Type 2 in a name such as Insulin Resistance Diabetes).

At the beginning of the twentieth century diabetes remained a single disease category and medical experts upheld the opinion that these patients had the same disease (Feudtner 2003). By the 1950s, however, technical advances made it possible to measure the amount of insulin in a person's body, and, clinicians were able to confirm that some patients with diabetes produced no insulin while others produced varying amounts. Attempts to standardize definitions, nomenclature, and diagnostic criteria around the world began around 1952 (Rock 2005). To grapple with developing nuances of the disease, including the recognition of the form of diabetes I have -LADA-, in 1995 an international Expert Committee was established to review the scientific literature since 1979 to determine whether or not these naming conventions remained valid (The Expert Committee 2002).

The recommendations of the committee were based on two years of collaboration between the American Diabetes Association (ADA) and the World Health Organization (WHO). A new classification system developed out of this committee's work which identified four types of diabetes: Type 1, Type 2, gestational diabetes, and "other" types.

These scientifically-based efforts to classify and re-classify diabetes bleed into public discourse in ways that impact identity work. An illustration can be taken from a *New York Times* article written by Richard Perez-Pena in 2006 in which the writer characterizes the types as follows:

> Most Type 1 diabetics develop the disease as children, without warning, on the basis of genetic factors. They are quite often thin. They come from all walks of life, neighborhoods and ethnicities. Their chief advocates are parents of children with Type 1, a group that includes skilled, upper-income professionals devoted to finding a long-sought cure, which many think is approaching. (para 9)

Type 1, in other words, is described as the end result of "bad luck." Type 2 identities, on the other hand, are associated with morality and are characterized as having "earned" their illness.

Such public discourse about Type 1 and Type 2 subjectivities have remained remarkably stable, along with the representations formed by them. As an example, historic narratives of the disease in the popular press detailed the suffering of people with diabetes. A 1915 headline in *The New York Times,* for example, announced that Indiana Senator Shively "suffers" from a septic form of diabetes. Others with diabetes in the news prior to 1920 also suffered, had "little hope of recovery," and often "succumbed" to the disease. People with Type 1 are still portrayed as victims and people with Type 2 are still portrayed as blameworthy. Almost a century later a 2012 *Washington Post* headline of an article written by a person with Type 2 diabetes gives a further example: "Diabetes affects millions; society should not stigmatize its victims" (Sklaroff). Perhaps one of the most vivid images of Type 1 diabetics as victims is in the movie *Steel Magnolias,* as Ferguson reports (2010). In the 1989 movie, Julia Roberts plays a young woman with Type 1 diabetes who is about to get married. In one scene she experiences a low blood sugar. The scene shows Dolly Parton holding her shaking head so that Sally Fields (Roberts's mother in the movie) can get Roberts to swallow some orange juice to counteract the low blood sugar. As depicted in this scene, Roberts is a victim of her own body and needs external help. In another movie, 2002's *Panic Room*, an adolescent Kristen Stewart acts out a similar dramatic hypoglycemia-induced scene. As Matt Paczkowski's chapter suggests, here, as in *Steel Magnolias*, the diabetic character is represented as a victim of her body and in need of someone else's help. Although approximately 5–10% of people with diabetes in the United States have Type 1 and the remaining 90–95% are Type 2 (CDC 2020),[3] representations of Type 2 diabetes are fewer. Perhaps the most famous representation being that of Michael Corleone (played by Al Pacino) in *The Godfather, Part III*. In this film, Michael, who is approaching 60-years-old, has a diabetic stroke. Still, identities associated with guilt and shame attach themselves to people with all forms of diabetes.

This stigmatized representational identity is also present in the public discourse of people with Type 1 and Type 2 diabetes across social media platforms. Deardorff's *Chicago Tribune* article points to a blog post on diabetesdaily.com in which the seriousness of Type 2 Diabetes is described. In response to the blog post one person comments:

> Worst article I've ever read. I cannot believe that you want to make people believe that Type 2 is worse than Type 1. I've been living with Type 1 for years, and maybe I'm biased one way more than the other, but one fact remains: I CAN'T FIX MY PROBLEM. Whereas most Type 2's CAN. I HAVE ideal body weight, I DO work out every day, I TRY and better myself and my situation, but it doesn't matter. Know why? Because I have a TERMINAL illness. Type 2 is hardly terminal. JUST EXERCISE AND STOP BEING FAT. I don't care if you think that what I'm saying is a little rough around the edges. You need to be told the truth, not "oh let's not fight about it, why can't we agree that Diabetes is all the same." WELL IT'S NOT. I have Type 2 relatives and they would all agree with me. I have it much worse than they do. Know what else I can't do? Get good insurance! I wonder why? Is it because America LIKES fat?

Another example can be seen in a comment made by a person with Type 1 on the petition site:[4]

[3] Although other forms of diabetes (including LADA, MODY, and gestational diabetes) are recognized, most public tracking of the disease by agencies such as the CDC and the organizations such as the American Diabetes Association focuses on Type 1 and Type 2.

[4] These comments are publicly available at https://www.change.org/p/revise-names-of-type-1-2-diabetes-to-reflect-the-nature-of-each-disease/c

> This is important to me because when I tell people I have diabetes they always think of type 2 and they don't think it is as serious as it is, and they think that I got it from eating a lot of junk food, and sweets. it upsets me because I never did, and I still don't.

These examples show that the stereotyped identities for Type 1 and Type 2 are inhabited by the participants in this public dialogue. In the first quote we see blatant body shaming and a nod to the idea that Type 2 diabetes is self-inflicted and maintained. In the second quote we see a milder distancing from the stereotype, but again a validation of type-specific stigmatization. Both users distance themselves from stigmatizing characteristics publicly associated with diabetes, and neither dispel those characteristics as myths for all people with diabetes regardless of type. Much as the cultural metaphors for diabetes seep into the online patient community (Arduser 2013), the stigma from cultural representations of the disease have filtered into this deliberative public sphere, reinforcing a hierarchy of impairment (Deal 2003). Based on his reading of disability literature regarding attitudes toward disabled people, Deal argues that a hierarchy of impairments exist for both disabled and non-disabled people toward "different impairment groups" (906). Within this hierarchy lies the potential of intra-group stigmatization.

While the claims of the Change.org petition writers suggest that the name change they are advocating is for scientifically accurate, the topoi used in creating their arguments and the counterarguments, insinuate that people with Type 2 are to blame for their disease and, therefore, do not deserve empathy. As I discuss in the next section, these public identities continue to attach themselves to people with diabetes in ways that complicate their relationship with an expert identity and the relationship with each other.

Expert Patient Ethos

Along with definition and classification, people also draw on their status as expert patients to make their argument in the diabetics' civil war. Aristotle stressed that a central means of persuasion is a rhetor's perceived character or ethos (Cooper 1932). To inspire confidence in claims advanced discursively, a rhetor must display the qualities of intelligence, moral character, and good will that are held in esteem by an intended audience. In the field of science, rhetors are also subject to the constraints of ethos (Prelli 1997).

In presenting his case study for the way science and scientists construct ethos, Prelli argued the ethos of scientists was based on the following norms: universalism, community, disinterestedness, organized skepticism, originality and humility. Expert patients similarly employ norms that rely on a certainty of numbers, medical knowledge of the disease, and what I call expert testimony.

Certainty of Numbers

Numbers are the currency in diabetic practices and discourse. We use them to assess our health through A1C percentages and time-in-range principles, make decisions about how many grams of carbohydrate to eat and how many insulin units to take. We weigh and measure ourselves and our food. Elsewhere (Arduser 2011) I have argued that the certainty of numbers and our use of them is also cultural capital, giving online community members both access to the community and an ethos of ***a smart diabetic.*** In the public sphere investigated here, however, numbers have a different function, as the following examples illustrate:

> They're Alike, yes? Like a Man and A Woman Is...How long can a t1 live w/o taking Any Insulin?How soon do Adult Onset T1's Get Complications vs Adult Onset T2's?And My favorite? Of the 2 Million T1's? What is the Ave. Weight for Each in 10 yr Increments? Vs the T2'sTothe Best of my Reserach? over 85% of T2's Are Obeise and Got it or Accelerated getting it by being obeise... (comment on 2010 diabetesdaily.com blog post "Which Is Worse: Type 1 or Type 2 Diabetes?")
>
> America is such a horribly obese nation the distinction needs to be made between a 'non' blame disease and a disease mainly caused by diet and lack of exercise. (comment of Change.org petition from 2017)

The first two excerpts illustrate how numbers can be used to other and stigmatize, declaring a percentage of people with Type 2 who are obese, though no reference is offered. This sentence links a high percentage (85%) with the stigma of having Type 2 drawing out the stigmatized representation of diabetes as fatness as it relates to lack of willpower.

> Type 2 occurs to a much greater % of our population today than ever before. How can you explain that in 1977, we had 6 million dx diabetics with about 10% of them type 1 and a US population of about 235 million people. today, we have over 24 million type 2 diabetics (about 1.5 m type 1) and a Us

> population of 305 million (est). This means the rate of type 2 has gone up from 6 to 24 million (4 × or 200%) though our US population went up from 235 tro 305 million today, or a rate ofalmost 30% (comment on 2010 diabetesdaily.com blog post "Which Is Worse: Type 1 or Type 2 Diabetes?")
>
> Something like 90% of "diabetics" are Type 2. Yet little research efforts were going to Type 2 research. I felt that the fundraising was somewhat fraudulent. It was written to give the impression it would help all diabetics, but that wasn't true, and they weren't forthcoming when asked directly. (comment on 2013 on *Diabetes Self Management* blog Rename Diabetes?

The third and fourth examples use numbers much in the way Aristotle discusses as an argument of size or degree. In *Rhetoric* (Cooper 1932) Aristotle states that these are arguments about "something expedient, something honorable, or something just" (146). Here, using numbers the writers are making the argument of size, stating the importance of understanding the forms of diabetes and the subsequent implications for medical treatment and potential research money devoted for a cure. The latter comment prioritizes Type 2 based on issue of degree.

Medical Knowledge

Displaying medical knowledge, whether in the form of knowing about or participating in clinical trials, reading medical journals or simply "talking like a scientist," is the second theme of an expert ethos in this situation. And while expert ethos claims based on medical or scientific knowledge are more prevalent within diabetes online communities, these claims still surfaced in the texts examined from this project as the following excepts suggest.

> This stomach fat begins to act like an endocrine organ by releasing a hormone that makes it even easier to store more internal stomach fat. The blood pressure begins to elevate at this point and our underused muscles begin to become insulin resistant. This is referred to as metabolic syndrome, a set of conditions that if left untreated will lead to type II diabetes... Both types are permanently life altering. Without Insulin a type I will die. Without insulin and or the plethora of other medications, such as: Dipeptidyl-peptidase 4 (DPP-4) inhibitors, Glucagon-like peptide 1 (GLP-1) agonists, Glucagon-like peptide 1 (GLP-1) agonistsm etc...(the list goes on) a type II will have many sever complications and ultimately die. (comment on 2010 diabetesdaily.com blog post "Which Is Worse: Type 1 or Type 2 Diabetes?")

> We ought to learn from diabetes name-change history, which isn't pretty. It began back in 1979, when jettisoning the terms "juvenile onset" and "adult onset" was proposed by an international task force sponsored by the NIH's National Diabetes Data Group. The ADA, Australian Diabetes Society, British Diabetic Association, and the European Association for the Study of Diabetes (EASD) signed on. With provisos, the World Health Organization eventually signed on as well (although they went farther and actually "created" five types of diabetes, of which only the first two had numbers). (excerpt from a 2018 blog post on Diabetes Mine)

The first example, from someone with Type 2, uses objective language (other than the use of the pronoun "we" when referring to people with Type 2). Given that and the use of specialized terminology the post takes on an ethos of someone that might be considered a medical professional. The second example from 2018 not only alludes to the ongoing civil war but draws on the use of name change classification discussed earlier in this chapter to convey historical knowledge.

"Expert" Testimony

Much more prevalent in the petition comments, blog posts, and comments examined for this study were reliance on what I describe as expert testimony.

> I'm a type 1 and it is very frustrating to fill out paper work and being just asked if I have diabetes and then get rejections and advertising or even doctor's just assuming I'm type 2. I'm sure type 2s are just as frustrated to always be assumed they need insulin. Only thing we have in common is that neither of us can tolerate carbs without some sort of intervention. (comment on 2010 name change petition on Change.org)
>
> My best friend is a tri-athlete with type 2. Perfect weight and everything else. Eats healthier than me and I am a type 1.5 and he has type 2 from his genes, not his lifestyle.Type 1 is not juvenile diabetes any longer just like type 2 is adult onset diabetes. Many children are now being diagnosed with Type 2 just as adults are getting diagnosed as type 1. Things are changing and we are still learning about this disease and its devastation on our world. (comment on 2010 diabetesdaily.com blog post "Which Is Worse: Type 1 or Type 2 Diabetes?")

Largely investigated as a topic of law, claims made through expert testimony exert a great deal of influence over the outcome of a trial (Redington 2017). According to Jo Mackiewicz's (2010) framework, when coupled with the expert patient identity, expert testimony falls within two categories: (1) regular experience using a product and (2) association with someone whose experience is relevant to the product. In language more relevant to this study, this testimony arises out of individuals' experience with diabetes and/or their association with someone with these experiences (similar to the mothers who started the Change.org petition).

Taken together, these appeals (i.e., classification, numbers, medical knowledge and expert testimony) to an expert patient ethos work to support the Change.org petitioners' argument for a name change based on seemingly objective criteria. However, combined with the ramifications of classification in and of itself, the ethos developed by expert patients "is not merely the production of eloquence, but also the cultivation of a set of habituated attitudes toward fellow citizens." (Terrill 2011, 297). And while he suggested that is an especially productive resource for citizenship, Robert Terrill also argued that these attitudes cultivate a form of duality. I argue that such duality encourages stigma reproduction related to the hierarchy of impairments and that from this reproduction comes a classification system built in the online deliberative spaces described here. Much as Kafer asks, "How is the category of disability used to justify the classification, supervision, segregation and oppression of certain people, bodies, and practices?" (2013, 9), we must ask how the push for name differentiation is doing so within these communities.

Concluding Connections

The argument between Type 1 and Type 2 diabetes that Deardorff (2010) described and the discourse surrounding the article and the Change.org petition is an ongoing, recurring rhetorical activity within diabetes patient communities, as the similar 2018 name-change petition on Change.org petition suggests. Understanding this activity as a system of exclusions that stigmatize human differences (Garland-Thompson 2005), we can challenge several assumptions made by both the medical community and general public about the disease. First is the assumption that the diabetic community is a singular or monolithic one. As I have argued elsewhere (Arduser 2017), diabetes—nor the complicated work people with diabetes undertake to care for their bodies—can be represented as a simple, singular process.

Using a disability studies perspective, this chapter has been able to highlight the diversity of this illness community and illustrate a glaring instance of community-generated reproduction of social stigma. Such social stigma of a disease by others is well recognized in scholarly literature (see Peel et al. 2005; Schabert et al. 2013) and the mass media (see Perez-Pena 2006). And more recent work has also examined perceptions of being stigmatized by lived experiences of stigma in people with diabetes (Basinger et al. 2020). Such work makes it clear that language has been "used to arrange people in ways that are socially and economically convenient to the society" (Linton 2006, 161). But the focus in these works is for the most part contained to the binary between non-disabled and disabled bodies, thereby missing the process of how people with disabilities/chronic illness stigmatize others with disabilities/chronic illness.

Despite the calls for unity in the comments I examined related to the Change.org petition, the defensive othering occurring in these texts results in supporting the belief system of the dominant group, namely people without diabetes. Returning to the metaphor of a civil war, deeply embedded prejudices continue to surface because of the discursive actions related to othering. The implications of the diabetes civil war include the reinforcement of stereotypes about Type 1 and Type 2 identities. These stereotypes can impact "built environments" such as research funding that includes developing new technologies, such as the artificial pancreas, and public health funding that can have impacts for people with Type 2 diabetes.

References

Arduser, Lora. 2011. Warp and Weft: Weaving the Discussion Threads of an Online Community. *Journal of Technical Writing and Communication* 41 (1): 5–31.

———. 2013. The Care and Feeding of the D-Beast: Metaphors of the Lived Experience of Diabetes. In *Rhetorical Accessibility: At the Intersection of Technical Communication and Disability Studies*, ed. Lisa Meloncon, 95–113. Amityville, NY: Baywood's Technical Communication Series.

———. 2017. *Living Chronic: Agency and Expertise in the Rhetoric of Diabetes*. Columbus: The Ohio State University Press.

Aristotle. 1932. *The Rhetoric of Aristotle*. Translated by Lane Cooper. London: Prentice-Hall, Inc.

Asen, Robert. 2000. Seeking the "Counter" in Counterpublics. *Communication Theory* 10 (4): 424–446.

Atwood, Molly E., Aliza Friedman, Brad A. Meisner, and Stephanie E. Cassin. 2018. The Exchange of Social Support on Online Bariatric Surgery Discussion Forums: A Mixed-Methods Content Analysis. *Health Communication* 33 (5): 625–628.

Bakke, Abigail. 2019. Trust-Building in a Patient Forum: The Interplay of Professional and Personal Expertise. *Journal of Technical Writing and Communication* 49 (2): 56–182.

Basinger, Erin D., Molly Farris, and Amy L. Delaney. 2020. Investigating the Experience of Diabetes Stigma in Online Forums. *Southern Communication Journal* 85 (1): 43–57.

Bowker, Geoffrey C., and Susan Leigh Star. 1999. *Sorting Things Out: Classification and Its Consequences*. Cambridge: The MIT Press.

Centers for Disease Control. 2020. National Diabetes Statistics Report. Centers for Disease Control. https://www.cdc.gov/diabetes/data/statistics/statistics-report.html.

Deal, Mark. 2003. Disabled People's Attitudes Toward Other Impairment Groups: A Hierarchy of Impairments. *Disability & Society* 18 (7): 897–910.

Deardorff, Julie. November 22, 2010. Diabetes' Civil War: People with Type 1 Diabetes, Outnumbered and Overshadowed by Type 2, Fight for Recognition, Resources—and a New Name for Their Disorder. *The Chicago Tribune*. http://articles.chicagotribune.com/2010-11-22/a-z/ct-met-diabetes-rift-20101122_1_diabetes-insulin-lifestyle-changes-and-medication

Dijk, Van, and A. Teun. 2018. Critical Discourse Analysis. In *The Handbook of Discourse Analysis Critical Discourse Analysis*, ed. Deborah Tannen, Heidi E. Hamilton, and Deborah Schiffrin, 466–485. United Kingdom: John Wiley & Sons.

Ferguson, Kevin L. 2010. The Cinema of Control: On Diabetic Excess and Illness in Film. *Journal of Medical Humanities* 31 (3): 183–204.

Feudtner, Chris. 2003. *Bittersweet: Diabetes, Insulin, and the Transformation of Illness*. Chapel Hill: The University of North Carolina Press.

Field, Stephanie J. 1994. Becoming Irish: Personal Identity Construction among First-Generation Irish Immigrants. *Symbolic Interaction* 17: 431–435.

Fraser, Nancy. 1990. Rethinking the Public Sphere: A Contribution to the Critique of Actually Existing Democracy. *Social Text* 25 (26): 56–80.

Garland-Thomson, Rosemarie. 2002. Disability, Transforming Feminist Theory. *NWSA Journal* 14 (3): 1–32.

———. 2005. Feminist Disability Studies. *Sign* 30 (2): 1557–1587.

Gee, James Paul. 2011. *How to Do Discourse Analysis: A Toolkit.* New York: Routledge.

Ghiaciuc, Susan. 2011. Invisible Credibility: Ethos and the E-patient. *Disability Studies Quarterly* 31 (1). Accessed December 14, 2020. https://dsq-sds.org/article/view/1372/1502

Goffman, Erving. 2017. Selection form Stigma. In *The Disability Studies Reader*, ed. Lennard J. Davis, 5th ed., 133–144. New York: Routledge.

Goodnight, Thomas G. 1982. The Personal, Technical, and Public Spheres of Argument: A speculative Inquiry into the Art of Public Deliberation. *Journal of the American Forensic Association* 18: 214–227.

———. 1987. Public Discourse. *Critical Studies in Mass Communication* 4: 428–431.

———. 2012. The Personal, Technical, and Public Spheres of Argument: A Speculative Inquiry into the Art of Public Deliberation. *Argumentation and Advocacy* 48 (4): 198–210.

Habermas, Jürgen. 1974. The Public Sphere: An Encyclopedia Article. *New German Critique* 3: 49–50.

Hughes, Bill. 2009. Wounded/Monstrous/Abject: A Critique of the Disabled Body in the Sociological Imaginary. *Disability and Society* 24 (4): 399–410.

Johnstone, Barbara, and Christopher Eisenhart. 2008. *Rhetoric in Detail: Discourse Analyses of Rhetorical Talk and Text.* Amsterdam: John Benjamins Publishing Company.

Kafer, Alison. 2013. *Feminist Queer Crip.* Bloomington: Indiana University Press.

Keränen, Lisa. 2014. Public Engagements with Health and Medicine. *Journal of the Medical Humanities* 35 (2): 103–109.

Linton, Simi. 2006. Reassigning Meaning. In *The Disability Studies Reader*, ed. Lennard J. Davis, 2nd ed., 161–172. New York: Routledge.

Macagno, Fabrizio, and Douglas Walton. 2009. Argument from Analogy in Law, the Classical Tradition, and Recent Theories. *Philosophy and Rhetoric* 42 (2): 154–182.

Mackiewicz, Jo. 2010. Assertions of Expertise in Online Product Reviews. *Journal of Business and Technical Communication* 24 (1): 3–28.

McKee, Heidi, and James Porter. 2009. *The Ethics of Internet Research: A Rhetorical, Case-Based Process.* New York: Peter Lang Publishing.

McPherson, James M. 1989. *Battle Cry of Freedom.* New York: Ballantine Books.

Oliver, Mike. 1990, July 23. The Individual and Social Models of Disability. Paper presented at The *Joint Workshop of the Living Options Group and the Research Unit of the Royal College of Physicians.* https://disability-studies.leeds.ac.uk/wp-content/uploads/sites/40/library/Oliver-in-soc-dis.pdf

Peel, Elizabeth A., Odette Parry, Margaret Douglas, and Julia Lawton. 2005. Taking the Biscuit? A Discursive Approach to Managing Diet in Type 2 Diabetes. *Journal of Health Psychology* 10: 779–791.

Perez, Jamie. 2013. Revise Names of Type 1 & 2 Diabetes to Reflect the Nature of Each Disease. *Change.org*. Accessed 2013. http://www.change.org/petitions/revise-names-of-type-1-2-diabetes-to-reflect-the-nature-of-each-disease.

Perez-Pena, Richard. 2006. Beyond 'I'm a Diabetic,' Little Common Ground. *The New York Times*, online, May 17. http://www.nytimes.com/2006/05/17/nyregion/17diabetes.html?pagewanted=all&_r=0.

Prelli, Lawrence J. 1997. The Rhetorical Construction of Scientific Ethos. In *Landmark Essays on the Rhetoric of Science: Case Studies*, ed. Randy Allen Harris, 87–104. Mahwah: Lawrence Erlbaum Associates.

Redington, Luke. 2017. Methodology on Trial: The Rhetorical Function of Toulminian Warrants in Expert Testimony. *Journal of Technical Writing and Communication* 47 (4): 396–418.

Rock, Melanie. 2005. Classifying Diabetes; or, Commensurating Bodies of Unequal Experience. *Public Culture* 17 (3): 467–486.

Schabert, Jasmin, Jessica L. Browne, Kylie Mosely, and Jane Speight. 2013. Social Stigma in Diabetes: A Framework to Understand a Growing Problem for an Increasing Epidemic. *The Patient—Patient-Centered Outcomes Research* 6 (1): 1–10.

Schwalbe, Michael, Sanrda Dodwin, Daphne Holden, Douglas Schrock, Shealy Thompson, and Michele Wolkomir. 2000. Generic Processes in the Reproduction of Inequality: An Interactionist Analysis. *Social Forces* 79: 419–452.

Snow, David, and Leon Anderson. 1987. Identity Work among the Homeless: The Verbal Construction and Avowal of Personal Identities. *American Journal of Sociology* 92: 1336–1371.

Terrill, Robert. 2011. Mimesis, Duality, and Rhetorical Education. *Rhetoric Society Quarterly* 41 (4): 295–315.

The Expert Committee on the Diagnosis and Classification of Diabetes Mellitus. 2002. Report of the Expert Committee on the Diagnosis and Classification of Diabetes Mellitus. *Diabetes Care* 25 (1): S5–S20.

Warnick, Barbara. 2007. *Rhetoric Online: Persuasion and Politics on the World Wide Web*. New York: Peter Lange.

Zarefsky, David, Carol Miller-Tutzauer, and Frank E. Tutzauer. 1984. Reagan's Safety Net for the Truly Needy: The Rhetorical Uses of Definition. *Central States Speech Journal* 35: 113–119.

The #insulin4all Movement: A Few Committed Individuals Isn't Enough

Clair Irwin

Introduction

In 1996, Eli Lilly released the first rapid-acting analog insulin, Humalog (insulin lispro). This drug acted more swiftly within the body than its predecessors and thus promised greater flexibility in dosing. At the time of its release, Humalog cost $20 USD/vial ($33 when calculated for inflation). Four years later, Sanofi released an equally revolutionary analog insulin. When Lantus went on the market, it cost around $21 USD/vial. Hugely popular for its slow-release function, medical professionals continue to prescribe Lantus (insulin glargine) more than its competitors or analog alternatives (Sanofi 2020).

"A few committed individuals" is a nod to France and Schulman's work on *How to Survive a Plague*. If you're unfamiliar with the AIDS crisis, it is an excellent film for those interested in learning more.

C. Irwin (✉)
University of Illinois Urbana-Champaign, Champaign, IL, USA

B. C. Frazer, H. R. Walker (eds.), *(Un)doing Diabetes: Representation, Disability, Culture*, Palgrave Studies in Science and Popular Culture, https://doi.org/10.1007/978-3-030-83110-3_4

Between their respective market release dates and 2014, the list prices for insulin outpaced inflation. By the time of #insulin4all's launch in 2014, Humalog cost $204/vial, and Lantus, $222/vial. An "average" household could afford 3 vials of insulin per month because they cost 5% of the median monthly income, just shy of $54k/year (Bureau, "Income and Poverty in the United States."). Yet for the 2-million (Bureau of Labor Statistics, "Characteristics of Minimum Wage Workers, 2014") earning the federal minimum wage of $7.25/hour or less, three vials' insulin cost 48% of their monthly income (assuming a 40-hour work week). To put it another way: three vials of insulin required 87 hours of minimum wage labor. Today, the list price of *one* vial of insulin lies around $300 (42 hours' minimum wage labor). A month's supply costs more than a month of fulltime minimum wage labor can afford.

Beneath these statistics lie their impact on quality of life. While the cost of insulin has risen, the need for this life-sustaining medication has not. For many people with diabetes, myself included, the high cost of insulin forces us to choose between insulin and rent, insulin and groceries, insulin and heat. The high cost of insulin demands we sacrifice rest, joy, and dreams to afford our breath. These conditions represent what we refer to as "the insulin crisis." While recent legislation in the United States suggests this crisis is a product of the 2010s, in truth it has wrought havoc on low-income Americans for nearly two decades. Activists with diabetes have responded to the insulin crisis through online and in-person organizing. As I will discuss in this chapter, #insulin4all started as an online movement (hence the hashtag). For the purposes of this chapter, I will look at the movement as a whole through my lens as an activist within it.

In analyzing #insulin4all, I argue that the activist practices of the movement are directly influenced by and a natural progression forward from the activist practices of ACT UP. ACT UP (Aids Coalition to Unleash Power) laid the groundwork for much of our activism and continues strong today. #insulin4all founder, Elizabeth Pfiester, has spoken of looking to ACT UP for ideas about strategy and organization. In 2019, I listened with other activists as an ACT UP scholar-activist reflected on his own experiences of healthcare advocacy as wisdom and cautionary tales for our efforts. After listening to them speak, I began exploring further points of influence. I was motivated to understand ACT UP's history and successes in the hopes that I could infuse my activism with elements that worked for them.

In this chapter, I argue that the movements are linked, not just in activist practices, but in the circumstances with which each arose and gained traction with the general public. Because ACT UP has now had so many years of history and development, I limit my analysis to the first three years of ACT UP's work to draw the most impactful parallels between the two movements. In so doing, I also examine the strengths of looking to ACT UP for guidance on how to engage in political healthcare advocacy. At a few points within this paper, I acknowledge the situational and historical circumstances that seem to have brought both ACT UP and #insulin4all into the public eye, specifically regarding whiteness. Seeing as many frontline AIDS activists were white men, some scholars have questioned whether a similar movement would have gained attention had it been led by lesbians and/or people of color. I have the same questions regarding the #insulin4all movement. However, examining the racial tension in #insulin4all, including an in-depth analysis of the U.S. infrastructures that orchestrated the insulin crisis and their intersection with white supremacist policies, is beyond the scope of this essay.[1]

At the time of writing this chapter, I have lived with Type 1 diabetes for eighteen years and volunteered with #insulin4all ("our movement" or "the movement") for three years. I founded the Illinois chapter of #insulin4all and have carried on in an education leadership role since returning to academia. My critiques, thus, come from within the movement and carry suggestions for forward momentum. With that said, attempting to record a movement from within its surge falls short of the complex reality experienced by a multitude of activists propelling our cause forward. The additional accounts and perspectives found throughout this book add to what I offer here.

I use auto-historiography as a methodology for several reasons. First, because of my place within #insulin4all, as a person with diabetes who has been forced to rationed my insulin due to in affordability; I understand the embodied experience of activism under these conditions. Being an insider-researcher allows me not only to recognize nuances of our movement, but also to represent the movement from within.

In terms of process, auto-historiography requires a marriage of autobiography with history (Aurell and Davis 2019). I used detailed personal records from 2018–2020, such as Twitter logs and journal entries to

[1] I hope to publish a companion piece to this chapter focusing on #insulin4all's troublesome relationship with race, including recommendations for forward restorative movement.

account for my own in-real-time reflections of the events I'll discuss herein. I provide a rough sketch of our #insulin4all advocacy within the historiographical record of on- and offline diabetes activism.

Diabetes as Disability

Disability studies as a field has settled on mostly uniform definitions and treatment of the terms: *disability* and *impairment. Impairment* is what disability studies scholar, Eli Clare (2009), describes as "real lived physical limitations:" or, the body's deviation from species-typical functioning. For diabetes, atypical pancreatic function is the impairment. The body not using insulin efficiently is an impairment. "Disability" is the manifestation of societal prejudice and biases against impairment. Inaccessibility is *always* a case of disability, because it occurs when other people/groups create a situation that ignores impairment. Inaccessibility for people with diabetes manifest in rigid attendance policies, "no food allowed" signs, obscured nutrition facts, and the largest inaccessibility of all—unaffordable insulin. Physical inaccessibilities are additional layers of disablement.

According to Clare, humanity's deepest and most impossible wish is to live life without impairment, or at least, without disability. This desire, in diabetes, is striving for self-management that is so perfected that the body is as close to species-typical as is possible. Along its ridges lie glimpses of that perfection: euglycemic A1C, painlessness, "strong work ethic"—anything we do "despite" our disability of diabetes. These glimpses lie just out of reach, as with any form of perfection. What is worse, we often locate the blame for any metabolic irregularity and/or subsequent complication within ourselves. Our society treats diabetes as the ultimate consequence for bad behavior and we bear the side effects of that treatment—internalization. We internalize the ableist thinking that threatens further impairment if we end up with anything less than perfection. And so, we try relentlessly, even though we cannot "overcome" an incurable illness through resolve and determination. The diabetes will still be in our bodies, no matter how much activism we do and how much change we make.

Yet we keep going. Clare asserts that this "is another kind of supercrip story, a story about internalizing supercripdom, about becoming a supercrip in [his] mind's eye." As a genre, "supercrip stories" depict someone with an impairment/disability managing to "overcome" their disablement in spite of their impairment. Rarely realistic, these stories build on the deficit model of disability and its conception that there exists a universal "normal" human body. The deficit model takes this idea of a universal corporeal normate and eschews any bodies deviating from the ideal. For people with impairments, this places us in a precarious doublethink. Our bodies deviate from normalcy, yet we must continue living in a world that either denies disability or blames the disabled for their impairments. Failure to "overcome" our impairment—to behave as if it doesn't exist—opens us up for criticism, unwanted surveillance and advice, pity, and scorn.

My experience leading the Illinois #insulin4all chapter ("the Illinois chapter") illustrates one such supercrip story. I spent twelve months leading the Illinois chapter while at the same time I spent six months preparing to or rationing my insulin. Months before, I had left my job as an elementary teacher because of discriminatory actions underscored by ableism (e.g. school authorities forbidding me from taking breaks to test my blood sugar). My resignation resulted in financial insecurity, which of course, resulted in me rationing my insulin. I kept this story to myself for the most part because I feared my choice to leave a toxic work environment would justify my lowered quality of life to our political adversaries; even though my story has within it specific intricacies of capitalist exploitation (i.e. my insulin insecurity exists because of corporate greed made possibly only in capitalist economies). The possibility of critique and dismissal silenced me so effectively that not even those in my own home knew I was rationing my dosages. I pretended like I had it all together. Like I could not just survive, but thrive through the hardest of times. I know now that I was performing and representing that supercrip narrative. And I experienced the cost of internalized supercripdom and its counterpart, internalized ableism. Participating and leading the Illinois #insulin4all chapter was my first opportunity to take a step back and see those internalizations for what they were: a lie. I was learning to identify the insidiousness behind the lie that had dictated so much of my thoughts and behavior. I was learning not only that I wasn't to blame for my impairment but that there were healthy ways to live with disability outside the bounds of supercripdom. In other words, I was unlearning internalized self-expectations that my disability would lead to a superhuman ability to overcome significant discomfort, pain, and trauma. I had to unlearn this lie even though it was so engrained that I'd begun to metabolize it into a walking forgetfulness of my own corporeal truth.

What follows is an auto-historiographical analysis of #insulin4all and ACT UP. The story of #insulin4all is told through my lens as a person with diabetes who has had significant involvement in the movement. The story of ACT UP comes by way of a collection of perspectives and documentations from activists, scholars, and journalists who have written about, and in many cases experienced the movement firsthand. My goal will be to illuminate the ways in which our activism in #insulin4all was influenced by and, what I would argue, a natural progression from the activist practices of ACT UP.

Founding and Organization

#insulin4all Founding and Organization

In November 2014, frustrated by the hollow messaging around World Diabetes Day, Elizabeth Pfiester[2] led T1International (a UK-based non-profit) in launching #insulin4all. Pfiester hoped to use the launch to recenter discussions of accessibility and affordability within the diabetes community. Many in the diabetes community used World Diabetes Day to focus on educating non-diabetics about the more physical aspects of diabetes like injections or number of glucose tests per day (Farley 2019). At the time of the launch, Pfiester lived in the United Kingdom as a medical refugee—someone who fled the United States in search of affordable health care and medications. Born in Illinois, she moved to the UK to pursue her graduate education in International Development and Humanitarian Emergencies at the London School of Economics and Political Science (Van Ness 2018).

While completing her studies, Pfiester realized she could make lasting change in the diabetes community (Van Ness 2018). She founded T1International and continues to serve as their executive director. T1International and Pfiester have played a foundational role in #insulin4all. Nevertheless, both quickly insist state volunteer activists have shaped the movement.[3] Though #insulin4all originated and continues as a world-wide effort, this essay focuses on the actions of US-based volunteer-activists like myself.

Unpaid volunteer activists put in both in-person and online labor for the US branches of #insulin4all and receive administrative support from T1International. At the time I was writing this chapter, nearly forty states

[2] Elizabeth Pfiester and Elizabeth Rowley are the same person.

[3] T1International, "USA Chapters—T1International."

had an #insulin4all chapter. A chapter leader guides each chapter, and most have additional leadership roles within their ranks. For example, the Illinois chapter has a chapter leader (Jennifer Ladisch-Douglass, who also serves as our legislative lead),[4] a communities of color outreach lead (Alzahrra Almajid), and a research, resource, and education lead (myself). Alison Hiller, who led the chapter between Ladisch-Douglass's tenure and mine, also continues in an emeritus role. Some chapters have more robust leadership teams, but many have only the chapter leader. Clayton McCook, chapter leader of the Oklahoma chapter, has essentially led the entire state by himself since 2018.[5] To offset the administrative labor and social pressure of carrying forward activism on behalf of all people with diabetes in our respective states, state chapters collaborated on delicate political strategies, mutual aid, and other endeavors falling within the scope of the movement.

Angela Lautner formed the first American #insulin4all chapter. A Kentucky resident, she attended the inaugural Eli Lilly protest in September 2017 (Wofford 2017), where she spoke to a small group of protestors about her experiences struggling to purchase insulin. She voiced anger and frustration over stopgap measures like accepting familial support and switching medications. Lautner founded the KOI (Kentucky-Ohio-Indiana) chapter with other patient-activists in March 2018, almost exactly 31 years after ACT UP's genesis. The KOI chapter would eventually split into three separate chapters managing their own states, but not before making national waves through publicity and legislative lobbying (Sable-Smith 2019).

#insulin4all has relied heavily on patient testimonials to emotionally stir representatives and the public into action. A large part of this strategic reliance on personal story comes from the relatively unique relationship diabetics have with all components of biomedicine. Our relationship with pharmaceuticals is not one born of discomfort, but rather of self-preservation. That is, we go after them not because what they do offends us, but because our lives depend on it. To have diabetes means daily hurtling biological circumstances that were, indeed, a death sentence just one century ago. Our bodies exist in a constant cessation of entropy; our lives unwind and untether as blood glucose levels go up; our minds hold

[4] Thanks to Jennifer Ladisch-Douglass, Alzahrra Almajid, and Alison Hiller for allowing mention of their names and roles in this essay.

[5] Clayton McCook has approved discussion of his work in this way.

suspended biological processes that no longer automatically function. To be diabetic is to stave off death, and if you find that melodramatic, you've never rationed your insulin.

ACT UP Founding and Organization

In the 1980s, AIDS was a death sentence. It attacked the immune system with inhumane efficiency and left the body vulnerable to any manner of infection. Any definition of AIDS fails to encapsulate the corporeal nightmare the disease presented before experts began to take it seriously. Hospitals turned away those infected with and dying of AIDS or other opportunistic infections like Kaposi's Sarcoma (France and Schulman 2012). Survivors speak of needing friends with excellent makeup skills, because the characteristic lesions on those infected with Kaposi's sarcoma often prompted explicit discrimination (Carlomusto and Schulman 2002). Various institutions like the US government and the medical field *heavily* stigmatized AIDS,[6] as indicated by its earlier names: the CDC called the infection the "4H" disease, referring to Haitians, hemophiliacs, heroin users, and homosexuals (Gilman 1987). Journalism's term, GRID, wasn't much better, referring to "gay-related immune deficiency" (Altman 1982).

Over 20,000 people living in the US had died of AIDS at the time of ACT UP's formation (FACT 2005). Nearly every ACT UP activist has a story like Robert Vazquez-Pacheco. Vazquez-Pacheco said in 2012 of his deceased lover, "I went through the beginnings of the AIDS epidemic with him, nurses putting his tray of food on the floor outside his hospital room, the whole thing. And he died in 1986 in bed next to me." Stories such as these prompted members of the New York City LGBTQ+ community to form ACT UP in 1987, rallied by an impassioned speech by author and playwright Larry Kramer (France 2012)

Parallels and Influences

In this section, I outline and describe the parallels, differences, and influences between #insulin4all and ACT UP. The purpose of this section is not to directly compare the movements, but to explore social and cultural connections and activist responses to them. First, both movements were spurred in response to existing activism and advocacy efforts. Pfiester and T1International deliberately rolled out the insulin4all campaign to course correct existing diabetes advocacy and activism perceived of as too soft and

[6] A stigma that continues today.

gracious (and too "in the pocket" of the pharmaceutical companies creating the crisis to begin with). Similarly, ACT UP activism appears to have been a natural progression from Larry Kramer's organization, Gay Men's Health Crisis (GMHC), which itself was formed in response to government inaction (History—GMHC 2021). Several accounts suggest that hundreds of individuals agreed to form ACT UP and begin their advocacy in a call-and-response style meeting. Larry Kramer refers to himself as the founder of the movement,[7] but it might be more accurate to describe him as the caller to whom the LGBTQ community responded. Thus, both movements built upon and shifted from community efforts who came before them.

The medium by which activists connected with the movement has changed with available technology, but this difference is, arguably, only superficial. #insulin4all began and primarily continues online, as evident in its hashtag. The flexibility of our digital activism has allowed even people sick from rationing their insulin to continue advocating for change despite significant physical and financial hardship. Though plenty of #insulin4all work exists on Instagram and Facebook, Twitter has served our movement as the primary mechanism of maintaining pressure on elected officials. Twitter's infrastructure has complicated elected officials' ability to completely ignore us when we speak (Holland 2020; Coburn 2020). Indeed, Twitter allowed the serendipitous interaction between Illinois Representative Will Guzzardi (D-39) and myself that marked the formation of the Illinois chapter (Irwin 2018). Organizing online has allowed a central feature of #insulin4all to thrive: an effective community structure of mutual aid. In our online communities, this looks like sending a vial of insulin or a set of pump supplies to others across the country who cannot afford or access them (Litchman et al. 2020). Though ACT UP formed during in-person community center meetings, they similarly happened between exchanges of mutual aid (i.e. helping those dying of AIDS write their wills and finding transportation to their doctor's appointments). While in-person activism may be less accessible than our cyber activism, ACT UP advocates never risked forgetting the consequences of failing to achieve their goals. They did what they could with what they had (e.g. using local media outlets and newsletters to publicize their stories and

[7] France, "The Men and Women Who Started ACT UP—New York Magazine—Nymag."

experience). And they took recordings to document the hundreds or thousands of ACT UP activists at their various protests.

Noteworthy documentaries like How to Survive a Plague demonstrate the theatricality with which HIV/AIDS activists took actions. Their visual protests and demonstrations were evocative, not just because of sheer crowd size (France and Schulman 2012), but because they addressed death. As if taking a page right out of the ACT UP handbook, #insulin4all activists have created and used tombstones and memorials in their in-person demonstrations (Raymond 2018). Thus, while the medium for and structures of connection was fundamentally different, both ACT UP and #insulin4all activists came together to produce mutual aid and to demonstrate their arguments with a theatricality worthy of media attention.

Noteworthy Departures

There are three areas of fundamental difference between ACT UP and #insulin4all that strengthen the impact of connection between them. First, ACT UP activists had considerable funds at their disposal. Meeting notes preserved in the New York Public Library's ACT UP special collection include treasury reports detailing thousands of dollars in funds. Activists used these funds for publicity materials like stickers, buttons, and posters, or for paying for members to attend legislative hearings. These funds came through the efforts of the fundraising branches of each ACT UP chapter (France and Schulman 2012). In comparison, #insulin4all chapters can expect roughly $100/year from T1International. Before T1International gained nonprofit status in the U.S., #insulin4all activists were actively discouraged from conducting fundraisers for chapter initiatives. This decision arose largely out of concern regarding misconduct reflecting poorly on the nonprofit with promises that once T1International 501C (3) status, chapters would receive more support. That #insulin4all activists have been able to remain a stable movement since its beginnings in 2014 is astonishing, given this difference.

Second, ACT UP disdains any hierarchical organization. Their website states, "All ACT UP members are leaders as we resist the traditional hierarchies and bureaucracies of other organizations."[8] #insulin4all, in comparison, has a heavily hierarchical structure in which each chapter falls under the jurisdiction of T1International. Somewhat predictably, as the movement grew, so appeared "shadow chapters" (groups claiming to be

[8] "Contact ACTUP New York | ACT UP NY."

official state #insulin4all chapters without the approval or oversight from T1International). Discussing the phenomena of shadow chapters and other oddities of the relationship between #insulin4all chapters and the nonprofit lies beyond the scope of this essay. However, it's notable that in many ways, the nonprofit expects #insulin4all volunteers to behave as employees without compensation. Examples of this expectation lies in branding and conduct guidelines, lack of funding, and communications. This is a particularly concerning aspect of #insulin4all, because it redistributes the power gained by grassroots organizing back into the hands of a nonprofit. As diabetics have seen time and again, nonprofits are often just as complicit in the insulin crisis. I say this not to levy judgement against T1International. However, the fact remains that we simply cannot trust organizations whose survival depends on our continued oppression, in this case, the insulin crisis.

Finally, and perhaps the most notable area of departure, the situational embodiment of HIV/AIDS in the 80s and diabetes today is fundamentally different. The antecedent conditions for each movement represent vastly different experiences of illness. People with insulin-dependent diabetes can expect to manage their health with injections for a typical lifespan, if they have the financial means to pay for it. People who contracted AIDS in the 1980s could not expect a typical lifespan, or even one lasting more than a few years.[9] We with diabetes have considerable privilege in comparison to early days AIDS activists because our condition isn't terminal.

Yet, as mentioned previously, diabetic people converse with death daily. When explaining the importance of insulin to those without my lived experience, I skip to the most important sentence: without insulin, I'm dead in three days. Considering the dynamics of structural privilege (i.e. being white) I benefit from, the condition of my life also differs from those who contracted AIDS in the 1980s because diabetes has a treatment by which it becomes chronic. Because AIDS in the 80s was considered terminal, it could be argued that ACT UP activists felt they had less to lose. While many HIV/AIDS activists, like Larry Kramer himself, survived until access to effective treatment was available, there was no way to predict who would survive and who wouldn't. We activists with diabetes,

[9] The development of pharmaceuticals changed mortality and morbidity for both AIDS and diabetes. The early mortality of AIDS was because there were no effective treatments. That changed drastically in 1996 with protease inhibitors.

though, must consider daily: will I lose my job because I said "Fuck pharma, but fuck Novo Nordisk, Sanofi, and Eli Lilly in particular"? How will I afford my insulin if I lose my job? Will I lose my child, because I can't afford *their* insulin? I told you we hold our lives suspended, and that's true, but we do so only through skilled use of *very* expensive tools. Our reliance on insulin has thus forced us into excessive caution.

Strategy and Milestones

ACT UP activists drove their advocacy using an "unapologetically confrontational" set of strategies. During their first protest in 1987, ACT UP activists gathered on Wall Street to protest the pharmaceutical industry's profiting off AIDS drugs. Of particular offense, activists focused on Burroughs Wellcome, the manufacturer of AZT. At the time, AZT was the only medication available to treat AIDS and tended to worsen quality of life after several weeks. Seven months later, ACT UP joined the March for Lesbian and Gay Rights on Washington, D.C. in October 1987 and demanded the Reagan administration prioritize fighting the AIDS epidemic (ACT UP 2012).

A year after their inaugural protest, ACT UP activists returned to Wall Street and for the first time, AIDS issues received major news coverage as the New York Police Department (NYPD) arrested over 100 activists. Chapters began forming around the country. Less than two months after their first major media coverage, ACT UP activists coordinated a series of protests focusing on specific intersections of the AIDS crisis like poverty and prison programs (ACT UP NY 2020). In October 1988, ACT UP activists swarmed the FDA to protest the extended drug testing timelines.

These actions sketch the first two years of ACT UP's existence. By late 1989, the FDA overhauled their entire pharmaceutical testing procedures to accelerate time between development and market debut. Despite this tremendous win, ACT UP activists maintained their pressure on those in power. On September 14, 1989, they invaded and stopped the New York Stock Exchange for the first time in history. On December 10, 1989, 4,500 protestors called out the Catholic Church for their "deadly, homophobic, and misogynistic AIDS and abortion policies" ('STOP THE CHURCH'). A month later, they halted Gov. Andrew Cuomo's State of the Union address to protest governmental inaction (ACT UP 2012). Other actions included "kiss-ins" (essentially sit-ins with gay couples kissing) and "the ever-popular (and very photogenic) die-ins" in which activists would lie down as if dead, holding posters with attention-grabbing images and phrases. ACT UP efforts included collaboration with artist collectives such as Gran Fury (d'Addario 2011).

ACT UP protestors refused to pull punches when calling attention to negligence perpetrated by the US government, the Catholic Church, medicine, and the pharmaceutical industry. At the same time, the depth of ranks within their organization allowed them to divert resources to support their community. People with AIDS often faced evictions, unemployment, and other forms of discrimination when their diagnosis became known ('Target City Hall'). ACT UP included in its organizational infrastructure committees devoted to helping members of their community advocate against insurers, landlords, and other wraparound issues related to AIDS (ACT UP NY 2020).

Before the US government passed the Americans with Disabilities Act,[10] people with AIDS had no legal protections from discrimination. The government passed a revised version of the ADA in 2008, increasing protections for people with disabilities using assistive devices, technology, or medication. I take time to mention this because #insulin4all coalesced in a world in which people with diabetes have had legal protection from disability-based discrimination for decades. The protections we enjoy have assuredly influenced our strategies in advocating for affordable and accessible insulin. We have not had to assault city hall with posters saying, "diabetics deserve a better place to live than your sidewalk." Many of us *only* know the privilege of legal protection, and thus we fail to manifest the same rage and fury ACT UP activists unleashed on the world. ACT UP activists had nowhere else to go. They had no legal protections to fall back on.[11] So, while members from both of our groups were/are dying due to ignorance and greed within the medical and pharmaceutical establishment, diabetic people, by and large, are not faced with the same sense of desperation and urgency. Instead, #insulin4all strategy has set its sights on the law.

[10] For more on the ADA, see "The Americans with Disabilities Act: A Brief Overview." Note that its passage did not immediately ensure people with disabilities wouldn't experience discrimination, but rather that they had allies should they choose to fight discrimination.

[11] With that said, many persons with AIDS were able to take advantage of an emerging structure of care largely led by the LGBTQ community at the time. See GMHC or MK Cerzwiez's comic narrative about Chicago.

The Legislative Goals of #insulin4all

#insulin4all strategy has emphasized passing legislation to achieve several goals. First, we've sought to increase transparency regarding the development, manufacturing, and pricing of insulin. In 2017, Nevada signed into law a prescription transparency statute, requiring pharmaceutical manufacturers to report to the state manufacturing costs, coupons, profits, and information regarding price increases (Sullivan 2019). While two pharmaceutical lobbying groups, PhRMA and BIO, initially sued the state regarding the law, they dropped the lawsuit in 2018 (Messerly 2018). Four other states (California, Maine, Oregon, and Vermont) have transparency legislation. These laws help demystify the drug pricing process, and as a 2019 report revealed, demonstrate unaffordability is a systemic issue spreading far further than one medication or state (Chollet et al. 2019). Notably, the trend of price-gouging insulin abruptly slowed in 2018, the year Nevada's law went into effect. In 2019, the state levied over $17 million in fines on companies "regarding noncompliance with the new price transparency law." (Sullivan 2019).

Secondly, activists have advocated for legislation providing emergency assistance in the event of expired prescriptions or other circumstances preventing adequate insulin access. Before #insulin4all gained momentum stateside, several states had already passed versions of "Kevin's Law"—emergency refill legislation, named after Ohio-based Kevin Houdeshell, who passed away after running out of refills over the New Year's holiday (Hoskins). In 2015, New Hampshire passed a law allowing a once-per-lifetime dispersal of a life-sustaining medication for no more than 72 hours. In 2017, Maryland passed an emergency refill law, with a once-per-lifetime limit and restricted to a 14-day supply.

Florida, Ohio, Arizona, Illinois, and Wisconsin have enacted similar laws, and many more states have passed this form of legislation since stateside #insulin4all activism began. Most recently, South Carolina Governor Henry McMaster (R) signed into law for immediate effect SB 16, which allows individuals to receive an emergency prescription refill once every year, covering medication for 14 days (30 if a 14-day supply is unavailable). This type of legislation has become even more vital given the increasing list of steps to obtain affordable insulin, a list that often takes days to complete. Consider Caiti Derenze's story: after her monthly prescription jumped from $50 to $300, she was ultimately instructed to talk to *four* different entities (the pharmacy, her insurance provider, Express Scripts, and her doctor) about the price increase (Talmadge). Should this process occur over a holiday weekend as it did with Kevin Houdeshell, it would prove deadly.

Third, activists have advocated for legislation focused on decreasing the cost of insulin, rather than increasing accessibility. Vermont, Florida (Anderson 2019), and Colorado (Rodriguez) have each passed laws allowing importation of prescription medications for resale within the state. These laws intend to bypass the bizarre difference in cost between insulins produced domestically and internationally (up to a 90% cost savings). Finally, Nicole Smith-Holt and James Holt Jr. have doggedly pursued legislation to create a safety net program in Minnesota in memory of their son, Alec, who passed away in 2017 from insulin rationing. Despite *significant* aggression from PhRMA, the Alec Smith Insulin Affordability Law went into effect July 1, 2020. The law allows Minnesota residents to buy a one-time supply of insulin for $35 if they have less than a week's worth of insulin (Edwards 2020). Less than a day before the law went into effect, the lobbying group PhRMA sued the state of Minnesota, claiming the act violates the Constitution. PhRMA's actions, though ultimately dropped, are noteworthy in that they mimic the group's reaction to the Nevada Price-Transparency statute. To date, #insulin4all activists have mobilized and successfully lobbied for over a dozen pieces of legislation improving access to insulin in the last two years. From what I could tell, in 2019, the movement consisted of roughly one hundred #insulin4all activists across the country. This group of committed individuals—less than the initial gathering of ACT UP activists—have passed over a dozen pieces of legislature in two years. Our success is remarkable, and worth celebrating.

It takes tremendous effort to pass a law. Here in Illinois, our one law to have passed—the Illinois Insulin Copay Price Cap law, formerly SB 667—did so without significant in-person effort from #insulin4all activists. We were simply too busy. We spent most of the legislative session leading up to SB 667's vote focusing on not one but *four* other bills. We worked with legislators before the Illinois House of Representatives and Senate convened; we attended committee hearings; we advocated for our community members to sign witness slips and call their representatives; we tracked down more people willing to tell their story. At the height of my work with #insulin4all in 2019 as the Illinois chapter leader, I spent at least forty (unpaid) hours a week advocating for change. I am not an exceptional activist within the movement.

Supercrip and the Human Cost of Activism

I take time to mention the labor I've invested to draw attention to one of the greatest examples of supercripdom within #insulin4all: strong work ethic. The praise we give each other is indicative of this. We speak about Smith-Holt and Holt Jr.'s "tireless" efforts. We weave it into the movement through our own expectations of ourselves. Lautner would spend hours before work each day, contacting senators and representatives, trying to get something, *anything* passed. Lautner, Smith-Holt and Holt Jr., and I each demonstrate in our actions a deep commitment to #insulin4all, but each of us has day jobs. Lautner and I both have diabetes, an additional full-time job. We have precious little time on our hands for rest, and the work we do is tremendously stressful—undoubtedly another point of similarity between activists of ACT UP and #insulin4all, though I digress.

Working ourselves to exhaustion has become such a movement norm that at least five chapter leaders have stepped down due to serious health complications. We share this norm with ACT UP activists, but the circumstances around our advocacy diverge from those around theirs. Unlike many diagnosed with AIDS, we don't have months to live; most of us living with diabetes expect long lives. The expectations of ourselves to labor without sufficient rest do not meet the reality of our limitations.

We #insulin4all activists perform and represent the supercrip narrative by continuing to call out corporate greed even when we need rest. We've passed legislation, been covered in hundreds of news articles, and tried to keep each other alive via mutual aid since 2018 when #insulin4all began in earnest. And yet, our bodies still need insulin, we are still impaired, and until insulin is free, we're still disabled by economic structures that favor wealth of a few over the lives of many. We live on life's needle-sharp edge: our life's sustenance too expensive to live with, too precious to live without. Our bodies unwinding as we try to save our lives by killing our bodies a little bit at a time (i.e. rationing). While death is not a forgone conclusion for us, as it was with many of our ACT UP activist predecessors, this crisis *is* killing us. When ACT UP formed three decades ago, nothing in the world could protect the body from AIDS' relentless attack. In 2021, now many years after #insulin4all began in the US, we have identified things that can protect the body from the slow unwinding of insulin rationing (e.g. mutual aid, state-by-state co-pay cap legislation).

Many of us #insulin4all activists seem to have steady access to those protective things. I, a grad student, have access to subsidized prescriptions; my insulin costs me $15 a month. Clayton McCook talks of his family's stability and its dependence on his wellness (Lieberman 2019; Konrad 2017; Siddons 2020). We care for our bodies as we work other jobs. Our lives rise from one blood sugar reading to the next, and so grows the list of what we may lose if we become too angry or radical within a given movement. Other, less tangible things protect us from the horrible unwinding death of insulin rationing. My educational background and professional connections helped me stay alive when I was in a position requiring I ration my insulin. In my experience, the institutions and providers of care in our medical system in the US listen to hetero-cis men more than anyone else; and to established adults more than 20-somethings like myself and a large portion of those who've died of insulin rationing. Education, professionalism (and its classist connotations), heteronormativity, and advanced age all protect against the insulin crisis because it is an issue that is inherently social and economic.

However, these privileges also push us toward more moderate forms of activism because we feel our socially constructed limitations even if we can't admit that truth. Too overworked to notice our inflexible expectations, too grateful for the tools we do have to harness the urgent rage of our predecessors—these are our limitations. We have so much awareness of our community—1 in 4 ration, 180 decisions a day, 8,000 hours spent thinking about diabetes in a year—so many numbers to quantify what *diabetic* means in the twenty-first century, and yet us #insulin4all activists haven't yet seen the needle move. As a society, we've done little to mitigate the daily crises of this illness. Diabetic people are still suffering, and they are still dying from the effects of rationing insulin. The primary public representation of diabetes still revolves around choice, lifestyle, and self-inflicted burden (Bock 2012). People with diabetes are still blasted across social media for being "fat" and for "choosing insulin over a healthy diet". However, it is my belief that not only has our cause been seen, heard, and even acted upon (i.e. legislation), our representational strategies have moved our community to see itself as a political one, instead of just individuals dealing with individual pains. Though, I'd also argue that we were lucky in the latter result. Without much pause to question our motives or logic, the #insulin4all movement gambled the entire community's welfare on our ability to pass laws and scream loudly enough into the void that the American public answered.

Looking Ahead

At the time of writing this chapter, activists, myself included, are still putting forth effort to make insulin affordable for everyone—which would supposedly (I am not convinced) end the insulin crisis. Here I feel compelled to echo critical disability theorist Michelle Fine in calling for us to "imagine structural transformations beyond inclusion." (Fine 2019). Why do we advocate for affordable insulin, but not for free insulin? Why do we advocate for better access to health insurance, but not universal health insurance? Why do we advocate for better access to insulin alone, and not for abolition of institutions—like prisons—that prevent reliable, self-directed access to insulin?

For my fellow advocates (including those interested but yet uninvolved) I have three recommendations. First, we must consider the most marginalized lives affected by the insulin crisis. If we are honest about insulin for *all*, then we must re-shift our advocacy to focus on abolitionist solidarity, among a myriad of other causes equally urgent. Secondly, we #insulin4all volunteers must distance ourselves from T1International, for our relationship with them encourages the very supercrip narratives I've warned against and because their enterprise relies on the highly skilled and unpaid labor of volunteers like me to feverishly work ourselves against our best interest. That they gain such tremendous power from us and fail to financially support us *during an economically fueled biomedical crisis* is unethical. Perhaps here is where we take a final que from ACT UP, which has lasted three decades with nonhierarchical structures, mutual aid, fundraising, and aggressive policy demands. Disbursing the responsibility and pressure across members better allows for personal self-care of the kind Audre Lorde asserts we must practice in order to change the world. The idea that a few committed individuals can change the world is perhaps true, but misguided. We need to release that pressure from ourselves, or the day will come when we lose one of our advocates to the very beast we fight.

Finally, we must resist the urge to distill our stories to facts and numbers, for these are things that oversimplify our experience. We focus on the statistics: 1 in 4 ration their insulin (Axios 2019). But the numbers don't work to shift the sort of public awareness we need to achieve our goals of affordable and freely accessible insulin. Thus far, we have focused on capturing the public's intellect, but this is a mistake. We must capture their hearts with our stories of diabetic struggle and *joy*. Instead of quantifying and calculating our pain, we must focus our work on creating.

Acknowledgements Many thanks to the following readers, editors, and moral support as I grappled with this bear of a project: John Asbill, Bonnie Mak, Bradley Irwin, Rachel Magee, Kiri Palm, Valerie Flynn, and Jodi Schneider. To my esteemed editors, this wouldn't be possible without your guidance and support.

References

ACT UP. 2012. ACT UP Accomplishments and Partial Chronology | ACT UP NY. https://actupny.com/actions/.

ACT UP NY. 2020. The ACT UP Historical Archive: ACT UP 1987 Wall Street Action—List of Demands. ACT UP NY Historical Archive. https://actupny.org/documents/1stFlyer.html.

Addario, John d'. 2011. AIDS, Art and Activism: Remembering Gran Fury. *Hyperallergic*, December 1. https://hyperallergic.com/42085/aids-art-activism-gran-fury/.

Altman, Lawrence K. 1982. New Homosexual Disorder Worries Health Officials (Published 1982). *The New York Times*, May 11, sec. Science. https://www.nytimes.com/1982/05/11/science/new-homosexual-disorder-worries-health-officials.html.

American Diabetes Association. Law Enforcement | ADA. Accessed October 13, 2020. https://www.diabetes.org/resources/know-your-rights/discrimination/rights-with-law-enforcement.

Anderson, Curt. 2019. Florida Governor Signs Bill for Foreign Drug Importation. June 11. https://apnews.com/article/d9692c759cde483da113ac9c21ea681e.

Aurell, Jaume, and Rocio G. Davis. October 2, 2019. History and Autobiography: The Logics of a Convergence. *Life Writing* 16 (4): 503–511. https://doi.org/10.1080/14484528.2019.1648198.

Bock, Sheila. 2012. Contextualization, Reflexivity, and the Study of Diabetes-Related Stigma. *Journal of Folklore Research* 49 (2): 153–178. https://doi.org/10.2979/jfolkrese.49.2.153.

Bureau of Labor Statistics. 2015. Characteristics of Minimum Wage Workers, 2014, 17.

Bureau, US Census. Income and Poverty in the United States: 2014. *The United States Census Bureau*. Accessed October 14, 2020. https://www.census.gov/library/publications/2015/demo/p60-252.html.

Carlomusto, Jean, and Sarah Schulman. 2002. Mix—The New York Lesbian & Gay Experimental Film Festival, 46.

Chollet, Deborah, William Mulhern, Jia Pu, and Mathematica. 2019. What Are We Learning from State Reporting on Drug Pricing?—The National Academy for State Health Policy. December 2. https://www.nashp.org/what-are-we-learning-from-state-reporting-on-drug-pricing/.

Clare, Eli. 2009. *Exile and Pride*. 2nd ed. Durham: Duke University Press.

Coburn, Morgan. 2020. Morgan Coburn on Twitter. *Twitter*, September 10. https://twitter.com/Morgan_Coburn/status/1304133116219420672.

Edwards, Kiya. 2020. 'This Fight Is Not over': Insulin Affordability Act Goes into Effect as Pharmaceutical Industry Sues. *kare11.com*, July 1. https://www.kare11.com/article/news/local/kare11-sunrise/alec-smith-insulin-affordability-act-in-effect-last-minute-lawsuit-filed/89-7e8d4bec-a6ee-4b77-8ff1-5971cf8a07ce.

FACT. 2005. AIDS Timeline. Fighting Aids Continuously Together. https://www.factlv.org/timeline.htm.

Farley, Audrey. 2019. Drug Prices Are Killing Diabetics. 'Walmart Insulin' Isn't the Solution. *Washington Post*, February 19, 5.

Fine, Michelle. 2019. Critical Disability Studies: Looking Back and Forward. *Journal of Social Issues* 75 (3): 972–984. https://doi.org/10.1111/josi.12344.

France, David. 2012. The Men and Women Who Started ACT UP—New York Magazine—Nymag. *New York Magazine*, March 23. https://nymag.com/news/features/act-up-2012-4/.

France, David, and Sarah Schulman. 2012. *How to Survive a Plague*. Documentary.

Gilman, Sander L. 1987. AIDS and Syphilis: The Iconography of Disease. *October* 43: 87–107. https://doi.org/10.2307/3397566.

Herman, Bob. 2019. Four Times as Many U.S. Diabetics Ration Insulin as Those in Other Wealthy Countries. *Axios*, June 18. https://www.axios.com/type-1-diabetes-rationing-usa-countries-survey-cbd86250-72f5-4177-8929-00ad933a0fcf.html.

History—GMHC. 2021. https://www.gmhc.org/history/.

Holland, Karlynn. 2020. New York #insulin4all on Twitter. *Twitter*. Accessed October 14, 2020. https://twitter.com/NYinsulin4all/status/1314248794922520577.

———. 2019. Diabetes Advocate Forces Arrest at Insulin Vigil. *Healthline*, September 19. https://www.healthline.com/diabetesmine/diabetes-advocate-arrest-insulin-vigil.

———. 2020. With Diabetes, Arrest and Incarceration Could Be Lethal. *Healthline*, August 20. https://www.healthline.com/diabetesmine/diabetes-endangered-arrest-and-incarceration.

Irwin, Clair. 2018. Renegade Librarian #insulin4all on Twitter. *Twitter*, July 24. https://twitter.com/RenegadeLib/status/1021797802630938624.

Konrad, Walecia. 2017. Black Market Insulin: What You Need to Know. *CBS News*. June 20. https://www.cbsnews.com/news/black-market-insulin-what-you-need-to-know/?intcid=CNM-00-10abd1h

Lieberman, Trudy. 2019. Canada, eh? Don't Fall for these Tired old Canards about Health Care Rationing. *Center for Health Journalism*. April 05. https://www.centerforhealthjournalism.org/2019/04/03/canada-eh-dont-fall-these-tired-oldcanards-about-health-care-rationing

Litchman, Michelle L., Tamara K. Oser, Sarah E. Wawrzynski, Heather R. Walker, and Sean Oser. November 1, 2020. The Underground Exchange of Diabetes Medications and Supplies: Donating, Trading, and Borrowing, Oh My! *Journal of Diabetes Science and Technology* 14 (6): 1000–1009. https://doi.org/10.1177/1932296819888215.

Messerly, Megan. 2018. Big Pharma Abandons Lawsuit over Nevada's Insulin Pricing Transparency Law after State Approves Trade Secret Protection Regulations. June 28. https://thenevadaindependent.com/article/big-pharma-abandons-lawsuit-over-nevadas-insulin-pricing-transparency-law-after-state-approves-trade-secret-protection-regulations.

Raymond, Jonathan. 2018. Parents Bring Ashes of Dead Children to Drug Company to Protest High Insulin Prices. https://www.cleveland19.com, November 17. https://www.cleveland19.com/2018/11/17/parents-bring-ashes-dead-children-drug-company-protest-high-insulin-prices/.

Sable-Smith, Bram. 2019. Americans Cross Border into Mexico to Buy Insulin at a Fraction of U.S. Cost. *FiercePharma*, February 12. https://www.fiercepharma.com/pharma/americans-cross-border-into-mexico-to-buy-insulin-at-a-fraction-u-s-cost.

Sanofi. 2020. Insulin Glargine | Lantus® (Insulin Glargine Injection) 100 Units/ML. home. https://www.lantus.com/.

Siddons, Andrew. 2020. Trump Assertions of Lower Drug Costs Mask Truth for Many Consumers. *Roll Call*. September 9. https://www.rollcall.com/2020/09/09/trump-assertions-of-lower-drug-costs-mask-truth-for-manyconsumers/

Sullivan, Thomas. 2019. Nevada Fines Drug Manufacturers for Failure to Comply with Drug Transparency Law. *Policy & Medicine* (blog), October 7. https://www.policymed.com/2019/10/nevada-fines-drug-manufacturers-for-failure-to-comply-with-drug-transparency-law.html.

Van Ness, Jonathan. 2018. Is There An Insulin Crisis Happening iyn the U.S.? With Elizabeth Pfiester, Founder and Executive Director of T1International, Episode #129 of Getting Curious with Jonathan Van Ness on Earwolf. Accessed September 22, 2020. https://www.earwolf.com/episode/is-there-an-insulin-crisis-happening-in-the-u-s-with-elizabeth-pfiester-founder-and-executive-director-of-t1international/.

Wofford, Karyn. 2017. Protesters at Eli Lilly's Headquarters Demand Transparency and Lower Insulin Prices. *ASweetLife*, September 13. https://asweetlife.org/protesters-at-eli-lillys-headquarters-demand-transparency-and-lower-insulin-prices/.

One or Many Voices: Narratives from #insulin4all

Valentina Sturiale and Guido Anselmi

Introduction

In 2014, as the price of insulin continued to rise in the United States, a social media campaign using #insulin4all was launched by T1 international and The Pendsey Trust. As the hashtag articulates, the campaign was designed to rally people with diabetes around the goal of making insulin affordable and accessible to all (which means free, according to some). The campaign, which quickly turned into a social movement, problematizes the fact that list prices per ml of Humalog and Novolog increased six-fold from 1998 to 2020 (Luo and Gellad 2020). In a non-socialized healthcare system, this means that people with diabetes who either do not have insurance, or inadequate insurance, face economic strain affording

V. Sturiale (✉)
Viralbeat srl, Milan, Italy

G. Anselmi
Università degli Studi di Pavia, Pavia, Italy
e-mail: guido.anselmi@unimib.it

B. C. Frazer, H. R. Walker (eds.), *(Un)doing Diabetes: Representation, Disability, Culture*, Palgrave Studies in Science and Popular Culture, https://doi.org/10.1007/978-3-030-83110-3_5

their life-prolonging medicine, which in turn pushed many to ration their insulin supply (Conner et al. 2019).

It is in this context that, from 2014, #insulin4all has been used as a vector for spreading awareness on the national health crisis connected to increased insulin cost by both activists and regular Twitter users. Perhaps because the crisis was so widespread and because healthcare reform had become a staple of liberal and progressive politics, the insulin crisis issue was featured in the beginning phases of the 2019 Democratic primaries. Both Bernie Sanders (Spalding 2019) and Elizabeth Warren (Warren and Blumenthal 2019) have extensively campaigned about the topic. As a demonstration of the far-reaching impact of insulin in-affordability, the issue also popped up on the federal policy agenda as a bipartisan topic when former President Trump proposed measures to control the price of insulin (HHS 2020). Though his effort was criticised by activists, it occurring at all indicates that the crisis was reaching a point of critical mass in the United States.

In this chapter, we investigate #insulin4all as a digital, hashtag based, social movement that raises awareness on the dramatic effects of the insulin crisis while promoting a specific representation of diabetes as a trigger for activism. We examine what kind of collective and individual frame is associated with the hashtag and which users act as influencers in spreading it. We came into this research after stumbling upon one of the many stories depicting the tragic consequences of insulin rationing. As researchers looking into social media analytics, who had previously explored the social media fallout of terror attacks and the emergence of the COVID-19 pandemic (in the global north), the stories of #insulin4all hit close to home. Being a diabetic and the partner of a diabetic living in a country with socialized healthcare, we have a semi-outsider lens on the #insulin4all movement. Going into this project, it was our aim to leverage our professional skills to fuel participation in a cause that is also ours.

Literature on digitally driven social movements starting from the 'Arab springs' (Meraz and Papacharissi 2013) up to #occupy (Beraldo and Galan-Paez 2013), #refugeeswelcome (Barisione et al. 2019; Siapera et al. 2018) and #blacklivesmatter (Ray et al. 2017) abound. Some studies intersect with critical research on disability studies, analyzing how the massive usage of social media platforms has fuelled collective self-identification of disabled people as activists (Ellis and Goggin 2015). Existing literature has analyzed how people have used digital networks to protest for their rights to citizenship (Mann 2018; Trevisan 2018), to receive adequate care (Pearson and Trevisan 2015), to alter mainstream representation of neurodiversity (Parsloe and Holton 2018) or the right of minorities to be seen and represented (Mulderink 2020) within overwhelmingly white and heteronormative mainstream representations of disability.

Digital networking has resulted in a radical re-intermediation in political participation. In order to influence the public agenda on a given topic, street-level activists exploit network affordances (Rogers 2013; Gerbaudo 2012). In other words, they exploit what the social media network offers the individual. Lowering the personal material costs of formal protest through engaging online enables a different form of action, termed *connective action* by scholars Bennett and Segerberg (2012). In essence, *connective action* is an unfolding mass action stemming from individuals rather than a group; it doesn't require formal organization (e.g. securing permits, paying for and making signs and flyers, etc). Unlike *collective action*, which is closer to what we think of when imagining traditional protesting, marches, and the like, *connective action* is relatively uncoordinated. At its most impactful, *connective action* depends on the capacity of activists to piggyback network affordances: to create a shared imaginary while fuelling affective (a la Meraz and Papacharissi 2013) identification. Fundamentally, a narrative of self-representation shared via tweet assures that each activist (referred to here and in the literature as a *node*) wants to and can contribute to an ongoing political effort, without the need of costly central coordination. *Connective action* functions through the sharing of *personal action frames*, which in the case of #insulin4all, looks like an activist personalizing a wide-spread position, argument, or ideology as a way to draw digital connections with friends or trusted others. Personal action frames often showcase high affect and justifications through a rights-based lens (e.g. 'we have the right to this'). *Connective action* as a strategy coexists (and eventually may enter in a positive feedback loop) with pre-existing collective action-based entities (e.g. formal organizations campaigning for something).

Though an active social movement unfolding across Twitter, #insulin4all lacks substantial coverage in digital movements research and disability studies.[1] Because of its growing size (we count 338,254 tweets at the time of publication) and because it sits at the intersection of lived experience, self-representation, and political economy, it ought to be documented and examined historiographically. We situate this chapter in a

[1] But see Ahne et al. 2020 for a similar twitter corpus.

social environment rife with market (dis)regulation, multinational pharmaceutical conglomerates who have monopolized the market of diabetes medications, and the willingness of public actors to fight against the influence of those pharmaceutical companies.

In this chapter, we do three things. First, we assess how #insulin4all has become 'visible' both within Twitter and in the traditional media ecosystem. To accomplish the latter, we charted the diffusion of the hashtag over the last 3 years. We also count news headlines mentioning #insulin4all or the insulin crisis, in order to better understand the evolution of the issue in the mainstream media. Second, to employ quantitative methods and a thematic analysis, we analyze how people have framed life experiences as a means of political participation and expression. Third, we explore potential gatekeepers involved in the movement.

Methods and Data

To analyze how #insulin4all has developed in the last three years, we aggregated 52,848 unique tweets from 7478 users. In order to account for retweets, we analyzed a total of 338,254 tweets using #insulin4all in the body of the tweet. Tweets were gathered through Twitter Search API via Python scripting. Furthermore, because we needed to ascertain whether #insulin4all, as a social movement, was penetrating into the mainstream news space, we also searched headlines of relevant US-based online news sources through Media Cloud, a free and open-source service to monitor online newspapers. We downloaded 2513 headlines through Media Cloud using the keywords 'insulin4all' or 'insulin' in order to exclude unrelated headlines. We manually reviewed the results of the search query isolating articles on price spikes or the insulin shortages; leaving us with 435 headlines, which we charted and thematically analyzed.

We know from network science (Barabási 2003) that social media platform engagement tends to favor concentration. This means that the main usage of Twitter involves sharing content produced by superconnected nodes. Superconnected nodes, which can be defined as 'influencers' with followers that greatly outnumber those of ordinary users, act as information spreaders (Wu et al. 2011). We measure retweet concentration through Gini index[2] in the context of a digital movement (Barisione et al.

[2]Originally developed to assess wealth inequalities in economics: the Gini index varies from 0 (everyone has the same amount of wealth) to 1 (one person has all of the wealth) in

2019), which can help us answer a central research question: how is influence distributed across the duration of the movement (Barberá and Rivero 2015; Aruguete and Calvo 2018).

For content analysis, we adopted a mixed methods approach: we detected peaks of activity on Twitter. Then we used a technique to detect 'typical' words (or hashtags or mentions) in subsections of our Twitter data—namely those that occur with simultaneous frequency within a single section and less frequency in the rest of the corpus. This technique is called "term's frequency and its inverse document frequency," or TF-IDF. Using TF-IDF allowed our analysis on words, hashtags and mentions to initially assess the contents of each peak (i.e. to have a rough idea of what topics were crucial in each peak date). In our case, we used TF-IDF to identify and analyze content on days with high activity (our 'peaks'). We perform thematic analysis examining the top ranked tweets for each peak (i.e. those whose total retweets are in the 90th percentile n = 5518). Then, using triangulation with the results of TF-IDF, we infer common themes (e.g. if the term 'caravan' is present we can connect that peak of activity to the 'caravan' to Canada initiative described in media articles).

Diffusion and Content Analysis

During the 957 days surveyed (from January 1st, 2018 to August 15th, 2020), we found that #insulin4all remained a constant presence amongst key sharers (even if low key when compared to hashtags connected to more famous social movements such as #blacklivesmatter or #refugeeswelcome). We identified six main peaks. Figure 1 demonstrates weekly trends and the six peaks we identified. The graph shows a black and white linear line-graph ranging from January 2018 to July 2020. Text on the graph identify peak 1 around July 2018, peak two (the highest of all) around February 2019, peaks 3 to 5 around July 2019, and peak 6 in July 2020.

Headlines mentioning #insulin4all, the insulin crisis or political debate offered further insights. Only nine headlines directly mentioned #insulin4all, however 426 more mentioned the insulin affordability crisis, crisis related deaths, and hardships or political initiatives connected to the price spike. As the following analysis will demonstrate, these peaks are

this case we use the same indicator to monitor how equally distributed are the retweets among different users.

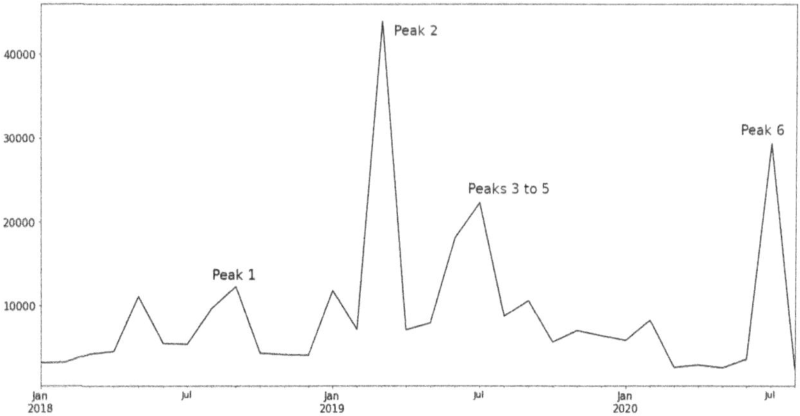

Fig. 1 Weekly Trends of #insulin4all

significant pieces of the unfolding #insulin4all story. Figure 2 shows the distribution of headlines per week using a black and white linear line-graph ranging from January 2018 to July 2020. The highest distribution of news articles peaks around 120 around July of 2019.

Despite a constant increase in insulin prices, this line-graph reveals that the #insulin4all movement reached a point of critical mass in 2019 on both Twitter and for the traditional media. This trend requires a deeper look. What has caused this surge of attention and mobilization? In essence why did this digital movement that has been active since 2018 peaked in this moment, at this time?

To understand the temporal evolution of issues we analyzed each peak by leveraging both the most topical words (TF-IDF), and thematic exploration of tweets. The first peak (13th to 19th of August 2018, Gini 0.96) is the smallest (5173 tweets) in terms of content. We found that it was connected to the annual conference held by the American Association of Diabetes Educators,[3] as #AADE18 is strongly associated with the peak. Tweets in this peak push a framing of the insulin crisis which stress the immediate need to move to action, as is demonstrated in these examples:

> I've used the same insulin (Humalog) since I was diagnosed with Type 1 diabetes at age 14. I'm 36 now and the price of my insulin has risen over

[3] now Association of Diabetes Care & Education Specialists (ADCES) https://www.diabeteseducator.org/

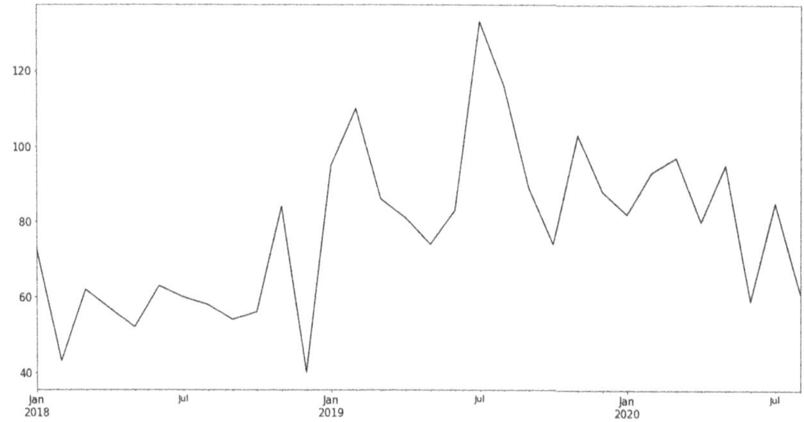

Fig. 2 number of headlines per week

1200% with no explanation other than greed to over $12k annually. I die in 1–2 days without it. #insulin4all #ShareATweetWithTheWorld—@ Kidfears99 (Laura Marston) on 14-08-2018

It makes absolutely no sense that a vial of insulin in Canada costs $34 and the same vial in the US retails for $320. This has to stop. #insulin4all #RTifyouagree—@AM_MacDonaldMD (Anne Marie MacDonald, MD) on 16-08-2018

It's pretty depressing as someone who loves a person with diabetes to see the many dollars that get thrown around conferences like #AADE2018. I'm feeling very much like our daughter is just a commodity to generate revenues right now. #insulin4all—@MelindaMWedding (Melinda Wedding) on 17-08-2018

Diabetic activists, here, frame the insulin affordability crisis as an intersection between biological existence and a lack of market regulation in a relatively clear and straightforward way. Melinda Weddings tweet, for example, leverages emotions (and collective identification) to introduce the conflict between profit and health. The conference to which she refers makes evident the commodification of diabetes by exposing the large financial investments in marketing and communication being made by pharmaceutical companies. This specific crisis point represents a core grievance of other activists and constructs a scenario in which the opportunistic agency of pharmaceutical companies is central: namely greed, monopolistic status, and regulatory capture are to blame. This is a key tactic used by activists to escalate matters from subjective experience (e.g. I have diabetes) to collective representation (e.g. our suffering comes from objective conditions) to action (e.g. something must be done to change material conditions).

The second peak in chronological order (4th to 10th of March 2019, 37,026 tweets, Gini 0.98) is subsumed by retweets of a tweet written by a diabetes activist who describes herself as an "unphunded insulin advocate" and regularly tweets using the #insulin4all hashtag. Her original tweet has been retweeted in total 34,144 times—thirteen of which came from verified Twitter accounts with a combined 1.01 million followers. Among those who contributed to its widespread diffusion by quoting the tweet are: Journalists Eoin Higgins (@EoinHiggins_), Josh Moon(@Josh_Moon), Paul Brandus (@WestWingReport); Attorneys Rabia Chaudry (@rabiasquared) and Max Kennerly (@MaxKennerly) and activist Ady Barkan (@AdyBarkan). The original tweet reads:

> picking up my insulin: Pharmacist: (finds rX, frantically reenters info in cash register, nervously steps back) Um, it's $728.40, did u want it? Me: yes, I *need* it.: (lowers eyes) Right. Insulin. I'm so sorry. We'll do this sad little dance again next month. #insulin4all—@msinsulindpndnt 9-03-2019

As we see from this very popular tweet, having to pay high prices for life-sustaining medication is a central tenet of the way diabetic activists perform self-representation. Many activists frame the insulin crisis in life-or-death-terms like this tweet shows. This framing serves as a counter-narrative. It shows a representation of diabetes as a serious and life-threatening condition that classic media can miss or make light of. Other tweets in this peak also share similar representations:

> We're not asking how many more people need to die of insulin rationing before action is taken. We're asking how many politicians need to lose their jobs because they did nothing to stop these deaths #insulin4all @jandeliott (James Eliott) 8-3-2019

> The pharmaceutical industry's price controls on life saving insulin for Type 1 diabetics is a shameful RACKET that should have every person of good-will outraged. Their greed & pursuit of profit at all costs is literally KILLING people. @AmandiOnAir (Fernand R. Amandi) 9-3-2019

Tweets from this peak de-naturalize diabetes and re-contextualize it as a byproduct of material economic and political conditions. Activists' tweet content argues that death does not come 'naturally,' but as a logical consequence of the U.S. government not proving healthcare. Tellingly, hashtags like #insulincartel and #medicare4all are strongly associated with this peak. Furthermore, activists flip the script of shame, blame and stigma by placing responsibility for death, diabetes-related complications and hospitalizations onto the political and corporate entities who organize and benefit from the rising cost of insulin.[4]

The third peak (24th to 30th of June, 11,591 tweets, Gini 0.93) corresponds to the in-person 'caravan' voyages taking place during the time of the peak. Caravan voyages involve many people with diabetes gathering together and taking trips across US borders (to either Mexico or Canada) to privately buy insulin in bulk (typical hashtags used simultaneously with #insulin4all are: #caravantocanada #affordableinsulinnow). The following two tweets demonstrate the caravan voyage theme:

> I bought some insulin in Canada today with no insurance. I paid $267 (USD) for insulin that would cost $4113 retail in the U.S. It's 15x more expensive in the U.S. Let's change this! (anonymous)

> I bought this vial of insulin today in Ontario, no prescription. Here's the problem with insulin pricing—what I paid today vs what's charged back home: $30 $275 We need pricing regulations. We need legislators to fight for the lives of T1D and T2D Americans. #insulin4all @hopekyra (Hope Charters) 29-06-2019

Not only do both tweets offer comparisons of insulin pricing based on location, but they also showcase the unfolding drama that, we argue, has propelled the movement forward. The practice of crossing borders to purchase affordable insulin became 'spectacular' and was featured in news media, which in turn furthered political mobilization (digital or otherwise). Hashtags related to formal politics (like democratic primaries) were strongly associated with this peak. For example: #taxtherich, #demdebate, and #warren2020.

[4] see Beguerisse-Díaz et al. 2017 for some examples

The fourth peak (15th to 21st of July, 5333 tweets, Gini 0.97) continues from the third in that the unfolding life and death drama is drawn out by activists by way of testimonies. The following two quotes exemplify this:

> Kayla was 28. Jada was 24. Jesimya was 21. All 3 died this past June because they couldn't afford insulin. In 2019. In the United States. This is why we fight for #insulin4all. @MsAllisonBailey (Allison Bailey) 17-07-2019

> Another death due to the high price of insulin: in Evansville IN, a 28-year-old woman died on June 5 when she couldn't get her insulin through her insurance & couldn't afford to pay the list price. #insulin4all @ferguriffic (Sarah Fergusson) 17-07-2019

Compared to the second peak, this fourth peak focuses more on the people who died due to forced insulin rationing whose stories were covered in mainstream and legacy media. Around the same time, the concept of forced insulin rationing—which involves people with diabetes using less insulin per meal to make it stretch over a longer period of time—grips the mainstream media. News stories of insulin unaffordability reaches an all-time high at this time. As such, it is fairly evident in this case how the #insulin4all movement is unfolding in a hybrid media system in which the stories being published by mainstream legacy media being framed by activists as a critical, urgent, and wide-spread problem. The activists, then, individually developed and deployed action frames that produced such affective engagement that the core tenets of the campaign got picked up and brought to audiences beyond twitter. Another notable difference, this peak (compared with previous ones) is slightly more aligned with national level political imperatives (e.g. #medicareforall) than other peaks seemed to have been.

The fifth peak (22nd to 28th of July 2019, 1168 tweets, 0.94) is quite similar to the third but more overtly aligned with U.S. political campaigning. It is nominally driven by tweets about caravanning to Canada as per following examples:

> There is no reason for a drug as simple as insulin, which costs $21 in Canada, to cost the equivalent of a mortgage payment.—@AOC #insulin4all #medicareforall @SSwork 26-07-2019

> I'm incredibly overwhelmed seeing all the tweets about this trip. I vividly remember dropping a vial of Lantus when I was 11 and the fear I felt of not

> knowing what I was going to do. We need #insulin4all. Thank you @BernieSanders—@oh_eyelean (Eileen Garcia) 28-07-2019

In these tweets we see activists in the movement using their digital activism via #insulin4all to play to and create dialogue with more formalized political campaigning. Other hashtags typically used in alongside #insulin4all are: #berniesanders2020 and #notmeus. Compared to previous peaks, representations of diabetes are deeply embedded into expectations for political change at the highest level (given the impending presidential elections). Activists in this peak, shift slightly away from individual action frames sharing hardship, and toward messages promoting and urging progressive change. A further indication that #insulin4all is operating in a hybrid media system, the issue of insulin affordability becomes actively promoted by progressive democratic politicians like Senators Elizabeth Warren and Bernie Sanders. In fact, Sanders publicly supported the caravans in person by joining a bus crossing the border (Grayer 2019) and through campaign twitter accounts. The following tweet exemplifies this:

> Three drug companies made $14.5 billion in profit last year, control 90% of the insulin in this country, it's just an amazing coincidence prices go up and and up and up, so what you do is you throw these people in jail if they engage in price fixing (@People4bernie 28-07-2019).

Around the same time Representative Alexandria Ocasio-Cortez made a public statement connecting stock buybacks and price inflation for lifesaving medications, explicitly mentioning insulin (Conti 2019). Rep. Ocasio-Cortez's statement was taken up and celebrated by activists during this peak.

The sixth and last peak in chronological order (6th to 13th of July 2020, Gini 0.98) is also one of the largest (24,476 tweets). Though, the vast majority of tweets in this peak (93%) are retweets of the following quote tweet shared by a 23-year-old woman with Type 1 diabetes:

> if you are rationing #insulin PLEASE reach out to the #insulin4all community and we will find some to send to you!!! we are in this TOGETHER. please please reach out—Emma, @Femmanisim on 6-7-2020

Emma's tweet here directly speaks to people with diabetes who are rationing due to insulin affordability. She opens a network of care and connection that much of the movement seems to have been built upon—a likely reason for its saliency with so many Twitter users. Emma's quote tweet linked to an article published on Al Jazeera that discussed a then-recent judicial controversy in which insulin manufacturers sued the state of Minnesota over the 'Alec Smith Law[5]'. The Alec Smith Law, named after a 26-year-old Minnesotan who died as a result of forced insulin rationing, was a piece of legislation enacted in April of 2020 that mandated affordable access to insulin for those who cannot afford it. The legislation being signed into law was heavily influenced by activists campaigning in-person and via social media. This peak, then, also contained outrage toward the drug manufacturers who sued the state over the Alec Smith Law.

Regarding mainstream media headlines, the main focus centred on federal level political initiatives to address insulin affordability. Such initiatives include: Senator Sanders' support to caravans to Canada (Grayer and Nobles 2019) as well as President Trump's plan to wholesale import insulin from Canada (4th week of July and 1st week of August 2019) (Abutaleb and McGinley 2019, Associated Press 2019), senate hearings on price spikes (Rowland 2019) (4th week of February 2019), and Eli Lilly's decision to release a 'half-price' generic version of Humalog in the US (1st week of March 2019) (Reuters 2019). If we look at these headlines, we begin to see how the issue mobilized by activists was taken up by local and national level politicians, initially as a 'bipartisan' issue. It is through looking at these in dialogue with Twitter activity, however, that we can truly appreciate how #insulin4all's digital mobilization used both individual action frames and broader anti-capitalist critiques as solutions to address insulin shortages (see peaks 4 and 5 especially).

Activists overarching story told through the ongoing life of #insulin4all is that the real-life threat to diabetic wellbeing and life is first and foremost a man-made one—politically and economically manufactured in an economic system that favors and rewards corporate greed and de-regulation. And the activists' message seemed to have been heard by some progressive democratic candidates and the journalists who cover them. With that said, many of the articles took a broader approach, which suggests that the

[5] The Al Jazeera tweet quoted by Emma read: "Drug makers sued Minnesota over a law requiring them to give low-cost insulin to people who can't afford it. 1 in 4 diabetics ration insulin due to skyrocketing cost. The law is named after Alec Smith, who died after rationing his insulin because he couldn't pay $1300/month. Author: @ajplus 2-07-2020.

radical anti-capitalist affect mobilized by activists on Twitter may have been lost.

Compared to the experiential perspective and frame deployed by Twitter users, mainstream media's portrayal of the crisis was relatively impersonal and bland. Mainstream media articles did not tend to cover individual deaths, or the day-to-day hardships that come from living with diabetes when access to affordable insulin is not available (45 headlines in total out of 426). Media articles tended to appeal to logic, rather than affect—a marked difference from activists' framing. Many articles used the position of devil's advocate to consider, for example, why proposed healthcare reform would work (or not), or the feasibility of this or that proposed course of action (e.g. importing insulin from Canada). It was in the articles that weighed pros and cons that the framing of the crisis painted by activists on Twitter faded into the background.

Discussion

Through our investigation, we uncovered how #insulin4all has become a social movement. It is evident how the emphasis on day-to day experiences and difficulties that come with diabetes have provided affective resonance and this, in turn, fuelled a collective (even if sporadic) mobilization. The experiential lens activists brought to the movement allowed the drama and suspense of living with diabetes and trying to afford insulin to be recognised at a public level. However, the questions of 'why now?' and 'who has driven the movement?' still stand. As it is often the case with digital movements (Barisione et al. 2019), #insulin4all is a mobilized effort springing from collective awareness of a shocking system-wide issue. While in other cases (eg, Siapera et al. 2018; Parsloe and Holton 2018; Al Nashmi 2018) awareness comes from an 'external event' (eg, a refugee child dies, a terror attack happens), in the case of #insulin4all, the movement grew from the sharing of individual *action frames* based on personal experience (or of someone very close).

Affective intensity, however, is just half of the puzzle. In order to function, a digital mobilization needs a target, something to mobilize against. #insulin4all finds its target in the economic-systemic conditions materially producing ill-health and even death for diabetic people. Examining representations of diabetes put forward by activists over Twitter shows us that the lines were quite clear from the beginning: greed and monopolies are to blame, politicians promoting dis-regulation are to blame, and the lack of an adequate healthcare system is to blame for the insulin affordability crisis. On the one hand, this provides further collective identification as the *personal frames* (e.g. "I have difficulties managing my diabetes") transforms into a community-level frame (e.g. "My difficulties managing diabetes come from present economical and political conditions"). In effect, this also provides an answer to the 'why now?' question. Because insulin costs continued to rise steadily, and because adequate health insurance became less and less accessible overtime, insulin affordability reached a point of critical mass for a majority of people with diabetes in the United States. Even individuals who had private health insurance through their jobs reported not being able to afford insulin (Litchman et al. 2020).

If we take a closer look at the compared trends of headlines vis-a-vis Twitter activity, we can appreciate how both have intense activity in the same period (roughly 2019). Understanding every bit of historical context that could explain why the insulin affordability crisis reached a point of critical mass in 2019 goes beyond the scope of this chapter, but we assume that a multicausal pattern is at work, as media narratives and digital activism seem to have entered a positive feedback loop with each fuelling the other. The worsening of economic inequalities combined with rising prices may be part of the explanation, but national level political entrepreneurship may be also a fairly cogent explanation. Progressive democrats were willing to push for an overhaul of healthcare towards a single payer model, generating interests and media attention that has provided a receptive environment for the issues raised by #insulin4all.

Regarding 'who has driven the movement,' we know from literature that *connective action* requires (and reproduces) radical reintermediation, namely producing agency out of digital networks, as individual users get magnified (even if for a brief period of time) to influencer status. Individual magnification, even if only from a single tweet, allows the experience of one individual to shape the affect of all connected nodes. However, the existence of radical reintermediation does not guarantee that the final outcome is plural, nuanced or even grassroots-led (Siapera et al. 2018). Measuring retweet concentration with the Gini index allowed us to reach some conclusions on this issue. The peaks we identified here sport quite high Gini values very close to 1 (for reference 0.75 are considered high values cf. Aruguete and Calvo 2018)—meaning that only a handful of accounts generate a majority of the retweets, we know that a small number of individual voices are being amplified.

Knowing that the movement is largely propelled by a few activists rather than many, a series of additional questions regarding internal community diversity in the digital movement arise: What about minorities? What about people with multiple disabilities? Is there a trade-off between a representation that emphasizes commonalities and one that produces an accurate nuanced testimony of what it means to be diabetic across multiple marginalities? Answering these questions is beyond the scope of this chapter, but we may have a glimmer of insight if we analyze what happens in different peaks. In general, peaks that have a strong 'political' frame (3rd and 4th for example) have a lower Gini index. This means that, comparatively, they host a more diverse pool of messages, including some (but very infrequent) conservative critiques aimed at the 'Medicare for All' project. Some of these different voices come from political agendas other than #insulin4all, ones that are more institutionalized and more reliant on collective action as opposed to connective action.

As the issue of insulin affordability becomes mainstream (namely as national level political entrepreneurs become interested in it as an issue), #insulin4all expands its reach. It must be noted, however, that there are some trade-offs that come with being an issue of interest in mainstream political discourse. There is a considerable loss of autonomy as political entrepreneurs and mainstream media step in and the unfolding story begins to be told by presumed outsiders. The representations of diabetic people and diabetes over Twitter may also become more representationally diverse than those involved in the initial core of #insulin4all. Along a similar vein, the agenda put forward by the movement may be co-opted by people and institutions who have a similar but slightly different agenda. This is clearly visible if we cross-reference the content which is widely shared over Twitter, which emphasizes personal difficulty as a trigger for action, with the kind of stories that circulate on mainstream media which emphasize political process (Rowland 2019; Thomas 2020) often with little recognition of bottom-up advocacy.

That said, this research has a limitation. A consequence of turning toward Twitter exclusively, is turning away from the effect of other platforms (eg Facebook, Telegram, Instagram) that may have widely divergent affordances and that may have enabled different mobilization strategies. However, to be fair, all platforms are subjects to the pitfalls of the attention economy. Nevertheless, additional research may find that other venues (Facebook groups) are more conductive to a plural narrative. Also, the COVID-19 pandemic has limited our capacity to verify the effect of institutional and media actors on the digital movement. As a matter of fact, the presence of such a large global news frame has all but obliterated the discussion on other medical emergencies. Further analysis on this topic with other qualitative and quantitative methodologies (ethnography or structural topic modelling comes to mind) would produce further insights and richer discourses both within Twitter and national news media.

With that said, this chapter contributes to what is known about the ways in which individual activists use #Isnulin4all to deploy *personal action frames* to locate the problem of the insulin affordability within a social and culture environment marked by greed and (dis)regulation. However, our study also brings up several questions regarding representation in diabetic activist spaces like the one on Twitter. For example, what makes an activist? What would empowered consciousness look like if the activists' action frames were to be taken up by the broader public? What would it mean then, to be diabetic?

References

Abutaleb, Y., and L. McGinley. (2019, July 31. Trump Administration Outlines Plans for Eventual Importation of Cheaper Drugs. https://www.washingtonpost.com/health/trump-administration-outlines-plans-to-allow-importation-of-cheaper-drugs-from-canada/2019/07/31/8df1fede-b390-11e9-8949-5f36ff92706e_story.html.

Ahne, A., F. Orchard, X. Tannier, C. Perchoux, B. Balkau, S. Pagoto, and G. Fagherazzi. 2020. Insulin Pricing and Other Major Diabetes-Related Concerns in the USA: A Study of 46 407 Tweets Between 2017 and 2019. *BMJ Open Diabetes Research and Care* 8 (1): e001190.

Al Nashmi, E. 2018. From Selfies to Media Events: How Instagram Users Interrupted Their Routines After the Charlie Hebdo Shootings. *Digital Journalism* 6 (1): 98–117.

Aruguete, N., and E. Calvo. 2018. Time to# Protest: Selective Exposure, Cascading Activation, and Framing in Social Media. *Journal of Communication* 68 (3): 480–502.

Associated Press. 2019, July 31. *U.S. to Set Up Plan Allowing Prescription Drugs from Canada.* https://www.nbcnews.com/health/health-news/us-set-plan-allowing-prescription-drugs-canada-n1037156?cid=public-rss_20190731

Barabási, A. 2003. *Linked: The New Science of Networks.* New York: Perseus.

Barberá, P., and G. Rivero. 2015. Understanding the Political Representativeness of Twitter Users. *Social Science Computer Review* 33 (6): 712–729.

Barisione, M., A. Michailidou, and M. Airoldi. 2019. Understanding a Digital Movement of Opinion: The Case of# RefugeesWelcome. *Information, Communication & Society* 22 (8): 1145–1164.
Beguerisse-Díaz, M., A.K. McLennan, G. Garduno-Hernández, M. Barahona, and S.J. Ulijaszek. 2017. The 'Who' and 'What' of # Diabetes on Twitter. *Digital Health* 3. https://doi.org/10.1177/2055207616688841.
Bennett, W.L., and A. Segerberg. 2012. The Logic of Connective Action: Digital Media and the Personalization of Contentious Politics. *Information, Communication & Society* 15 (5): 739–768.
Beraldo, D., and J. Galan-Paez. 2013. The# OCCUPY Network on Twitter and the Challenges to Social Movements Theory and Research. *International Journal of Electronic Governance* 6 (4): 319–341.
Conner, F., E. Pfiester, J. Elliott, and A. Slama-Chaudhry. 2019. Unaffordable Insulin: Patients Pay the Price. *The Lancet Diabetes & Endocrinology* 7 (10): 748.
Conti, A. 2019, July 30. *Pharma Companies Have Spent Billions Buying Back Their Own Stock Vice.* https://www.vice.com/en/article/a3x5jb/pharma-companies-have-spent-billions-buying-back-their-own-stock.
Ellis, K., and G. Goggin. 2015. Disability Media Participation: Opportunities, Obstacles and Politics. *Media International Australia* 154 (1): 78–88.
Gerbaudo, P. 2012. *Tweets and the Streets: Social Media and Contemporary Activism.* London: Pluto Press.
Grayer, A., and R. Nobles. 2019, July 11. *Bernie Sanders to Join People with Type 1 Diabetes on Canada Trip for Cheaper Insulin.* https://edition.cnn.com/2019/07/11/politics/bernie-sanders-goes-to-canada-prescription-drugs/index.html.
HHS. 2020, July 24. *Trump Administration Announces Historic Action to Lower Drug Prices for Americans.* https://www.hhs.gov/about/news/2020/07/24/trump-administration-announces-historic-action-lower-drug-prices-americans.html.
Litchman, M. L., Oser, T. K., Wawrzynski, S. E., Walker, H. R., & Oser, S. (2020). The Underground Exchange of Diabetes Medications and Supplies: Donating, Trading, and Borrowing, oh my!. *Journal of diabetes science and technology* 14 (6): 1000–1009.
Luo, J., and W.F. Gellad. 2020. Origins of the Crisis in Insulin Affordability and Practical Advice for Clinicians on Using Human Insulin. *Current Diabetes Reports* 20: 2.
Mann, B.W. 2018. Rhetoric of Online Disability Activism:# CripTheVote and Civic Participation. *Communication Culture & Critique* 11 (4): 604–621.
Meraz, S., and Z. Papacharissi. 2013. Networked Gatekeeping and Networked Framing on# Egypt. *The International Journal of Press/Politics* 18 (2): 138–166.
Mulderink, C.E. 2020. The Emergence, Importance of# DisabilityTooWhite Hashtag. *Disability Studies Quarterly* 40 (2).

Parsloe, S.M., and A.E. Holton. 2018. # Boycottautismspeaks: Communicating a Counternarrative Through Cyberactivism and Connective Action. *Information, Communication & Society* 21 (8): 1116–1133.

Pearson, C., and F. Trevisan. 2015. Disability Activism in the New Media Ecology: Campaigning Strategies in the Digital Era. *Disability & Society* 30 (6): 924–940.

Ray, R., M. Brown, N. Fraistat, and E. Summers. 2017. Ferguson and the Death of Michael Brown on Twitter:# BlackLivesMatter,# TCOT, and the Evolution of Collective Identities. *Ethnic and Racial Studies* 40 (11): 1797–1813.

Reuters. 2019. Eli Lilly to Offer Half-Price Insulin for People with Type 1 Diabetes. https://www.nbcnews.com/health/health-news/eli-lilly-offer-half-price-insulin-people-type-1-diabetes-n978981?cid=public-rss_20190304.

Rogers, R. 2013. *Digital Methods.* Cambridge, MA: MIT press.

Rowland C. 2019, February 25. Drug Executives Grilled in Senate Over High Prices. https://www.washingtonpost.com/business/economy/drug-executives-grilled-in-senate-over-high-prices/2019/02/25/abc89c04-393f-11e9-aaae-69364b2ed137_story.html?noredirect=on&utm_term=.d2b3ec7af3da.

Siapera, E., M. Boudourides, S. Lenis, and J. Suiter. 2018. Refugees and Network Publics on Twitter: Networked Framing, Affect, and Capture. *Social Media+ Society* 4 (1). https://doi.org/10.1177/2056305118764437.

Spalding, D. 2019, July 28. Bernie Sanders Visits Canadian Pharmacy, Talks Drug Prices. https://www.reuters.com/article/idCAKCN1UN0SV-OCATP?edition-redirect=ca.

Thomas, K. 2020, March 11. Insulin Costs May Be Capped in a Medicare Program. https://www.nytimes.com/2020/03/11/health/insulin-drug-prices.htm

Trevisan, F. 2018. Connective Action Mechanisms in a Time of Political Turmoil: Virtual Disability Rights Protest at Donald Trump's Inauguration. *Australian Journal of Political Science* 53 (1): 103–115.

Warren, E., and R. Blumenthal. 2019. Inaccessible Insulin: The Broken Promise of Eli Lilly's Authorized Generic. https://www.warren.senate.gov/imo/media/doc/Inaccessible%20Insulin%20report.pdf

Wu, S., J.M. Hofman, W.A. Mason, and D.J. Watts. 2011, March. Who Says What to Whom on Twitter. In *Proceedings of the 20th international conference on World wide web* (pp. 705–714).

PART II

Film, Television, Visual Art and Performance

Essays in Part II interrogate samples of art and entertainment, effectively challenging common representations of diabetes. These essays primarily critique media examples including film, television shows, visual art, and theatre. They also offer the reader evocative and unexpected portrayals of the diabetes experience.

In 1997, Stuart Hall's seminal text *Representation: Cultural Representations and Signifying Practices* argues that representations have the power to create meaning for the object they depict. Hall contends that rather than standing in for something else, representations themselves create meaning on their own. In a shared cultural space, representations create a conceptual roadmap for meaning-meaning. This notion contrasts with the intuitive assumption that representations draw meaning from what is "real" in the world. In this part, authors do not contend with whether or not a representation is accurate. Instead, they explore the implications of representations in their own right.

In the article, "Laughing to Keep from Dying: Black Americans with Diabetes in Sitcoms and Comedies," Phyllisa Deroze traces the representational pattern of linking diabetes and death for Black Americans in film and television comedies. Looking at *Soul Food*, *Boondocks*, *Madea's Big Happy Family*, *Madea Family Funeral*, *30 Rock*, and *Black-ish*, Deroze traces how African American characters use humor to "deflect, ignore, or silence their experiences with diabetes complications." Set against the background of her own diagnosis experience, Deroze critiques the representation for its power to shape and limit beliefs about life with diabetes.

Bianca C. Frazer examines the television series *Parks and Recreation* to explore how the show establishes a comedic relationship between government actions and diabetic people. In "'Diabetes, Yuck!': Comedy, Disability, and The Dangers of Parody in *Parks and Recreation* (2009–2015)," Frazer argues that by disregarding the politics of diabetes as a disability, the show's comedy "fails to invoke audience's critical thinking around government actions." Using cultural theories of parody and punching down comedy, Frazer contends that the show "re-injures diabetic people with its parody by solely focusing on diabetic individuals and exaggerating reckless choices."

In the piece, "Diabetic Data Art: Numbers Beyond Control," Samuel Thulin offers an innovative possibility for diabetic people to create Diabetes Data Art (DDA) with their diabetes data. Thulin considers two examples, Doug Kantor and Justus Harris, who use data in relatively normative ways. Thulin, then, identifies two examples, Shimon Attie and Robbie McCauley, who alternatively emphasize lived experience and community responses in their work. Thulin argues that Diabetes Data Art allows artists to focus on their lived experience, which "thickens" data. In an exciting call for diabetics to do "anything else" with their data, Thulin poses polyvocal, multiple ways for creators to engage with bodily difference.

Blending poetic narrative and theory, Matt Paczkowski provides an insightful critique of the popular film *Panic Room*. Blending his own experiences with diabetes and desire-frustration theory, Paczkowski outlines areas the film "gets right" and some of its flaws as well. Paczkowski pays extended attention to the mother-daughter relationship in the film, deeply exploring the caregiving and taking between the mother, Meg, and the diabetic daughter, Sarah. In his essay, "Panic Rooms: Suspense in Type 1 Diabetes" Paczkowski ultimately argues that everyday life with diabetes meets the metrics of the thriller genre of cinema.

"My Tale Told by a Woman: *Lucille* and The Dramaturgy of Diabetes" tells the story of playwright and scholar G. William Zorn. In 2007, Zorn was commissioned to write a play about diabetes, but at the time he had little to no knowledge of the illness. In an unexpected turn of events, Zorn was diagnosed with diabetes himself while writing the play. His diagnosis experience informed the writing of the play. Zorn argues that lived experience is necessary to create and capture important moments during a diabetes diagnosis, particularly to contrast traditional diabetes education that can infantilize those with diabetes. Additionally, the mode of theater combined with the playwright's lived experience contributed to a play that features engaging characters, models patient education that acknowledges full personhood, and demonstrates the importance of human connection.

This section bring togethers writes to provide insight in the following questions:

- What common representational troupes exist in media and entertainment about diabetes?
- What critical lenses might we apply to such representations to recognize their shortcomings and seek new representational strategies for the diabetes experience?
- How might the lived experience of diabetic people influence the creation of the work and expand possibilities for surprising and innovative representations?

Laughing to Keep from Dying: Black Americans with Diabetes in Sitcoms and Comedies

Phyllisa Smith Deroze

Because my mouth
Is wide with laughter
And my throat
Is deep with song,
You do not think
I suffer after
I have held my pain
So long?

Because my mouth
Is wide with laughter,
You do not hear
My inner cry?
Because my feet

P. S. Deroze (✉)
Pompano Beach, FL, USA

B. C. Frazer, H. R. Walker (eds.), *(Un)doing Diabetes: Representation, Disability, Culture*, Palgrave Studies in Science and Popular Culture, https://doi.org/10.1007/978-3-030-83110-3_6

Are gay with dancing,
You do not know
I die?
—Hughes 1994

The poem "Minstrel Man" by Langston Hughes appropriately applies to an issue I see permeating across America's television and film comedies—laughter operating as a tool to ignore, avoid, and escape the seriousness of diabetes. By reflecting society's values and modeling behavior, television and film are "politically charged commodities" that have a profound impact on the real world (Norden 1994). Like the comedic entertainer in Hughes's poem, Black American characters in sitcoms and comedies are often concealing diabetes complications while distracting their audiences with laughter. The repetition of rendering diabetes management invisible and simultaneously highlighting extreme diabetes complications and/or diabetes death through explicit and symbolic scenes of death and dying creates a stigmatizing diabetes narrative. Even when presenting an occasional serious moment about the reality of diabetes, the significance of diabetes management is drowned out by punch lines. Subconsciously, these repeated images of Black American characters ineffectively managing diabetes formulate misguided public knowledge about diabetes and can encourage medical bias. As Arleen Tuchman notes, "Casting those with Type 2 diabetes as responsible for their disease masks the structural inequalities that produce poor health and divides people with diabetes into those who are innocent and those who are guilty" (2020). This division is harmful to African Americans who have a history of experiencing racial inequalities in healthcare (Matthew 2015; Washington 2008).

When I was diagnosed with diabetes in 2011, the only thing I knew about the condition is that it would kill me and that I should keep it a secret. In fact, "I'm gonna die" were the first words I voiced to the triage nurse who told me that I had diabetes while pointing to the number "592" on the glucose monitoring device. My words were not a question; they were a statement that I saw manifest as truth many times on television. I believed a diabetes diagnosis meant that I had two options: a quick death or slow death accompanied by dismemberment one toe or foot or leg at a time. Because I did not know anyone who openly talked about living with diabetes, my perception of the condition came primarily from the news media, hearsay, and television shows and movies. When I became a diabetes blogger, I used an alias for nearly seven years because I was terrified of being stigmatized, but I wanted to fill a void and create a resource of inspirational diabetes content highlighting African American culture. I stopped writing under a pseudonym years ago and my work as a global diabetes activist, peer support group facilitator, and researcher writing about the intersections of health, race, and feminism have flourished since embracing my fears of diabetes stigma.

Over the years, I have witnessed the lack of culturally appropriate diabetes information create barriers for peer support group attendees, family, and friends to be able to decipher between diabetes facts and diabetes myths, such as diabetes being a curable condition. When I reflect on my own experiences, TV and film shaped my view of diabetes long before I was diagnosed. Therefore, I hope that by examining the representation of Black American characters we might better understand how these performances shape the public imagination. This chapter explores the film and TV comedies *Soul Food*, *Boondocks*, *Madea's Big Happy Family*, *Madea Family Funeral*, *30 Rock*, and *Black-ish* and provides an analysis of African American characters who appear frequently laughing and using humor to deflect, ignore, or silence their experiences with diabetes complications.

Blackness, Disability, and Comedy

My analysis is informed by theoretical frameworks on stigma, disability in film, and African American humor. Stigma, as defined by Erving Goffman is "an attribute that is deeply discrediting," and represents a "special kind of relationship between attribute and stereotype," that leads us to "believe the person with a stigma is not quite human. On this assumption we exercise varieties of discrimination, through which we effectively, if often unthinkingly, reduce his life chances" (Goffman 1963). Diabetes stigma "refers to the experiences of negative feelings such as exclusion, rejection, or blame due to the perceived stigmatization of having diabetes. Socially identifiable characteristics related to diabetes can include insulin injections, blood glucose monitoring, dietary restrictions, obesity, and hypoglycemic episodes, all of which can contribute to the experience of diabetes stigma" (Liu et al. 2017).

The disability scholars writing about crip humor provide a general understanding of how people with disabilities use humor to cope in the world; however, when looking at Black American characters, it was vital that my reading of these films and TV shows also be informed by theories about African American comedy and humor. Similarly to Chris Bell, author of the essay "Is Disability Studies Actually White Disability Studies," who remarks that the field "by and large focuses on the work of white individuals and is itself largely produced by a corps of white scholars and activists" (Bell 1997), I found the scarcity of diversity in essays on disability and humor problematic. The authors' racial makeup is not merely the point of the scrutiny, but rather the multiple moments of misunderstanding when blackness is ignored or discussed separately from disability.

For example, in the essay "Stepping Backwards with Disability Humor? The Case of NY Gov. David Paterson's Representation on Saturday Night Live," the authors write "In the big picture it appears that SNL pushed racial comedy to the back burner in favor of the easier 'sell'" (Haller and Becker 2014). They describe the skit as exclusively ableist because the Governor is legally blind. It is only when Armisen mentions Richard Pryor do the authors make a connection to race. What they fail to observe by only focusing on Paterson's disability is that Paterson is both blind and Black American and that the joke about him being a buffoon could still be used against him if he were not blind. As Mel Watkins, African American humor scholar, points out in *On the Real Side: A History of African American Comedy*, "Minstrelsy, with its buffoonish caricatures of blacks, enthralled an entire nation with its exaggerated image of the behavior of its underclass victims—behavior that, to a great extent, it has initially encouraged and often demanded" (Watkins 1999). Pioneering Black American comedians like Bert Williams were forced to perform in blackface and transform into coons for white audiences (Chude-Sokei 2006). Minstrelsy is the root of American comedy and a force that African American entertainers still must contend with when performing. It is imperative that this historical knowledge informs analyses of jokes aimed at African Americans like with the SNL skit because these jokes reside at the intersection of disability and blackness. The Paterson joke is not exclusively ableist, it is also racist. Another example of jokes located at the intersection of blackness and disability appears later in the paper when Tyler Perry's Madea brings diabetes into a joke about police brutality against Black people.

This paper does not distinguish between types of humor (satire or slapstick) or laughter (tone and physical movements) but rather focuses on how the humor reinforces diabetes stigma against Black Americans. I am cautious to label this an analysis of crip humor because a fundamental aspect of crip humor "often lies in having a disabled teller, as well as an audience who understands the teller's perspective and worldview and thereby 'gets' the joke" (Milbrodt 2018). Without knowing if the jokes being analyzed in this chapter are written by people with diabetes, I avoid the term "crip humor." As such, this chapter is not presenting a Black disability humor aesthetic, a project left for future endeavors, but it instead adds to disability scholarship that critiques "society's prejudice towards people with disabilities and ways of effecting positive change" (Smit and Enns 2001) by providing an overview of varied representations of African American characters with diabetes portrayed in television and film comedies and sitcoms.

Black Americans with Diabetes in Film and Television

I begin with the 1997 comedy-drama film, *Soul Food* because it is arguably the first Hollywood blockbuster that centers on a Black American woman with diabetes. Mama Joe, who is affectionally referred to as "Big Mama" (a name commonly bestowed to elderly African American women) represents the matriarch of her family. She expresses her love through weekly Sunday dinners consisting of soul food cuisine. Big Mama is the nucleus of a family that falls apart almost immediately after she is hospitalized and dies prematurely from complications of diabetes.

One Sunday while cooking, she burns her arm on the stove and the following conversation transpires between Big Mama and one of her three daughters.

MAXINE	You ain't been takin' your insulin? I bet you ain't been to a doctor, either.
MAMA	I don't need no doctor. There's nothing salve, turpentine and my herbs won't cure.
MAXINE	Except your diabetes.

This is how the audience is introduced to diabetes. It is serious enough to cause harm to the beloved matriarch, but Big Mama prefers to keep the conversation light and to focus on the main event, Sunday dinner. Her faith in homeopathic remedies instead of the insulin she is prescribed helps to build a foundation of diabetes stigma by signaling that Big Mama is insufficiently managing diabetes. Sadly, her inability to feel the stove's heat indicates that she has at least one severe diabetes complication and it also foreshadows Big Mama's death.

In a later scene at her youngest daughter's wedding, Big Mama appears dancing, laughing, and smiling throughout the entire event. When she uses her jovial spirit and wit to diffuse a tense moment between the bride and groom, it confirms that she is laughing while dying. Big Mama's health quickly deteriorates, and she undergoes a lower leg amputation.

MOTHER JOE	I'm not getting my leg cut off.
TERI	Mama, you have to. There's no blood circulating to that leg. You're diabetic.
MAXINE	You haven't been watching what you eat. (Tillman 1997)

As if the recommendation to have a lower limb amputation is not awful enough, her daughter blames Big Mama for being in poor health. The explanation "you're diabetic," leaves open the interpretation that an amputation is inevitable for people with diabetes. It also stigmatizes Big Mama and creates distance between her and her daughters and the audience. She is portrayed as a person that does not manage diabetes properly and because of that, she gets what she deserves.

Arleen Tuchman's, *Diabetes: A History of Race and Disease*, traces the creation of the "good" and "bad" diabetes patient caricatures back to the early twentieth century when Dr. Elliott Joslin emphasized personal responsibility. "Ultimately, then, if physicians and 'apostles' did their part and an individual's condition nevertheless grew worse, blame could be placed only on the choices the individual made, as though each and every person had the same obstacles and challenges to overcome" (Tuchman 2020). Big Mama's daughters fall in line with this way of thinking demonstrated by their scolding of Mama Joe. The bad diabetic is problematic for many reasons and for African Americans it can be especially harmful given the racial disparities in American healthcare systems. Irby Jones, President of the National Medical Association, chastised the secretary in one of her 1986 President's Column. She wrote, "Well, as black Americans, we know it is not as simple as all that. Blaming the patient will not cure the ills of America's underserved minorities. The diseases correctly identified by HHS (Health and Human Services) as affecting the health of the black community so devastatingly are in large measure the result of poverty, neglect, underlying prejudices, and the resulting stress ... We all know that while health education indeed may be helpful, as Mrs. Heckler suggests, what we really need is better nutrition in early life, better housing, and more and better jobs" (Tuchman 2020). These socio-economic factors are not mentioned by Big Mama's daughters who represent varying economic and social classes. Unfortunately, none of the daughters ask if their mother can afford the insulin they berate her for not taking.

Shortly thereafter, Big Mama has the surgery, suffers from a stroke, and remains in a coma for five weeks. *Soul Food* demonstrates Kevin Ferguson's point that "... diabetes only exists [...] as a breakdown and never as a lived experience. This tends to be true of the diabetic filmography, which is filled more with gangrene, amputation, kidney failure, sweat, and comas than it is with glucometers, insulin, healthy eating, or exercise routines" (Ferguson 2010). Because the audience is not privy to Big Mama's lived experiences with diabetes before developing complications, empathy for her is not cultivated. Peter Longman remarks that "What we fear, we often stigmatize and shun and sometimes seek to destroy" (Longmore 2001). In *Soul Food*, Mama Joe this point when she is stigmatized and is "destroyed" through a death scene removing her promptly from the plot. This short-lived diabetes subplot perpetuates the misconception that diabetes attacks the body quickly and brings unavoidable doom.

To further demonstrate the harmful effects of stigmatizing Big Mama's diabetes in *Soul Food*, we can examine the African American, adult-animated, socio-political, satirical series *The Boondocks*. In season 1, episode 10, *Soul Food* is parodied by Huey Freedman—a revolutionary, politically conscious, semi-militant teenager.

> *Soul Food* is a movie about a big, humongous, black grandmother, aptly named Big Mama. Big Mama demonstrates her love by feeding herself and her offspring enormous amounts of pig lard. Then get this, Big Mama's arteries are so clogged, they gotta amputate her arm … Right, okay, whatever, leg. Then, she dies from a heart attack or another stroke or somethin. And what does the family do after she dies? They get together for a Sunday dinner and eat the same food that just killed Big Mama. The same food. They didn't learn a lesson, nobody went on a diet, and that's the end of the movie. (McGruder 2006)

The satirical summary demonstrates the main points that many audiences gathered from the movie. The diabetes subplot moves so rapidly as a silent killer that it is easily forgotten. *The Boondocks* episode as well as numerous film reviews do not mention diabetes as being central to her death because Mama Joe is stigmatized for eating soul food and holding her responsible for causing her own death remain the pot liquor that audiences extract, not diabetes (Ebert 1997; O'Neal Parker 1997).

By creating opportunities to blame Big Mama's love for soul food as the root cause of her development of diabetes, *Soul Food* perpetuates diabetes stigma. A similar conclusion is also reached by Ferguson who reviews thirty-six films with diabetes characters in "The Cinema of Control: On Diabetic Excess and Illness in Film." He writes, "Clearly, Big Mama's traditional Sunday dinner was what kept the fractious family together. The film bizarrely suggests, however, that such familial closeness can only come from a sacrificial refusal to self-govern. [...] Big Mama's no-nonsense, unmeasured approach to living is the major reason her health is poor, but it is hard to see how this privileging of tradition fits with the narrative, since Big Mama's death is a major blow that nearly ends the family" (Ferguson 2010). The blame is placed on Mama Joe without any inquiry into the quality of the diabetes education, treatment, or care she received. As Paul Longmore points out in, "Screening Stereotypes: Images of Disabled People," "disability is a punishment for evil" (Longmore 2001) and Big Mama's evil was eating African American cuisine. Unfortunately, *Soul Food* and *The Boondocks* fail to acknowledge that Big Mama could have incorporated soul food into her diabetes management.

The matriarch in African American films is a character that transcends the individual woman and symbolizes the epicenter of love, wisdom, and respect. Losing the matriarch of the family to complications of diabetes is something that many Black Americans experience. Some entertainers have openly shared their anguish around watching diabetes claim their mother's life including Pattie LaBelle, Sherri Shepheard, and Tyler Perry (LaBelle and Randolph 2003; Shepherd and Fitzpatrick 2013; Perry 2014). Perry uses Mabel Earlene "Madea" Simmons, an elderly woman he transforms into in his plays, films, and television shows, as an opportunity to keep the black matriarch alive. Madea, the embodiment of his mother and aunts, is so popular that Perry has built a billion-dollar empire largely with the Madea series (LionsGate n.d.).

Tyler Perry's Madea collection avoids many of the pitfalls in *Soul Food* because Madea lives a thriving life with diabetes, albeit with complications. Additionally, Madea is not the only main character living with diabetes and this allows Perry to discuss diabetes from multiple angles. For example, *Madea's Big Happy Family* begins to dispel commonly held myths about diabetes within the first ten minutes of the movie. As Cora enters the hospital to check on her father, she sees a familiar person, Aunt Bam.

AUNT BAM	Baby, what are you doing here?
CORA	Mr. Brown wasn't feeling well last night. Well, you know he has diabetes, right?
AUNT BAM	He does?
CORA	Yep.
AUNT BAM	Lord, that's gonna kill him.
CORA	Don't say that.
AUNT BAM:	Lord, he's gonna die. He's gonna die.
CORA	He's not gonna die with that.

The trope of connecting diabetes with death appears here, but as a point to be contended with and highlighted for being misunderstood. The humor is turned towards Aunt Bam who ignorantly believes that diabetes is synonymous with Mr. Brown dying. While this myth-busting moment suggests a more positive trajectory of the diabetes narrative in the comedy, it is short-lived.

In the subsequent scene, Cora joins her father as they await the doctor's update. Dr. Evans provides the following details,

DR EVANS	See, the problem with a lot of people is they think diabetes is just a little sugar. It isn't. Now you have to eat right .... You have to exercise .... And let me tell you something, there are people who have lost their eyesight, their limbs, and even died from this disease. Now you gotta get serious about this, lose some weight, start exercising, or things could get worse. (Perry 2011)

The physician is well-intended and demonstrates an ability to use culturally specific language to communicate with Mr. Brown; however, he falls into the trap of using scare tactics to inform Mr. Brown about the importance of proper diabetes management. Hence, the misappropriation of diabetes to death and dying is made again. Tyler Perry's fans adore Mr. Brown's ability to rival Madea for comedic relief through his singing, jokes, and outlandish attire. When Cora reveals to the doctor that Mr. Brown is not managing diabetes well, his similarity to Hughes's "Minstrel Man" is revealed to the audience. Mr. Brown has been making audiences laugh for years while suffering in silence.

Moreover, Perry often uses Madea's diabetes as a means to intensify the comedic moment. In *A Madea Family Funeral*, when police officers pull Brian over while escorting Madea and other elderly family members to an anniversary party, a conversation about police brutality erupts.

MADEA	You put that camera on 'em, they start acting different.
HATTIE	Well, get yours out and let's go live.
MADEA	Hell, no. I ain't finna reach up in there. Hell, I done had too many bullet holes and stab wounds. I done got old, they don't heal the same no more. I got diabetes. (Perry 2019)

Madea reminds everyone that she has diabetes by strategically positioning "I got diabetes" in a statement about wounds. It is not merely a consequence of age that causes her to heal slower, but rather a combination of time and diabetes that have caused this effect. A serious diabetes complication—slow healing wounds from elevated glucose levels—is merged into Madea's joke about police brutality against Black Americans. Madea, like Mr. Brown, applies humor to evade the reality of the diabetes complications she endures. When Madea reveals her wounds do not heal quickly, she simultaneously discloses that she is also suffering from diabetes complications while maintaining her position as the series preeminent comedian.

Similarly, the television sitcom *30 Rock* starring Tracy Morgan exploits severe diabetes complications as comedic relief. While diabetes is a leading cause of death, it is also manageable and not everyone suffers from diabetes complications, but audiences will not know these facts if death and dying are the only recurring tropes of diabetes characters in these television shows and sitcoms. Tracy Jordon, the show's protagonist is diagnosed with prediabetes during a doctor's visit in season 3, episode 9.

DR. SPACEMAN	Now we know what we're dealing with. Unless you make some serious lifestyle changes, you're in danger of becoming diabetic.
TRACY	So, how bad is diabetes really?
DR. SPACEMAN	It's quite serious. If left untreated you could lose a foot.
TRACY	Can I replace it with a wheel, like Rosie from the Jetsons?
DR. SPACEMAN	I suppose. But then you'd have to register as a motor vehicle. (Fey 2009)

Tracey's pre-diabetes diagnosis is immediately connected to an extreme negative health outcome, an amputation. Because the doctor does not explain what he means by "serious lifestyle changes" Tracey and the audience are left only with the vivid image of "you could lose a foot" to understand diabetes. Without any guidance as to how Tracey might be able to circumvent an amputation, it comes across as an unavoidable consequence of a diabetes diagnosis.

The joke referencing an imagined wheel is made into a reality in the next scene as the camera focuses on Tracy's feet. He has one foot on a homemade skate as he wheels into the workplace relying on his bodyguards for assistance.

KEN	Good Morning Mr. Jordan, what's that on your foot, Sir?
TRACY	It's a practice wheel for when I lose my foot to diabetes.
KEN	You can't eat candy if you have diabetes
TRACY	There's no link between diabetes and diet. That's a white myth, Ken.
KEN	It's not a myth. Gentleman back me up.
DOT COM	I don't know. My dad had diabetes and he ate whatever he wanted until he died on the day I was born.
KEN	How do you not see the connection? (Fey 2009)

30 Rock's extended joke with Tracy could underscore the importance of Black Americans getting proper treatment because they are three times more likely to have an amputation than their counterparts; (Control 2014) however, the educational moment is undercut by a joke that serves to maintain diabetes stigma and maintain a strong tie between diabetes and death and dying. Likewise, Dot Com's statement about his father eating whatever he wanted before he died paints the father as a "bad diabetic" who caused his own death because he lacked self-control. Furthermore, Tracy's diagnosis episode is most memorable for seeing him prepare for an imaginary inevitable amputation by putting a skate on his foot and mock the impending physical disability assumed to be aligned in his destiny after developing prediabetes.

Lastly, the most recent television sitcom to bring diabetes centerstage is *Black-ish*. Dre Johnson, the protagonist, is diagnosed with Type 2 diabetes in season 4, episode 9. Unprecedentedly, the episode begins with acknowledging racial disparities, revealing socio-economic and environmental risk factors, and discrediting harmful myths about diabetes. Before the opening credits emerge, cartoon illustrations bring Dre's voiceover to life,

> ... But as easy as we seem to have it, we're twice as likely to get diagnosed with diabetes. While genetics are a factor, diabetes has also been linked to obesity, poor diet, and inactivity. But don't get it twisted, it's not all our fault. For a lot of us it's hard to be fit living in a food desert with no decent healthcare or gyms. And let's be honest, who has time to exercise when you're working two jobs to make ends meet. Even if you can make time, it's dicey because if someone sees you running in the hood, they'll give you

> something to run from. Despite our best efforts, 'the sugars' is super common with black folks. 1.3 million Black Americans are currently living with it today. In fact, it's so common that I already have it. (Barris 2017)

Dre's monologue offers important pushback against diabetes stigma that places all the blame of a diagnosis on the person with diabetes. Researchers have noted that African Americans in poorer neighborhoods have an increased number of health conditions, including Type 2 diabetes, that are directly related to the lack of access to fresh food, an overabundance of fast-food restaurants, and the lack of sleep (Reitzel et al. 2016; Chaput et al. 2007).

The episode also engages directly with the use of homeopathic remedies to manage diabetes. Convinced by a documentary that his father shows him, Dre embarks upon a journey of curing his diabetes by fasting, detoxing, going to sweat lodges, reading wellness blogs, getting colonics, and hiring an online certified health coach. Similarly, to Mama Joe, Dre wrongfully puts faith in alternative medicine to effectively remedy diabetes. Dre fails to cure his diabetes, faints at a work function, and dreams he died from diabetes complications. Albeit in a dream, the recurring theme of death emerges. Dre awakens frightened about dying before he is ready and vows to follow the doctor's guidelines for managing diabetes in hopes to prevent his nightmare from coming true.

Black-ish is an example of progress in the representation of African American characters with diabetes. In the episode, the audience observes Dre checking his blood sugar, something not seen in the other comedies, and he comes to understand that diabetes is not a death sentence. *Black-ish* was able to combat many myths, maintain its comedic tone, educate its viewers, and give hope to people who are managing diabetes. However, since that episode, Dre's diabetes management has fallen into the silent margins only coming up once again two seasons later. If *Black-ish* fails to maintain a healthy diabetes subplot it risks Dre becoming another African American sitcom character who entertains at his peril and embodying the Minstrel Man who is laughing while dying.

Toward a New Diabetes Narrative

In closing, the representation of Black American characters in sitcoms and comedies has improved since *Soul Food*, but these characters are still stigmatized and silenced. The most harmful message—blaming people with diabetes for causing their diabetes—remains prevalent. Producers and writers have the power to change this diabetes narrative by showcasing characters eating soul food in moderation, discussing diabetes in neutral or positive scenarios, and demonstrating daily diabetes management. Diabetes complications might be discussed as a possible progression for some people rather than a swift inevitable outcome for everyone. Creators could avoid using diabetes as a tool to intensify a character's connection to death and dying. I am not suggesting that diabetes humor is unacceptable, there are far too many disability comedians and crip humor enthusiasts to make that claim. My point is this: laughter in TV and film should not come at the expense of showcasing people living well with diabetes. The lack of diversity in representation only re-enforces damaging stereotypes. It is possible to display scenes where characters are counting carbs and taking insulin or oral medication for the soul food dinner on Sundays. If these types of changes are embraced in film and TV, a new diabetes narrative can be created and, in time, no one newly diagnosed with diabetes would utter, "I'm going to die" as their first words—as I did when I was first diagnosed.

References

Barris, Kenya. 2017. *Black-ish*. Performed by Anthony Anderson. American Broadcast Company.

Bell, Chris. 1997. "Is Disability Studies Actually White Disability Studies." In The Disability Studies Reader, by Lennard J. Davis, 402-410. New York: Routledge.

Chaput, J.-P., J.-P. Després, C. Bouchard, and A. Tremblay. 2007. Association of Sleep Duration with Type 2 Diabetes and Impaired Glucose Tolerance. *Diabetologia* 50 (11): 298–304.

Chude-Sokei, Louis. 2006. *The Last 'Darky': Bert Williams, Black-On-Black Minstrelsy, and the African Diaspora*. Durham: Duke University Press Books.

Control, Diabetes In. 2014, October 17. African-Americans More Likely to Have Amputations. Accessed 1 Oct 2020.

Ebert, Roger. 1997. *Soul Food*, September 27. https://www.rogerebert.com/reviews/soul-food-1997. Accessed Aug 2020.

Ferguson, Kevin L. 2010. *The Cinema of Control: On Diabetic Excess and Illness in Film*. Vol. 31. New York: Journal of Medical Humanities.

Fey, Tina. 2009. *30 Rock*. Directed by Tina Fey and Alec Baldwin. Performed by Tracy Morgan.

Goffman, Erving. 1963. *Stigma: Notes on the Management of Spoiled Identity*. Englewood Cliffs: Prentice-Hall, Inc.

Haller, Beth, and Amy B. Becker. 2014. Stepping Backwards with Disability Humor? The Case of NY Gov. David Paterson's Representation on 'Saturday Night Live'. *Disability Studies Quarterly* 34 (1).

Hughes, Langston. 1994. "Minstrel Man." The Collected Poems of Langston Hughes, by The Estate of Langston Hughes. New York: Alfred A. Knopf.

LaBelle, Patti, and Laura Randolph. 2003. *Patti LaBelle's Lite Cuisine*. New York: Gotham Books.

LionsGate. n.d. *Tyler Perry's Madea*. https://www.lionsgate.com/franchises/tyler-perrys-madea. Accessed 12 Sept 2020.

Liu, Nancy F., Adam S. Brown, Michael F. Younge, Susan J. Guzman, Kelly L. Close, Richard Wood, and Alexnadria E. Folias. 2017. Stigma in People With Type 1 or Type 2 Diabetes. *Clinical Diabetes* 35 (1): 27–35.

Longmore, P.K. 2001. Screening Stereotypes: Images of Disabled People. In *Screening Disability*, ed. C.R. Smit and A. Enns. Lanham: University Press of America.

Matthew, Dayna Bowen. 2015. *Just Medicine: A Cure for Racial Inequality In American Healthcare*. New York: New York University Press.

McGruder, Aaron. 2006. *Boondocks*. Directed by Joe Horne. Performed by Regina King.

Milbrodt, Teresa. 2018. "Today I Had an Eye Appointment, and I'm Still Blind": Crip Humor, Storytelling, and Narrative Positioning of the Disabled Self. *Diability Studies Quarterly* 38 (2).

Norden, Martin F. 1994. *The Cinema of Isolation: A History of Physical Disability in the Movies*. New Brunswick: Rutgers University Press.

O'Neal Parker, Lonnae. 1997. *Washington Post*, September 1997. https://www.washingtonpost.com/wp-srv/style/longterm/movies/review97/soulfood-parker.htm. Accessed 15 Aug 2020.

Perry, Tyler. 2011. *Tyler Perry's Madea's Big Happy Family*. Directed by Tyler Perry. Performed by Tyler Perry.

———. 2014. *Facebook*. February 12. https://www.facebook.com/TylerPerry/photos/my-mother-at-age-40-before-diabetes-destroyed-her-quality-of-life-so-tragic-for-/10152374503268268/. Accessed 16 Aug 2020.

———. 2019. *Tyler Perry's A Madea Family Funeral*. Directed by Tyler Perry. Performed by Tyler Perry.

Reitzel, Lorraine R., Hiroe Okamoto, Daphne C. Hernandez, et al. 2016. The Build Food Environment and Dietary Intake Among African-American Adults. *American Journal Health Behavoir* 40 (1): 3–11.

Shepherd, Sherri, and Billie Fitzpatrick. 2013. *Plan D: How to Lose Weight and Beat Diabetes (Even If You Don't Have It)*. New York: HarperCollins.

Smit, Christopher R., and Anthony Enns. 2001. *Screening Disability: Essays on Conema and Disability*. Lanham: University Press of America.

Tillman, George. 1997. *Soul Food*. Directed by George Tillman. Performed by Irma P. Hall.

Tuchman, Arleen. 2020. *Diabetes: a History of Race and Disease*. New Haven: Yale University.

Washington, Harriet. 2008. *Medical Apartheid: The Dark History of Medical Experimentation on Black American From Colonial Times to The Present*. New York: Random House.

Watkins, Mel. 1999. *On the Real Side: a History of African American Comedy*. New York: Lawrence Hill Books.

"Diabetes, Yuck!": Comedy, Disability, and the Dangers of Parody in *Parks and Recreation* (2009–2015)

Bianca C. Frazer

Every time I find myself on the phone with a health insurance agent, I am eventually on the verge of laughing, screaming, and/or crying. One particular morning in late January 2021, I begin by dialing a new company for the first time. I punch through an extensive maze of auto-generated questions. I wait on hold for 15 minutes. Finally, a real person answers and recommends that I order the generic version of insulin [insert my silent scream]. The agent puts me on hold again while I rage-text a colleague about this suggestion. I am taken off-hold and told that because there are no generic versions of insulin this order will cost me hundreds of dollars. The agent needs to call the pharmacy, so can I please hold again? While that music, you know the music, plays in the background, I ridicule myself

B. C. Frazer (✉)
Department of Disability and Human Development, University of Illinois Chicago, Chicago, IL, USA
e-mail: bfrazer@uic.edu

B. C. Frazer, H. R. Walker (eds.), *(Un)doing Diabetes: Representation, Disability, Culture*, Palgrave Studies in Science and Popular Culture, https://doi.org/10.1007/978-3-030-83110-3_7

for electing to pay *more* money this year for what I thought would be better coverage. Eventually, after an hour on the phone and for reasons I never learn, the order does not go through. Weeks later I bitterly wonder where I can find the comedy treatment of this absurd exchange, one which I know occurs frequently in diabetes communities.

Unfortunately for me and other insulin-dependent diabetics, television portrayals of diabetes frequently focus on the individual and their poor choices as the fodder for comedy. Writers on one such comedy, *Parks and Recreation*, make frequent use of this representational strategy. After Greg Daniels and Michael Schur's successful work on the American version of *The Office*, they conceived of *Parks and Rec*. Adopting a similar mocumentary and talking-head camera style as *The Office*, *Parks and Rec* follows the relationships and workplace shenanigans of local government employees in Pawnee, Indiana. As the Parks and Rec department works to better the lives of Pawnee residents, they often focus on the problem of diabetes in their town. In this essay, I explore the comedic relationship the show establishes between government actions and diabetic people. By not considering the politics of diabetes as a disability, the show's comedy fails to invoke audience's critical thinking around government actions. Instead, the show re-injures diabetic people with its parody by solely focusing on diabetic individuals and exaggerating reckless choices. Ultimately, the comedy perpetuates beliefs that United States government has no role addressing systemic harm to people with diabetes.

Diabetes and Television Comedy: Background and Context

Pop culture representations of diabetes regularly recycle simplified notions about those who have it for comedy. Particularly in the television sitcom genre, references to diabetes and stereotypes about it appear ubiquitously: from *The Office* ("Michael Scott: "Why don't you go outside and take a shot of insulin and have a nap ok?"), to *New Girl* (Jessica Day: "You just hang out with jerks like Gavin. Oh, I'm sorry, DJ Dia-beat It"), and *Big Bang Theory* ("Penny Hofstadter: "Well, as a waitress, sales was a big part of my job, and believe me I convinced a lot of very large customers who should not be eating cheesecake to have more cheesecake ... one of those chubbsters had an insulin pump"). As these lines illustrate, comedy writers assume that their audience already imagines a natural link between poor choices, fat embodiment, and diabetes. Though many shows make use of this seemingly obvious correlation, *Parks and Recreation* incorporates this assemblage into the show on several occasions, from reoccurring jokes to full episode plot lines.

The central character on the show, Leslie Knope, played by Amy Poehler, works as the Parks and Recreation deputy director. Knope regularly tries to improve the lives of Pawnee citizens. Knope believes that her job includes at times intervening and regulating the residents' worser impulses. Leslie's views often conflict with Ron Swanson, portrayed by Nick Offerman, who acts as the director of the department and identifies as a libertarian. Ron works to actively undermine the goals of the department to improve, or intervene, on citizen's lives. In Season 2, Episode 15, titled "Sweetums," Leslie wants to prevent a local candy manufacturer from selling sugary products in local parks. Ron tells the camera, "Leslie needs to butt out. The whole point of this country is if you wanna eat garbage, balloon up to 600 pounds and die of a heart attack at 43, you can! You are free to do so! To me, that's beautiful" (Daniels 2010c). Meanwhile, Leslie Knope has set up public forums to inform the public of how sugary the Sweetums bars are, believing that government should provide services and protect the public from its most base instincts.

The tension in the show over Ron and Leslie's governing philosophies are often played out through diabetes narratives, which commonly focus on individual's failure to self-govern.

With its commentary on the nature of local politics, *Parks and Rec* frequently follows its government employees outside the office and into the lives of the residents. While department employees attempt to promote "healthy," outdoor activities, their conflict with local residents written as careless, large, and loud people who are obsessed with fast food and sugary sodas. In the Season 5, Episode 10, named "Two Parties," Leslie battles with a local fast-food chain over their attempts to build a Paunch Burger on an empty lot where Leslie would like to build a new park. A local resident walks by and notices that a sign has gone up on the lot that reads, "Future home of Paunch Burger: Start drooling, fatties." The resident points to the sign and says, "Aw, sweet! A new Paunch Burger!" Leslie shouts at him facetiously, "Their burgers will kill you! They're full of wasps!" but the person retorts, "Yeah, but they taste real good." In this interaction, the writers create a parody of a resident so enamored with fast food that he totally disregards the mean-spirited Paunch Burger advertising and Leslie's warning. The scene exaggerates how these residents lose all sense of reason and coherence at the promise of fast food.

Punching Down and Nonperformativity

In this essay I explore two related concepts. First, I reflect upon what I call the 'politics of punching down,' referring to the form of comedy that mocks marginalized groups. Contemporary television comedy writers avoid punching down comedy with people with disabilities. I argue that writers do not conceive of diabetic people as a marginalized group and the punching down comedy remains morally justified. In particular, I will examine episodes of *Parks and Rec* that mine comedy from mocking Pawnee residents with diabetes. While the show aims to parody the notion that people who do not "control their diets" are foolish, the writers choose to punch down, thereby not evoking critical thinking of this concept.

Typically, parody evokes critical thinking in the viewer and opens up the potential to generate social change. In parody a creator presents an audience with a familiar subject with exaggerations. As creators parody a subject, they point audience attention to areas that require critical thinking and thereby generate potential for change (Hutcheon 2000). For example, *Parks and Rec* exaggerates depictions of Pawnee residents' relationship to food in order to parody the stereotype of middle-America's love of fast food and sugar. However, the danger of parody emerges when such depictions reanimate the stereotypes that focus on individuals and do not examine systemic forces that require critical thinking to change. I argue that the ideological underpinnings of 'punching down' produces serious consequences for people living with diabetes including the maintenance of an individualized view of diabetes.

Second, I turn to a form of 'punching down' comedy in the show that also has the effect of excusing the audience from critical thinking: the nonperformativity of government efforts to "fix" the problem of diabetes. Sara Ahmed coined the term *nonperformative* to define speech acts, such as promises or apologies, that do *not* do what they say they are doing (2006). Ahmed developed this idea to critique institutional speech acts (including words, written materials, and images) such as a university releasing a statement condemning a racist incident on campus. Ahmed notes that while the speech act may state that the university values diversity or promises future action, such speech acts are actually *nonperformatives*, as they work by "not bringing about the effects that they name" (2006,

105). Ahmed argues that these speech acts themselves can be read by the public as taking an action, but the speech acts do not enact anti-racism by merely existing. Entrenched systemic problems are left intact. While the audiences encountering such statements understand them as the moral response to racism, Ahmed notes that statement may promise but does not necessarily produce material effect.

I argue that a similar dynamic occurs with the show's treatment of government employees' attempts to "do something" about diabetes in Pawnee. The show assumes it's audience will understand the moral justification of a local government taking action to help diabetic people, but the show portrays these efforts as ineffectual and humorous, particularly when actions are directed towards changing Pawnee residents' behaviors. By centering individual behavior in its efforts to curb instances of diabetes, the show does not draw audience's attention to systemic conditions. This comedy occurs at one of the central contradictions of the show between Leslie's interventionist beliefs and Ron's dedication to free-market capitalism. However, with discussions of diabetes, Leslie and Ron's views are not in tension at all: they both further the logics of individual responsibility as the basis for health while reproducing the existing stigmas and undesirability of diabetes identity. Ultimately, comedy that punches down at marginalized groups reproduces oppression. There is also a missed punch that leaves those who hold power unscathed and limits the potential for systemic change.

Representations of diabetes as a stigmatized identity alongside nonperformative government actions are not just fodder for comedy, but concepts with real-world consequences for people with diabetes. First, the representation of diabetes as a condition caused by foolish and reckless individuals contributes to 7.3 million U.S. adults with undiagnosed diabetes (Centers for Disease Control and Prevention 2020). For example, when the National Institutes of Health released a report that noted one third of adults with diabetes do not know they have it, the chair of the National Diabetes Education Program recommended that "you should talk to your health care professional about your risk" (2006). However, someone might resist disclosing their risk to their healthcare provider if it means acquiring such a highly stigmatized identity.

Representations of nonperformative government actions further medicalized and individualized notions of diabetes while concealing the role government might take in regulating systemic issues, such as insulin prices. Unaffordable insulin has cased the deaths of many people, with and without insurance, who rationed their insulin (Alliance 2020). When lawmakers seem to step in with language and legislation to prevent such tragedies, their nonperformative speech acts often do not create the policy changes that audiences think they do. For instance, when state-level lawmakers introduced insulin co-pay cap bills, #insulin4all activists spoke out about how few people the legislation would actually assist. Upon pointing this out, activists noted that lawmakers got "defensive and hostile" (Johnson 2021).

By parodying individuals, not the faulty programs or pay-for-use healthcare systems, the creators of *Parks and Rec* miss an opportunity to evoke critical thinking in audiences. Although the creators frequently parodied real-world political events, including the 2013 U.S. government shut down, the critical lens remains on the foolishness of diabetic people. In other words, writers failed to draw attention to politicians and legislators with power over diabetes-related policy. I argue that the moralizing and individualizing of diabetes prevents the most compelling part of parody from working. Rather than produce a social critique that moves and transforms audiences, the writers punch down, thus affirming the status quo for the audience.

Punching Up, Punching Down: Considering Disability and Television Comedy

Here, I situate representations of diabetes within frameworks established by scholars of disability, comedy, and American television. Disability studies scholars Beth Haller and Amy Bree Becker contend that in the era of modern television, "discerning TV viewers know the shows that trade in cheap laughs by making fun of people with disabilities are not tapping into much creativity" (2014). When TV writers avoid mocking people with disabilities for humor, they are avoiding *punching down*, or "the act of picking on marginalized groups for laughs" (Cohen 2018). *Punching up* refers to a form of comedy where creators aim their critiques at those with power.

Forms of comedy like satire allow their creators to wield their punch with the purpose of hitting those with power in society and exposing their irrationality. G. K. Chesterton writes that the role of satire is to "perceive some absurdity inherent in the logic of some position, and … draw the absurdity out and isolate it, so that all can see it" (Gray et al. 2009, 12). With political satire, the comedian specifically *punches up* by calling audiences' attention to the absurdities of those in positions of governing power.

Writing about TV comedy, David Marc observes that while political satire makes fun of public actions and structures, sitcoms "tend to flatter their viewers by ridiculing personal behavior rather than the people who run things" (2009, x). Sitcoms focus on magnifying and making fun of individual behaviors. With representations of diabetes in television comedies, writers seem to believe that people with diabetes fail to follow common sense and do not take care of themselves in simple ways like eating healthy and exercising (Boero 2007; Bock 2012). While writers parody characters' behaviors, they reenforce the underlying belief that many people in middle America disregard common-sense health imperatives.

Literary theorist Linda Hutcheon notes that "parody signals how present representations come from past ones and what ideological consequences derive from both continuity and difference" (1989, 93). Her point about *continuity* means that parody must in some way recreate the original. However, Hutcheon points out the danger of re-injuring the targeted group when recreating a stereotype for exaggeration. In terms of the *difference* Hutcheon notes, parody relies on the audience understanding there are differences which make the representation funny. *Parks and Rec* exaggerates the idea that people with diabetes lack common sense and do not care about their health. It may be that the show intended to evoke an audience's critical thinking around diabetes and awaken "common sense," which is often the perceived corrective for "lifestyle" diseases (Boero 2007). Viewing diabetes solely through the medical model, or an individualized lens, justifies such mockery of individual behavior.

Jerry Gergich: The Schlemiel and the Schlimazel

Early on in the series, the creators mark the character Jerry Gergich as the target of much ridicule in the office. In Season 2, an episode titled "Park Safety," Ron Swanson shares this story to characterize Jerry: "David Myers, the Jewish guy who works at City Hall, once told me something: a schlemiel is the guy who spills soup at a fancy party. A schlimazel is the guy he spills it on. Jerry is both the schlemiel and the schlimazel of our office" (Daniels 2010a). Ron characterizes Jerry as the one who makes blunders, as well as the person who suffers the consequences, in the same episode that we learn Jerry has diabetes.

Later in that episode, Jerry tells the office that he was mugged in the park, and Leslie goes on a local TV broadcast to let the town know the government is failing to keep citizens safe. On the show, Leslie introduces Jerry: "Diabetic. Sloppily out-of-shape. Friend" (Daniels 2010a). In an office meeting, Jerry accidentally delivers a series of physical gags included malapropisms, pants ripping, and farting while his colleagues attempt to hold back their jokes. Leslie learns that Jerry was not mugged but fell in the park while reaching down to pick up a half-eaten burrito. He lied to the office for fear of being bullied about his behavior.

Writers use diabetes as one marker among many to show that Jerry deserves bullying and mockery. This individualized approach to diabetes reenforces the narrative that those with diabetes are worthy of punch-down comedy, as their own irresponsibility and blunders render them the target of jokes. In Sheila Bock's analysis of diabetes-related stigma, she found that notions of "healthy living [are presented as] simple, common sense behaviors" (Bock 2012, 157). If one's health is the product of following common sense, then diabetes is the effect of willfully disregarding behaviors that are obvious and simple.

Audiences reading diabetes as non-compliance with common sense encourages moral superiority towards those who seemingly choose not to comply. Martha Balshem wrote that lifestyle diseases tend to construct the sick as "foolish, morally flawed, or ignorant" (1993, 24). Constructing diabetes as such a spoiled identity makes sense of the subsequent dehumanization, discrimination, and reduced life chances (Goffman 1963). This representation of Jerry as unendingly foolish and disgusting also erases systemic conditions around diabetes. For example, the show never examines complex insurance bureaucracy, unaffordable medication and supplies, or patronizing clinical interactions. Comedy creators view diabetes as an individual moral failing, so the punch needs to land on these people and their perceived bad behavior. Characters make fun of Jerry based on his failure to pursue better health, but their actions to address diabetes in the community are comedic nonperformatives.

Nonperformativity and the Pawnee Cares Diabetes Research Telethon

Ahmed defines *nonperformatives* as speech acts that "do not do what they say: they do not, as it were, commit a person, organization, or state to an action" (2006, 104). I use Ahmed's term to discuss *nonperformative* government actions related to diabetes. I argue that politicians use nonperformatives seeming to help with the "crisis" of diabetes, but in fact there is no bite to their bark. Characters on the show express concern about diabetes incidence in the town while also chastising diabetic residents. Because both happen simultaneously, their efforts to "fix" the "problem" of diabetes are humorously inconsequential. While writers on the show use nonperformatives to create comedy, the consequences are more severe when U.S. politicians utilize nonperformatives in their efforts to address diabetes issues.

Consider Episode 22 of Season 2 on *Parks and Rec*, titled "Telethon." In the episode, Leslie commits the entire office to work an all-night telethon event meant to raise money to find a cure for diabetes. The context of a telethon places the episode in the history of the non-disabled culture framing of disability as pitiable and in need of charity (Longmore and Kudlick 2016). Disability scholars have long critiqued and analyzed the telethon as an example of the charity model of disability that situates disabled people as needy and non-disabled people as moral and good for giving generously to support them. When read in the context of structural and cultural access to resources, the charity model is propelled and sustained by the paucity of government resources afforded to disabled people. Theoretically, if governments provided equitable tools and resources, disabled people would not be in need.

The most famed and regularly critiqued example of such a telethon would be Jerry Lewis' efforts to raise money for the Muscular Dystrophy Association (MDA) with the MDA Kids Telethon. Disability rights activists who called themselves Jerry's Orphans gathered at telethons to protest the paternalizing and demeaning effects of the television spectacle. While the MDA discontinued the event in 2015, the conversation around telethons reignited in 2020 when Kevin Hart, eager to be welcome in the public space again after homophobic tweets resurfaced, was invited to host a re-vamped MDA Telethon.

At least vaguely aware of the legacy of such telethons, the Telethon episode features a similar set-up to the legendary MDA telethons: a bank of volunteers sits at telephones ready to take donations, a series of hosts present short video segments relating the urgency of the problem, and a celebrity guest presents a large check for research at the end of the show. Leslie explains why she signed up fellow employees to work at a Telethon raising money for diabetes: "every year Pawnee Cares teams up with the local cable access station to raise money for diabetes research, and its important because Pawnee is the fourth fattest town in the U.S" (Daniels 2010d). With this comment Leslie conflates fatness with diabetes, and clearly states that it is significant issue in Pawnee.

As the evening gets underway, the Parks and Rec crew take various on-camera roles to keep the telethon going. Local newswoman Joan Callamezo kicks off the event by looking at the camera and cheerfully declaring, "Diabetes, Yuck!" I admit that I laugh at such a blatant and simplified statement about diabetes as a *spoiled identity* (Goffman 1963). As an insider, privy to what it is like to live with diabetes, I agree with the sentiment that diabetes sucks. But Joan is not talking about the nature of living with diabetes. She is talking about diabetic people as disgusting. In contrast with the established patronizing ideology of the charity model inherent to telethons, this is an example of a telethon where pity shifts into blame. It's not 'oh poor diabetic people', it's 'yuck diabetic people'. Enacting another parody of the disgust felt by diabetic people, this segment misses the opportunity to give any agency to diabetic people in Pawnee. The show relies on the original disgust and makes it funny by exaggerating that perspective towards the people who they are raising money for. As the show progresses, it becomes clear that diabetic people make their own town look bad, so there is inherently a self-serving mechanism that furthers the nonperformativity and comedy of these government actions. In keeping with the effect of the MDA telethon, the telethon reenforces the need for non-disabled people's pity, generosity, and a high-ground morality to care for diabetic people.

As the telethon progresses, various hosts introduce small segments meant to educate and induce moral panic about diabetes. At one point the telethon co-host introduces a segment by saying, "Coming up a very special video presentation called, "Even my Tongue is Fat: The Story of Pawnee." Repeatedly, characters simplify the relationship between fat embodiment and diabetes, using them interchangeably. Leslie introduces the next piece: "For now, please let's take a look at this moving video entitled, "One Butt, Two Seats: The Widening of America." In her efforts to help, she comedically reproduces the stigma associated with diabetes.

Natalie Boero terms "obesity" as a post-modern-epidemic, which media outlets aim to cure through "a rapid spread of fear and calls for vigilance" (2007, 43). Again, these jokes seem like they are meant to parody such media coverage of fat embodiment or diabetes that the media often frames as epidemics, but the show never complicates that stereotype or looks to the contradiction of social conditions to weight or diabetes. It only draws audience attention to the simplified and degrading media coverage and reinjures diabetic people with reminders of the underlying notion that diabetes is disgusting. Boero suggests that "moral panic together with the location of the problem within the individual precludes a more macro level approach to health and health care delivery at a time when health care services are being dismantled or severely cut back" (2007, 41). This point is essential to understanding the sleight of hand taking place through jokes about diabetes like the ones in the Telethon episode. While it seems that government actors must intervene on individual behaviors, they do not discuss the burden of endless insurance bureaucracy, unaffordable healthcare, or the structures of for-profit pharmaceutical companies.

Again, the stated goal of the Telethon is to raise money for diabetes research. Leslie creates shirts for the telethon staff that read, "Diabetes! Let's Dia-beat-this." This joke embeds overcoming and individual efforts into diabetes narratives. During the telethon, a banner in the background features white cursive lettering with the phrase, "Working for a cure." The event itself is held to raise money for diabetes research, and the culminating moment occurs when guest celebrity Detlef Schrempf presents a check for $5000 to the camera for diabetes research. Raising money to support research and a cure seem strangely incongruent with stereotypes about diabetes. We are led to believe through the gags that diabetes is a problem caused by individual overconsumption of food. It seems nonsensical and strange to raise money to research a problem when we as the audience have already been given the answer.

As media reproduces stigmatized representations of diabetes, it means that people working in healthcare also traffic in nonperformatives as well, leaning on individuals to change while concealing the position of those in power who maintain systemic barriers. Sociologists at the University of California San Francisco studied staff who work with low-income people with Type 2 diabetes and confirmed that there are "well-documented structural causes of poor health (e.g., precarious employment, inadequate housing, unaffordable healthy foods)" (Chaufan et al. 2013, 145). While staff workers were aware of these systemic conditions, they still believed:

> the ultimate source of poor health and health inequalities [was] within clients … Put another way, they believe that individual characteristics of *clients make the difference* in their health, such that if these changed, clients' health would substantially improve and likely be no different from that of higher income groups. (Chaufan et al. 2013)

Entertainment re-enforces bias and stigma held by staff and internalized by clients. Media circulates stereotypes in public discourse while minimizing or erasing other contextualizing factors that are difficult to undo once internalized.

The Nonperformativity of Public Heath Campaigns: The "Dia-Beat-It" PSA

Parks and Rec incorporates the role of public health on the TV show because of the department's recreation projects and Leslie's friendship with a local nurse, Ann Perkins, played by Rashida Jones. Perkins takes a job in the Pawnee government as a part-time public relations director for the Health Department. In Season 4, Episode 2, Ann Perkins approaches the city-budget auditor Chris Traeger, played by Rob Lowe, to film a Public Service Announcement to fight diabetes (Daniels 2010b). In the broader context of the show, the character Chris Traeger was born with a rare-blood disease. This start to his life has motivated him to exercise aggressively and adhere to a strict natural and organic diet. Entering the show as an Indiana State Auditor hailing from Indianapolis to fix the town budget, Chris provides a stark contrast with the culture of Pawnee. In short, Chris focuses solely with his physical health, nutritious food and exercise, and also providing government oversight and responsible management.

In Ann's effort to get Chris to do the ad, she plays him the older PSA. The PSA shows Walt Morphling, a middle-aged, fat, white man speaking directly to the camera. Walt says, "You can prevent adult-onset diabetes by getting an annual check-up, exercising, praying …" Chris asks Ann who the person in the footage is, and Ann tells him:

Ann: That was Walt Morphling, he was the Director of Public Health, before he had to retire at 46 because he had diabetes.
Chris: That is sad. And in this town, understandable.
Ann: I would like to shoot a new PSA, and I think it would be good to get someone is healthy and telegenic, and I thought you would be perfect.

Ann's words assert that there is power in Chris' appearance as thin and athletic to have an effect addressing instances of diabetes.

In this episode, the show uses the nonperformativity of Ann's Public Health campaign to humorous effect. As they shoot the PSA, Chris says the line, "Diabetes Can't be cured, but it can be prevented. Make a choice. Make a change. And together, we can make a difference." Chris wants to film the PSA again, telling Ann, "this is important to me because it is important to you. I mean, you spent a lot of time and energy on writing this," to which Ann responds, "Not really." In Ann's admission that she did not spend much time on the ad, she communicates that the messaging around diabetes prevention is simple. It does not require much more than a thin, white, male person telling others to individually make better choices. Perhaps this PSA and its simplicity parodies existing diabetes PSAs meaning to point out and exaggerate how simple public health makes out diabetes prevention to be: individuals just need to make better choices (Walker and Frazer 2021).

Eventually, the humor comes from Chris taking the simple idea and making it almost nonsensical. He jumps in front of the camera several times repeating the line, "Diabetes, fight it!" Ann laments how strange Chris' repetition and effort seem: "I cannot believe I dated him. For a long time. He broke up with me!" In the background, Chris can be heard brainstorming new lines for the PSA: "Fat equals splat as in you're dead! There's something there." Chris' efforts to simplify the message and make it rhyme become absurd, but they do not draw an audience's attention to anything further than the simplicity of the overall message.

In later seasons, the Parks and Rec team are rarely taking up the issue of diabetes anymore. In Season 6, Leslie brokers a merger with the formerly ultra-wealthy, but now bankrupt neighboring town, Eagleton. In the end of Episode 3, "The Pawnee-Eagleton Tip Off Classic," Leslie announces the merger and members of both towns disapprove. During a press conference, a Pawnee resident protests: "Why should I bail them out with the hard-earned money from my unemployment check?" By exaggerating the lack of charity and reciprocity from someone receiving government support, the joke punches down at people receiving government support. To calm the uproar, Eagleton representative Ingrid de Forest, played by Kristen Bell, persuades Eagleton residents to accept the merger offer: "They're a town of angels- greasy, denim-clad angels." Here the writers mock Eagleton's upper-class disdain of Pawnee, parodying coastal elites' disdain towards mid-west and low-income cultural sensibilities. Still, as the show exaggerates and parodies Pawnee's citizens cultural norms, including the love of fast food and high rates of diabetes, the writers do not address the systems that prevent low-income diabetic people from accessing the resources they need. In the show, the in-flux of other classes and cultural sensibilities erases the problem of diabetes in Pawnee.

Concluding Thoughts

Turning back to my January phone conversation with the insurance agent, I found myself rage texting a colleague. As a former resident of Illinois, she might know about the celebrated Illinois price caps for insulin that I had heard about. How can my insulin cost hundreds of dollars with this famed Illinois insulin co-pay price cap? How is this possible? When one looks past the good press and more closely at these recent pieces of popular legislation, they are very limited in who they serve and very limited in what they do (Emerson 2021). Such legislation only applies to the limited number of people who have federal insurance plans. This legislation will not help the most underserved people—those without insurance.

In Montana, a #insulin4all advocate exchanged messages with her representative over the bill HB222, intended to become a $35 a month copay cap. When the advocate challenged Representative Jessica Karjala over the limitations of the bill, the advocate noted: "it appeared she just wanted to move the bill forward with the idea she would help a population of people without actually taking our input into consideration" (Johnson 2021). This bill exemplifies real world nonperformative government action with diabetes. The bill and subsequent speech acts declaring the "lifesaving effects" of such a bill does not do the action it says it will do, and representatives balked at critiques to their efforts (Johnson 2021). Such nonperformatives in the real world are preceded by representational strategies in the world of television and comedy that insidiously normalize and morally justify punching down comedy.

In the post-Trump era, many comedians are reckoning with their past jokes about marginalized groups, particularly if their jokes relied on reanimating harmful content. In a review of Bo Burnham's 2021 comedy special *Inside*, TV critic Gabrielle Sanchez registers Burnham processing with his own past in the song "Problematic." Sanchez observes that *Inside* arrives "at a time where comedians find themselves reckoning with the fact that not every joke they've made has been in good taste, and that racism, misogyny, ableism, and homophobia peddled out by comedians is no longer taken lightly" (Sanchez 2021). In a 2021 conversation between comedian Sarah Silverman and film critic A.O. Scott, Silverman reflects on Scott's critiques of her 2005 comedy special *Jesus is Magic*. Scott had criticized punching down comedy from liberal comedians and Silverman admits that at the time she believed, "I'm liberal, so I'm not racist, so I can say the N-word, because I'm illuminating racism" (Scott 2021). Silverman realizes that performances of racism from a white comedian with the intent to mock racists still reanimates racist language and causes harm.

Acknowledging his own problem as a critic, Scott implicated himself within similar liberal sensibilities thinking that it was permissible to punch down with marginalized groups, assuming audiences "get" that he feigned the punch: "I have these oven mitts of irony on that, so no one's here going to get burned" (2021). As television comedies use humor to illuminate the contradictions, complexities, and absurdity of living with diabetes in the U.S., they must consider diabetes as a disability with its social and political implications. If they do, they might stop burning diabetic people with moral certitude and instead bring the punch to those with power, where creators and audiences alike are capable of achieving transformational change.

References

Ahmed, Sara. 2006. The Nonperformativity of Antiracism. *Meridians* 7 (1): 104–126. https://www.jstor.org/stable/40338719.

Alliance, Right Care. 2020. High Insulin Costs Are Killing Americans. Rightcarealliance.org. https://rightcarealliance.org/actions/insulin/.

Balshem, Martha. 1993. *Cancer in the Community: Class and Medical Authority.* Washington: Smithsonian Institution Press.

Bock, Sheila. 2012. Contextualization, Reflexivity, and the Study of Diabetes-Related Stigma. *Journal of Folklore Research* 49 (2): 153–178. https://doi.org/10.2979/jfolkrese.49.2.153.

Boero, Natalie. 2007. All the News That's Fat to Print: The American 'Obesity Episdemic' and the Media. *Qualitative Sociology* 30 (1): 41–60.

Centers for Disease Control and Prevention, CDC. 2020. *National Diabetes Statistics Report, 2020: Estimates of Diabetes and Its Burden in the United States.* https://www.cdc.gov/diabetes/data/statistics-report/index.html.

Chaufan, Claudia, et al. 2013. 'You Must Not Confuse Poverty with Laziness': A Case Study on the Power of Discourse to Reproduce Diabetes Inequalities. *International Journal of Health Services* 43 (1): 143–166.

Cohen, Sascha. 2018. A Brief History of Punch-Down Comedy. *Mask Magazine*.

Daniels, Greg. 2010a. Park Safety. In *Parks and Recreation*, ed. Michael Trim. NBCUniversal Television Distribution.

———. 2010b. Ron and Tammys. In *Parks and Recreation*. NBCUniversal Television Distribution.

———. 2010c. Sweetums. In *Parks and Recreation*, ed. Dean Holland. NBCUniversal Television Distribution.

———. 2010d. Telethon. In *Parks and Recreation*, ed. Michael Trim. NBCUniversal Television Distribution.

Emerson, Jakob. 2021. Illinois capped insulin costs, but most people can't take advantage of it. https://newschannel20.com/news/local/illinois-capped-insulin-costs-but-most-people-cant-take-advantage-of-it.

Goffman, Erving. 1963. *Stigma: Notes on the Management of Spoiled Identity.A Spectrum Book*. Englewood Cliffs, NJ: Prentice-Hall.

Gray, Jonathan, Jeffrey P. Jones, and Ethan Thompson. 2009. The State of Satire, the Satire of State. In *Satire TV : Politics and Comedy in the Post-Network Era*, ed. Jonathan Gray, Jeffrey P. Jones, and Ethan Thompson, xiv, 283. New York: NYU Press.

Haller, Beth, and Amy Bree Becker. 2014. Stepping Backwards with Disability Humor? The Case of NY Gov. David Paterson's Representation on 'Saturday Night Live'. *Disabiilty Studies Quarterly* 34 (1). https://doi.org/10.18061/dsq.v34i1.3459.

Health, National Institutes of. 2006. *One-Third of Adults with Diabetes Still Don't Know They Have It.* U.S. Department of Health & Human Services. https://www.nih.gov/news-events/news-releases/one-third-adults-diabetes-still-dont-know-they-have-it.

Hutcheon, Linda. 1989. *The Politics of Postmodernism. New Accents.* London and New York: Routledge.

———. 2000. *A Theory of Parody: The Teachings of Twentieth-Century Art Forms.* Urbana: University of Illinois Press.

Johnson, Madison. 2021. *Insulin Pricing: Co-Pay Caps.* The Beta Cell Foundation. https://betacellfoundation.org/resources/advocacy/insulin-pricing/co-pay-caps/.

Longmore, Paul K., and Catherine Jean Kudlick. 2016. *Telethons: Spectacle, Disability, and the Business of Charity*. New York: Oxford University Press.

Marc, David. 2009. Forward. In *Satire TV: Politics and Comedy in the Post-Network Era*, ed. Jonathan Gray, Jeffrey P. Jones, and Ethan Thompson, xiv, 283. New York: NYU Press.

Sanchez, Gabrielle. 2021. *Bo Burnham 'Fesses Up in Comedy Special Inside*. The AV Club. https://www.avclub.com/bo-burnham-owns-up-to-his-problematic-origins-in-come-1847053881.

Scott, A. O. 2021. How a Review Changed Both Sarah Silverman and Our Critic. *The New York Times*, May 19. https://www.nytimes.com/2021/05/19/movies/how-a-review-changed-both-sarah-silverman-and-our-critic.html.

Walker, Heather, and Bianca Frazer. 2021. The Metanarrative of Diabetes: Should You Be Eating That? In *Metanarratives of Disability: Culture, Assumed Authority, and the Normative Social Order*, ed. David Bolt. Routledge.

Diabetic Data Art: Numbers Beyond Control

Samuel Thulin

Introduction

Diabetic data is big. And it's getting bigger. As medical device companies develop more and more wearable sensors and increase the accessibility of networked devices, the diabetic body becomes a rich extraction site for the collection of this vital data. Guest editing a special section in a recent issue of Diabetes Spectrum, Aaron J. Kowalski (2019) writes: "Diabetes, by its nature, is a data-driven disease" (179) and envisions us at the beginning of a "diabetes data revolution" (179). With the improvements in data collection for individual patients and in the aggregation of data sets, many people hope these developments will fortify diabetes management. As an example, by February 2020, over 10,000 people had donated their de-personalized data to the Tidepool Big Data Donation Project, a research initiative with the aim of making the data associated with diabetic self-management more intelligible and actionable to users, health care teams, and researchers. Few people contest the centrality of diabetes data, and it

S. Thulin (✉)
Montreal, QC, Canada

B. C. Frazer, H. R. Walker (eds.), *(Un)doing Diabetes: Representation, Disability, Culture*, Palgrave Studies in Science and Popular Culture, https://doi.org/10.1007/978-3-030-83110-3_8

is continually rallied in support of better understanding and controlling the condition.

In this brief chapter, I take a different approach to diabetic data. This approach draws inspiration from my daily, lived experiences with and reflections on data as a Type 1 diabetic, from my conversations and collaborations with critical disability studies scholars, activists, and artists, and from my own media arts practice. Rather than arguing for the utility of data in diabetes management, I ask how diabetics might use their data to creatively engage in critical conversations about how we understand and experience our bodies and relationships with devices and data. I argue for the importance of art as a space for exploration, critique, and reflection in an era of ever-proliferating data, and I imagine the possibilities of diabetic data art.

Data Orientations

Diabetic self-management, "the cornerstone of care" for diabetes (Clark 2008), involves fundamental orientations to data—ways of understanding data, its value and purpose. Perhaps most crucially, the predominant orientation to data rests on the idea that data orients us to our disease—in the past, in the present, in the future. It indicates how well or poorly we've been managing our condition, it suggests what we should do now—what action should be taken (injecting insulin, exercising, eating something etc.)—and it warns of future outcomes both short-term (as in the trending arrows of Continuous Glucose Monitor (CGM) displays) and long-term (as in statistical data showing the association of diabetic complications with "uncontrolled" diabetes). In this context, a biomedical perspective understands more data as meaning better orientation, and the problems that data might pose—whether these involve accuracy, privacy, or other concerns—are viewed as hurtles that will sooner or later be overcome. Within this "technological ethos," which Chris Feudtner (2003) argues dominates American medicine (4), the ultimate ideal would be that data orientations function so perfectly that we no longer need to be consciously aware of them. This is the endgame of "closed loop" or "artificial pancreas" systems, for example, where data and hormones would interact so seamlessly that we can forget about them and get on with our lives.

But while these data orientations might hold an appeal, not dissimilar to the appeal of a cure, they are also undergirded by more troubling cultural orientations towards bodily difference. Our current predominant diabetic data orientations reinforce the privileged status of fully able, "normal" bodies in multiple ways. Such bodies are the benchmark for the promise of improved diabetic care. Target blood sugar ranges are derived from the bodies of non-diabetics, an approach that on the one hand seems reasonable enough, but on the other hand becomes troubling when it involves a data-assisted disciplining of the bodies falling outside the target range. Such disciplining is complex, and varies from overt scolding by doctors, nurses, family members, and friends to internalized self-reprimands even in the presence of compassionate others. It also entails the cognitive dissonance of wanting to be gentle towards oneself while feeling the disappointment of bad numbers. The body's refusal to be "normal" in these circumstances, its difference, determined through data, is treated by medicine and prevailing cultural attitudes as a problem to be solved rather than as a difficult yet valuable way of being in the world.

At the same time as such data orientations draw diabetics into the ongoing struggle of attempting to match the numbers of people without diabetes, they orient us to "normal" bodies in another way. As Stephen Horrocks (2019) points out, the technological development of diabetic devices means that diabetic practice becomes less and less externally visible. That is, a CGM and insulin pump hidden by clothing require less obvious bodily interaction than pricking and drawing blood from one's finger or injecting a dose of insulin with a syringe or pen. As devices become increasingly networked, people with diabetes can perform their self-management duties even more covertly through smartphone apps—meaning that bystanders, friends, and family members need not be confronted with an overt display of bodily difference. Horrocks writes: "the shift toward constant and concealed treatment practices is emblematic of a much broader system of biomedicalized control that devalues non-normative bodies, and thereby devalues a life lived with(in) one" (3).

Diabetes has long had a complicated relationship with disability, with many diabetics preferring not to identify as "disabled" (Forlano 2017, 4; Kafer 2013, 14). Even before the recent technological advances in diabetes care, diabetes could be largely made invisible by slipping to the bathroom or by delaying blood sugar testing and insulin injection until a private moment (though potentially suffering the consequences). Now, without the need for diabetics to perform visible acts of drawing blood and injecting foreign fluids—with everything tightened up onto the body via wearables—diabetes can become more invisible than ever, and diabetics can even more readily pass as "normal." The diabetic body's transgressive connections with the "outside" world can more easily than ever be kept under wraps, even as these connections multiply beyond the circulation of physical materials (blood, insulin) and into data flows. An affront to the ideals of autonomy, self-determination, and wholeness, the diabetic body resonates with Rosemarie Garland-Thomson's (1997) disabled figure, representing "the incomplete, unbounded, compromised, and subjected body, susceptible to external forces" (p. 45). It is not surprising, then, that medicine puts diabetic data in the service of better orienting diabetic bodies towards "normal." Garland-Thomson critiques how "the myriad structures and practices of material, daily life enforce the cultural standard of a universal subject with a narrow range of corporeal variation" (24). What we lose through the predominance of normative diabetic data orientations are more expansive and generative orientations towards bodily difference—orientations that do not foreclose what a body should be, how it should be present and represented in the world.

More Data Orientations

I suggest that although diabetic data might be necessary for diabetes management and treatment, it can simultaneously operate as a resource for critique and for opening up other possibilities for reflecting on bodily difference. A source of inspiration comes from work in critical data studies that shows that data is not neutral and not raw—that it is always cooked and always oriented (Gitelman and Jackson 2013). As Craig Dalton and Jim Thatcher (2014) put it: "in both its production and interpretation, all data—'big' included—is always the result of contingent and contested social practices that afford and obfuscate specific understandings of the world" (Data Is Never Raw section, para. 1). Different ways of working with data consequently provide different perspectives on the world. Catherine D'Ignazio and Lauren F. Klein's (2016) call for feminist data visualization is instructive as it asks us to consider all the practices that go into constructing a visualization and the possible outcomes it might have, rather than focusing on the visualization as an isolated object simply presenting data to the viewer. D'Ignazio and Klein's (2020) recent book, *Data Feminism*, highlights the workings of power in data science and the importance of critically examining and challenging existing data practices, always attending to how such practices and the knowledge they involve are situated. Similarly, Yanni Loukissas' (2019) insistence on "how local conditions matter for understanding data in everyday practice" (p.11) asks that we consider not only how we are oriented by data but how it is that we orient data—what meaning do we attribute to it and how? In what contexts? The work of D'Iganazio and Klein and of Loukissas emphasizes the value in working hands-on with data both to arrive at deepened understanding and to develop more equitable data practices. The questions and approaches raised by critical data studies help in breaking out of habitual understandings of diabetic data and offer potential for envisioning the data differently.

While critical approaches to diabetic data remain rare, there are nevertheless inklings of projects that begin to suggest opportunities for rethinking our diabetic data orientations. Doug Kanter, founder of Databetes, for instance has designed imaginative visualizations of his own blood glucose levels over a year-long period. Eschewing the bar graphs typically offered for making sense of data through diabetic management software, Kanter's colourful, creative visualizations offer another lens on his data collection. Going a step further in terms of novel data manifestation, Justus Harris has developed what he calls Diabetes Data Sculptures, using people's blood sugar readings to produce 3D printed objects. Here, Harris collapses the usual linear temporality of diabetic data into a complexly textured object that can be held in one's hands. But while Kanter and Harris' innovative approaches to the presentation of data break away from the utilitarian visualizations prevalent in clinical practice, they are still ultimately oriented by the ideals of diabetic management. Kanter notes how his visualization helped him to have the best year of blood sugar control of his life (Kanter 2013). Harris sees the benefits of Diabetes Data Sculptures in how they might bring people to better understand their condition and make necessary changes to their self-management (Tenderich 2016). Thus, while Harris and Kanter embrace art and design as alternative ways of knowing and understanding, they simultaneously gravitate toward the impulse to use the artwork or design object for pedagogical purposes and improved outcomes. Although the object provides a welcome opening for re-imagining our relationships with data, it also maintains the goals and values attached to the data orientations of diabetic self-management, where clinical results are what matter most.

My intention is not to suggest that the desire to improve one's numbers or to better understand one's condition (with the purpose of improving one's numbers) is misplaced in and of itself. Rather, I argue that the pervasive data orientations that dominate diabetic self-management might foreclose other rich possibilities for the ways people with diabetes relate to their bodies and their data. On a social level, the predominance of particular data orientations, informed by normative views on bodies, risks undermining an appreciation of difference necessary for transforming attitudes towards chronic illness and disability. One way we can incorporate appreciation of difference is through the adoption of an approach to diabetes data art that draws on the best of what diabetes art already has to offer.

Diabetes Art

If, for a moment, we suspend the conversation about data gathering and control, we see that there exist rich artistic strategies for communicating about diabetic experience beyond a focus on improved clinical outcomes. Although the following artworks do not deal directly with diabetic data, they suggest some refreshing possibilities for approaching diabetes that might help to expand the ways we orient and are oriented by our data. Indeed, works like Shimon Attie's *White Nights, Sugar Dreams* and Robbie McCauley's *Sugar* turn attention to the complexity of diabetic experience and focus on the lives and stories of those who have diabetes.

In *White Nights, Sugar Dreams*, Attie, a Type 1 diabetic, presents abstract videos of continually shifting interactions between sugar and red liquid accompanied by audio recordings of interviews with eight people on their personal experiences living with diabetes. The video installation was exhibited in 2000 at the Rhode Island School of Design Museum, following a residency within the Art ConText community-based arts series. The work offers a rendering of diabetes that is at once phantasmagoric, highly personal, and polyvocal as Attie's imagery, spread across three screens, meets the oral stories of his interviewees. In her analysis of the work, Petra Kuppers (2007) stresses the importance of multiplicity, writing: "A different sense of cause and effect, physicality and diagnosis, living-in-time emerges from this communal work: no one way of living with diabetes puts itself at center stage" (50). Such work does not offer insights on how to better treat one's condition, nor is that Attie's intention. Instead, Attie explores multiple registers of difference—that people with diabetes are not only different from people without diabetes but are also different from each other—while fostering a sense of solidarity that does not depend on the eradication of those differences. The work is both an intimate, dreamlike, imagination of bodily processes and a social forum where the complexity of diabetic experience is shared and reflected upon.

Robbie McCauley's solo performance work, *Sugar*, offers another social and community-based exploration of diabetes. The work was first performed in 2006 at Ohio State University, with subsequent performances, including those at ArtsEmerson in Boston (2012) and New York Live Arts in New York City (2018), receiving significant media attention; the script is included in the anthology *solo/black/woman* (2013). In this one-woman play, McCauley presents her own story and commentary on diabetes, with multiple perspectives woven in from participatory story sharing circles. Like Attie, McCauley grounds her work in her own experiences living with diabetes while also embracing a multiplicity of ways of understanding the illness. As Sheila Bock (2015) puts it: "Rather than presenting a coherent illness narrative, then, *Sugar* disrupts generic conventions and presents McCauley's experiences in an intentionally fragmented way, shifting attention from *her* story to the diversity of ways in which people draw upon and evaluate multiple ways of knowing in their attempts to make sense of diabetes" (128). Focusing particularly on the links between contemporary experiences of diabetes in the African American community and Black history in America, "her performances of *Sugar* open up discursive spaces for marginalized perspectives to enter into the conversation" (132). As Bock explains, McCauley deftly weaves a variety of points of view and sources of knowledge together resisting a reductionist opposition of local, community knowledge vs expert institutionalized medical knowledge. Emphasizing a dialogic and processual approach, McCauley's work highlights the negotiations that go into living with and making sense of diabetes on an individual and social level (135).

Artworks like Attie's and McCauley's reveal and make space for considering aspects of diabetes that are simultaneously personal, social, and cultural, and that extend beyond the logistics of daily testing and treatment. How might we extend our approach to data in such a way that it too reveals a kind of multiplicity? How might we fully acknowledge and explore the ways in which data is personal, social, and cultural? What would diabetic data art look like?

Possibilities for Diabetic Data Art

In advocating for diabetic data art, I seek to draw out the polyvocal and relational qualities of data and our experiences with data. The numbers we collect and calculate on a daily basis are more than remote abstractions dwelling in a realm apart from the experiential aspects of diabetes. For many people with diabetes, numbers have complex physical, emotional, and affective registers developed through years of hourly engagement with them. For instance, I experience low numbers simultaneously as weakness, irritability, desperation, hunger, and inability to think, as spoonfuls of honey and crumpled juice-boxes, as frustration and disappointment for falling below my target range, and as a sense of relief at there being an explanation for why I feel so bad. Numbers are intimately woven into ongoing diabetic practices, part of how we understand our illness, and sense and make sense of it to ourselves and others.

Thus, it is not just the numbers. It is the host of embodied practices, activities, and affects that go into producing the numbers. Data comes from decisions, labour, maintenance, protocols—all of which might fade into the background due to their repetition, but which exert a steady influence on the lives of those who undertake them. To draw attention to these aspects of working with data is to follow critical data studies' call to remember that "data are local" (Loukissas 2019) and "require our participation" (Gitelman and Jackson 2013, 6). It is also to explore what Laura Forlano (2017) has referred to as the *intimate infrastructures* of diabetic practice, involving human-machine relations and the ways these affect understandings of our bodies. Forlano, for instance, talks about the iPhone apps she uses to manage her diabetes as part of these intimate infrastructures, highlighting the fragility of these networked technologies and her complicated relationships with them as they produce particular materialities, meanings, affects, and ways of relating to space and time (3). In these intimate infrastructures, "the world collapses onto the body and, at the same time, the body expands out into the world" (3). Forlano's discussion of intimate infrastructures, anchored in a world of apps, continuous glucose monitors, and insulin pumps, among other contemporary networked technologies, resonates with Anne Marie Mol and John Law's (2004) discussion of diabetes and "doing hypoglycaemia" from 13 years earlier. Mol and Law emphasize the work that goes into keeping a body together (57) and note how diabetic bodies both *incorporate* their surroundings and *excorporate* bodily actions (52–53). Through this work diabetics challenge conventional body boundaries, as processes that once seemed contained within the body and its organs weave the body into myriad relations with human and non-human others.

When the main focus of attention for diabetics and their health care providers is the data itself in the form of numbers and their clinical interpretation, then the labour, the expanded and permeable body, and the multiplicity of relationships involved in producing and working with the data become obscured. Diabetic data art's orientation to data could be something akin to that elaborated through Forlano's discussion of "data rituals." Forlano advances the notion of "data rituals" to underline "the lived experience around data (rather than merely the transmission of data)" (12). She draws on James Carey's distinction between transmission and ritual views of communication, where transmission involves extending a message across space for the purposes of control, and ritual involves drawing people (and non-humans, as well) together in fellowship. Diabetic data rituals change depending on the situation, but they always involve humans and non-humans coming together in the production and circulation of data, whether this is testing one's blood sugar before eating dinner with friends or uploading one's CGM data to TidePool. Whereas our data orientations are typically centered on transmission and control, the concept of "data rituals" provides an opening for attending to the many other aspects of doing data.

It is possible to imagine at least two broad approaches to diabetic data art: 1) one that takes up the lived experiences associated with diabetic data, using any artistic resources preferred by the artist; and 2) one that takes up the lived experiences associated with diabetic data by using data itself as vital artistic resource. It is the second approach that is perhaps the most challenging, as it involves not only dwelling on different orientations to data, but also re-orienting the data, making it do something other than what the biomedical perspective commonly assumes it is supposed to do. This double intervention is critical because it suggests not only that experiences of data are multiple, but that what we habitually take to be objective, stable data is itself also multiple in how it can be used and made to mean. People with diabetes, whether identifying as artists or not, can creatively engage with the production and sense-making of data. Such interventions are critical in that they offer possibilities for re-appropriation of the data that seems to dictate the diabetic body. Anthony Ryan Hatch (2019) describes what he refers to as diabetic numerology, which is "an approach to clinical medicine that sees numbers as essential for the management of bodies" (231). Hatch asserts that numbers such as blood sugar values, insulin doses, grams of carbohydrates, and dates of appointments mean "*nearly* everything for my life as a diabetic person" (231). Indeed, the pervasiveness of numbers only seems to increase with technological change, as Horrocks (2019) refers to what he calls Datafied Body Doubles. He argues that the current biomedical perspective not only understands the body through numbers, but also understands numbers through other numbers, to such an extent that diabetics and their health care providers undertake practices that "attempt to recreate the dynamic nature of T1D bodies' physiologies in data form" (14). In the midst of such deterministic and abstracted approaches to data, how might the creative strategies I align with diabetic data art offer ways of living with data differently?

A first intervention might simply be to do something else—anything else—with one's data. Not necessarily instead of, but in addition to its habitual uses. This at once enacts its potential multiplicity and creates a new lived experience with data through an out-of-the-ordinary interaction with it.[1] I view this doing-something-else-with-data as a way of making space for us (diabetics and those who are close to them, as well as the art-going public and researchers interested in social aspects of diabetes) to understand the relationships between data and bodies differently. It makes space for us to think of numbers beyond control, beyond diabetic numerology, beyond the objectives of self-improvement and bodily mastery. It focuses attention on the data rituals of diabetic practice and suggests a kind of "thickening" of data (Wang 2016), where the local, contextual, and embodied dimensions of data are given their due. In other words, it makes space for making sense of data other than as a diagnostic tool. Writing on personal digital data assemblages, Deborah Lupton (2018) notes that "They are not separate entities from people's bodies and selves, but rather are materialisations and extensions, alternative ways of knowing and enacting bodies and selves" (9). If this is true, then a proliferation of exploratory and experimental practices using the data assemblages we are inevitably entangled with contributes to new ways of sensing and making sense of our human and non-human relationships.

And yet, to focus too much on "making sense," in terms of "making data intelligible and knowable" (Lupton 2018, 8) might inadvertently restrict the possibilities of diabetic data art. Making sense of data is what diabetics and health care professionals already constantly do—looking for patterns and trends in the data is central to our current data orientations. Yet despite the tremendous push to make sense of diabetic data, it just does not always make sense to us the way we want it to. Sometimes my blood glucose readings are high for no apparent reason. Even when

[1] I have been experimenting with these ideas in my artistic practice, particularly my works *Hemo-resonance #1* and *Hemo-resonance #2*. More information on these artworks at: https://samuelthulin.com/.

patterns are identifiable, they seem to be constantly in the midst of changing, becoming no longer a pattern. Instead of pursuing the never-ending quest for meaning, diabetic data art might make space for this lack of making sense. Freed from the calculus of diabetic control, the numbers might do a multiplicity of things that do not need to be intelligible in terms of transmitting clinically interpretable results. The numbers might be creatively translated into sounds, lights, text, vibrations, visuals, tastes, or smells that affect the body without the need for telling the body how well or poorly it has been doing or what it should do next to optimize its health. In other words, they might explore the sensuousness of human-non-human relationships without a concern with making things interpretable and actionable. In doing so, diabetic data art makes a world in which the idea of "fixing" a "malfunctioning" body no longer seems to make sense—either to us or to audiences—as the body and its interactions with data become the sources of experiences that value different bodies rather than working towards an idealized, narrowly-conceived "normal" body.

This redirection from the usual sense-making associated with diabetic data opens up possibilities for making it make sense in new ways. On the one hand, allowing the data to be nonsensical can create a valuable space apart from forced intelligibility. On the other hand, it can suggest other avenues for re-attaching the data to meaning in new ways. The data might now provoke reflections on how we understand the boundaries of the human body in an era of rapidly advancing networked health technologies. Or it might provide an opportunity to consider the temporalities of the body and how these relate to the technologies we design and rely on for measuring and treating chronic illness. Or it could offer resources for understanding how bodies are converted into data according to particular systems and protocols that involve myriad levels of decision-making. While I have been focusing largely on personal bodily data, diabetic data art could also examine larger aggregated data sets and statistics—for instance the landmark 1993 Diabetes Control and Complications Trial that continues to inform diabetic orientations to data. It could probe, from a critical perspective, the association of certain types of diabetes with certain types of bodies (such as associations between Type 2 diabetes, obesity, and ethnic minorities (Zheng et al. 2018), for example), unravelling habitual readings and orientations to statistical data and looking at the assumptions that go into its production, circulation, and interpretation. It could help raise awareness of the racialization processes that have historically informed, and that continue to inform, scientific research on diabetes (Hatch 2016, Hay 2018, Montoya 2011). By enacting a suspension of taken-for-granted data orientations, diabetic data art could contribute to making space for critique of those orientations and for fostering a greater sense of diabetes' complex and long-standing relationships with social justice.

Conclusion

Diabetic data art challenges what should be done with diabetic data. In doing so, it opens itself to criticism. After all, don't we all know what should be done with diabetic data? Don't we all recognize its centrality to keeping us alive and healthy? Why bother making art with it when its purpose is so well-established? Isn't such a pursuit not only pointless, but also irresponsible? To some extent, these questions have to do with the value of art in society, which is a much larger issue than I can adequately address here. But assuming a shared recognition of art's value, the questions also raise issues concerning how we parcel our lives and experiences. Are there things that should remain firmly in the realm of science and medical treatment? If we accept that there are, what are the implications of this belief?

I argue that to restrict data to instrumentalism is to adhere to entrenched habits of understanding not only what data should be and do, but also, and most critically, what bodies should be and do. Diabetic data art asks how diabetes can provide new insights on and ways of understanding bodies in the midst of technological change, rather than taking data and technology simply as correctives to misbehaving or malfunctioning bodies. This might constitute another "diabetes data revolution" (Kowalski 2019), where there is not only a proliferation of data, but also a proliferation of ways of approaching relationships between data and bodies—not in antagonism to medicine, but as another avenue of practice. Both Kuppers and Bock, in their respective analyses of the artworks of Attie and McCauley, point out that while these artists make space for multiplicity, polyvocality, and relationality in understandings of diabetes, they do not do so in order to produce a binary between art and medicine. Rather their works dwell in negotiations of meaning, dialogue, and richness of experience, including a range of experiences connected to medical practice. Approaches to diabetic data art might build on the inventive data practices already developed by designers and artists such as Kanter and Harris, putting them into dialogue with the multiplicity central to Attie and McCauley's works.

To approach data as something that we create and collaborate with allows for deepened sensitivity to the complexity of diabetic relationships with the world, our entanglements and negotiations within changing technologies and practices. Diabetic data art can offer space for much needed engagement with difference, chronic illness, and disability that values the multiplicity of bodies, the multiplicity of data, and the multiplicity of their interconnections. In doing so, it can offer avenues for shifting away from a focus on data as purely diagnostic or statistical resource and towards a recognition of living with diabetes as a valuable way of being in the world. Such an affirmation and approach to data is not meant to deny the many different kinds of struggles we face as diabetics—quite to the contrary, it is meant to give a fuller respect to those struggles and to the insights we gain from our embodied experiences with diabetes. As diabetes continues to become more and more intimately intertwined with data practices, making data itself experiential in ways that communicate valuing bodily difference as vital to a just society becomes all the more relevant.

References

Bock, Sheila. 2015. 'Grappling to Think Clearly': Vernacular Theorizing in Robbie McCauley's Sugar. *Journal of Medical Humanities* 36 (2): 127–139. https://doi.org/10.1007/s10912-015-9326-8.

Clark, Marie. 2008. Diabetes Self-Management Education: A Review of Published Studies. *Primary Care Diabetes* 2 (3): 113–120. https://doi.org/10.1016/j.pcd.2008.04.004.

D'Ignazio, Catherine, and Lauren F. Klein. 2016. Feminist Data Visualization. In *Workshop on Visualization for the Digital Humanities (VIS4DH)*. Baltimore.

———. 2020. *Data Feminism. Strong Ideas Series.* Cambridge, MA: The MIT Press.

Dalton, Craig, and Jim Thatcher. 2014. What Does a Critical Data Studies Look like, and Why Do We Care? *Society and Space*, no. 29. http://societyandspace.org/2014/05/12/what-does-a-critical-data-studies-look-like-and-why-do-we-care-craig-dalton-and-jim-thatcher/#.

Feudtner, John Christopher. 2003. *Bittersweet: Diabetes, Insulin, and the Transformation of Illness*, Studies in Social Medicine. Chapel Hill: University of North Carolina Press.

Forlano, Laura. 2017. Data Rituals in Intimate Infrastructures: Crip Time and the Disabled Cyborg Body as an Epistemic Site of Feminist Science. *Catalyst:*

Feminism, Theory, Technoscience 3 (2): 1–28. https://doi.org/10.28968/cftt.v3i2.28843.

Garland-Thomson, Rosemarie. 1997. *Extraordinary Bodies: Figuring Physical Disability in American Culture and Literature*. New York: Columbia University Press.

Gitelman, Lisa, and Virginia Jackson. 2013. Introduction. In *'Raw Data' Is an Oxymoron*, ed. Lisa Gitelman, 1–14. Cambridge, MA; London, UK: The MIT Press.

Hatch, Anthony Ryan. 2016. *Blood Sugar: Racial Pharmacology and Food Justice in Black America*. University of Minnesota Press.

———. 2019. Against Diabetic Numerology in a Black Body, or, Why I Cannot Live by the Numbers. In *Body Battlegrounds: Transgressions, Tensions, and Transformations*, ed. Chris Bobel and Samantha Kwan, 231–233. Nashville, TN: Vanderbilt University Press.

Hay, Travis. 2018. Commentary: The Invention of Aboriginal Diabetes: The Role of the Thrifty Gene Hypothesis in Canadian Health Care Provision. *Ethnicity & Disease 28* (Suppl. 1): 247–252.

Horrocks, Stephen. 2019. Materializing Datafied Body Doubles: Insulin Pumps, Blood Glucose Testing, and the Production of Usable Bodies. *Catalyst: Feminism, Theory, Technoscience* 5 (1): 1–26.

Johnson, E. Patrick, and Rivera-Servera, Ramón H., eds. 2013. *solo/black/woman: Scripts, Interviews, and Essays* (Pap/DVD edition). Northwestern University Press.

Kafer, Alison. 2013. *Feminist, Queer, Crip*. Indiana University Press.

Kanter, Doug. 2013. *The Healthiest Year of My Life*. Doug Kanter. https://cargocollective.com/dougkanter/The-Healthiest-Year-of-My-Life.

Kowalski, Aaron J. 2019. Realizing Better Diabetes Outcomes Through a Diabetes Data Revolution. *Diabetes Spectrum* 32 (3): 179–181. https://doi.org/10.2337/ds19-0004.

Kuppers, Petra. 2007. *The Scar of Visibility: Medical Performances and Contemporary Art*. 1st ed. Minneapolis: University of Minnesota Press.

Loukissas, Yanni Alexander. 2019. *All Data Are Local: Thinking Critically in a Data-Driven Society*. Cambridge, MA: The MIT Press.

Lupton, Deborah. 2018. How Do Data Come to Matter? Living and Becoming with Personal Data. *Big Data & Society* 5 (2): 205395171878631. https://doi.org/10.1177/2053951718786314.

Mol, Annemarie, and John Law. 2004. Embodied Action, Enacted Bodies: The Example of Hypoglycaemia. *Body & Society* 10 (2–3): 43–62. https://doi.org/10.1177/1357034X04042932.

Montoya, Michael J. 2011. *Making the Mexican Diabetic: Race, Science, and the Genetics of Inequality*. University of California Press.

Tenderich, Amy. 2016. Diabetes as an Art Form: Glucose Data Sculptures Inspire. Healthline. June 7. https://www.healthline.com/diabetesmine/diabetes-data-art-therapuetic.

Wang, Tricia. 2016. Why Big Data Needs Thick Data. *Medium.Com* (blog). January 20. https://medium.com/ethnography-matters/why-big-data-needs-thick-data-b4b3e75e3d7.

Zheng, Yan, Sylvia H. Ley, and B.Hu. Frank. 2018. Global Aetiology and Epidemiology of Type 2 Diabetes Mellitus and Its Complications. *Nature Reviews Endocrinology* 14 (2): 88–98.

Panic Rooms: Suspense in Type 1 Diabetes

Matt Paczkowski

In my senior year of my undergraduate degree, I was driving home from a friend's house. Alone in my Jeep, I felt a familiar shakiness in my leg. I hadn't eaten in a couple of hours, and I knew that the added insulin delivered through my pump would eventually catch up with me. Having lived with Type 1 diabetes since the age of four, I found the sensation both familiar and striking. I checked the time; it was just after midnight.

The empty roads that night were illuminated by a few passing headlights along the service road. Since I was about ten miles from my home, I decided to pull over and check my glucose levels. I watched my hand tremble while holding the meter.

Shakiness: symptom number one of hypoglycemia.

The meter beeped, as it does to warn against dangerous levels: 68. The number was low—not catastrophic, but low—68 milligrams of glucose per deciliter of blood. The last time I checked, I was at 110. At 68, my brain is still functioning as expected—I feel weak, tired—but cognizant. Once I dip below 60, my cerebral functions will deteriorate until I get that number back up. It's the reason I keep packs of glucose tablets in my-

M. Paczkowski (✉)
The City College of New York, New York, NY, USA

B. C. Frazer, H. R. Walker (eds.), *(Un)doing Diabetes: Representation, Disability, Culture*, Palgrave Studies in Science and Popular Culture, https://doi.org/10.1007/978-3-030-83110-3_9

That's right, I realize. I switched to jeans before leaving the house and forgot to bring the glucose tablets with me. *Well, that's okay, I always have backups in my....* I open the glove box and pull out the clear jar of watermelon flavored glucose tablets. It feels light, and I can see through the packaging. Empty. I forgot to refill them after the last episode. I watch my hands, which now shake with force.

I check again, quickly: 61. In a few minutes, I won't be thinking clearly, and if my numbers dip below 50, it'll be too late. I might be in seizure territory. I had a hypoglycemic seizure several years prior, and my mind flashes to myself in that bed, the phone pressed against my ear, the pain in my back and in my mouth. I estimate my remaining time. Probably six minutes or so.

I look at the clock: 12:18. By 12:24, I won't be me.

I know not to panic, so I switch over to logic. My brain runs calculations, calculations that will not be possible in a few minutes. Fifteen minutes to home. Probably don't have fifteen minutes. Can call someone. Police? Takes too much time. By the time they arrive, I'll be unconscious. Family? They'll panic.

12:19.

My brother spilled a large soda in my car a few weeks ago; I might be able to suck some sugar out of the carpeting, but I know that's dubious, at best. At worst, it wastes time. I can get out of my car and find a house. Knock on a door. Explain. Ask for juice, food, something, but who will answer the door after midnight for a stranger?[1] And if they do answer, and my numbers are too low, I won't even be able to explain without appearing incoherent.

I shouldn't be driving—I know I shouldn't—but sitting and doing nothing is more dangerous. And, if a 911 operator doesn't understand me, or can't find me, I risk lying unconscious on the side of the road all night.

If I get to that 24-hour Burger King around the corner, I'll be back to normal.

[1] This line of thinking was based on personal perceptions of my appearance and identity. On that night, I was a twenty-something, well-dressed, white man in a moderately wealthy neighborhood. Had I differed in age, race, gender identity, and/or economic status, this scene may have played out very differently. Would I have considered knocking on a stranger's door asking for food? Would this search for salvage have even crossed my mind?

"Large Coke. Whopper." It sounds like someone else is speaking, and I don't remember getting here. Completing the transaction is a blur. I'm in the 40s. Definitely in the 40s. Can feel it, that underwater feeling. The night sky, the stars, the trees, the moon all exist without me.

I think I use my credit card because it's faster, but I do not recall. I shove the straw in, pull my car into a handicapped spot out front, and inhale the sugary liquid, drinking faster than I know I can. Drink. Drink. Drink. Gulps flowing down my esophagus. I swoosh the sweetness around my mouth like Listerine, allowing beautiful diffusion to pull glucose in through my veins. There's a convalescent ecstasy as I feel my thoughts return, like coming up for air. I breathe it in, watching my hands steady. I gaze out at the trees swaying against the night sky, and I recall how beautiful the world can be. I open the windows to allow the cool, dark air in.

I devour the Whopper in a carnivorous manner that would disgust me on any other day, but this primal consumption means consciousness returns. There's a part of me that knows this binge will shoot my blood sugar way up, and I'll have to spend most of the night adjusting insulin levels until I resolve the high numbers. But for now, I don't mind because I can think again. I am me again. I can see the trees, I can smell the air, I can feel the night.

* * *

This narrative is emblematic of living with Type 1 diabetes, which in daily life is often characterized by suspense. Action and suspense in cinema, however, typically features nondisabled characters as the protagonists. I used to think that having Type 1 diabetes excluded me from vicarious living because I did not see James Bond insert an insulin infusion set or the Black Panther count his carbohydrates. The suspense genre, in particular, just seemed incompatible with chronic illnesses. How could one survive an external threat on top of the internal one?

However, I often think of the 2002 film, *Panic Room,* which depicts a character living with Type 1 diabetes thrust into extraordinary circumstances. The plot features eleven-year-old Sarah Altman, played by Kristen Stewart, and her mother, Meg, portrayed by Jodie Foster. On the very night Sarah and Meg move into their new Upper West Side brownstone, the home is broken into by three central villains. A cat-and-mouse game ensues, in which the mother and daughter hide in the eponymous panic room, which also holds the millions of dollars in bearer bonds the villains are after. With plummeting glucose levels and no access to her glucagon kit, Sarah eventually succumbs to an on-screen hypoglycemic seizure while trapped in the panic room.

Viewed through the lens of Aaron Smuts's desire-frustration theory of suspense in cinema, *Panic Room* emerges as a case study. Smut argues that "suspense results when one's desire to affect the outcome of an imminent event is frustrated" (Smuts 2008, 289). In *Panic Room,* the viewer vicariously experiences Sarah's powerlessness to stop her plummeting glucose levels upon which her life depends. That "frustration," or lack of agency, yields suspense. It may seem like filmmakers use diabetes as a plot device for dramatic effect in the thriller genre in a way that does not give these characters agency; however, I argue that life with diabetes has striking similarities to the thriller film constructs in daily life where we in fact do have both agency and suspense. Whereas Sarah's situation in the panic room can be deemed "extraordinary," diabetics experience the same suspense—or "panic"—in "ordinary" circumstances, such as my routine drive home where the desire to arrive home safely was frustrated by a hypoglycemic episode. The same panic is imbued in America's insulin crisis, where deep disparities in health care and insurance have resulted in insulin rationing and increased mortality (Fralick and Kesselheim 2019).

In hypoglycemic "panic rooms," like Sarah, diabetics enter a world of suspense fueled by desire and frustration to control our blood sugars, and by extension, to live. Yet in our regular lives, a trip to the supermarket, a walk around the block, or an elevator trip at work can suddenly become laced with the high-stakes dangers of a blockbuster thriller with a disabled person with agency at its center. And the ensuing panic is not contained to one room: it's an omni-present plot device built of our bodies and in our collective life stories.

In this essay, I explore both the accurate and flawed representations of lived experience present in *Panic Room*'s model of suspense. This analysis will demonstrate ways in which media can both capture and conceal the persistent suspense of disabled main characters, as well as how we can communicate this reality with others.

Representative of Lived Experiences: Scene Analysis

My friends and I rented *Panic Room* from Blockbuster Video in 2004. I recall watching it in a stuffy basement and the thrill of seeing Humulin R insulin vials stacked in Sarah's bedside refrigerator. I knew at once that the character was Type 1 diabetic, and that she was in a danger that transcended the home invasion. My friends struggled to follow the plot, and they questioned me about the disease and its risks.

Panic Room introduces diabetes covertly; that is, the disease is shown without ever being named. Critic Kevin L. Ferguson notes that "*Panic Room*'s emphasis on vision and technology necessitates a paternalistic, monitoring attitude towards the diabetic character" (2010, 196). This storytelling choice not only rewards observant viewers, but it is emblematic of nonvisible disabilities in general. Type 1 diabetics do not wear signs. The disease is often camouflaged, except to keen-eyed observers familiar with the trimmings of an insulin pump, a glucometer, dietary choices, and regimented exercise. It is not uncommon for diabetics to "pass by default," a concept explored in Ellen Samuels's essay, "My Body, My Closet: Invisible Disability and the Limits of Coming-Out Discourse" (2003, 240). Samuels provides the stark example of a deaf-blind woman, Megan Jones, who notes the significance of nonverbal signs with her own nonvisible disabilities: "Jones became so frustrated with strangers not believing in her visual and hearing impairments ... that she began to use a white cane she did not need: 'I find that when I use a cane people leave me alone ... people go right into their Blind-Person-With-A-Cane-And-Guide-Dog Red Alert mode'" (241). *Panic Room* also uses nonverbal signs, like Jones's white cane, to clue viewers into Sarah's nonvisible disability. The glucometer watch, the red glucagon box with its thick glass needle, the insulin vials, and the bedside orange juice bottles—all are representative of how filmmakers reveal diabetes in a cinematic setting.

Watching the movie with a group of friends was a notable experience, as it opened a discussion around Type 1 diabetes. Passing was common in my teenage years, as there was little desire to reveal and discuss the nuances of living with diabetes with a group of friends who were in the midst of discovering their own identities. But, while watching *Panic Room,* the discussion was forced into public. My friends asked about low blood sugar levels, the difference between insulin and glucagon injections, how food affects glucose levels, and how long an episode of hypoglycemia lasts. And, when I saw the seizure on screen—Sarah's arched back and curled toes—I felt relief instead of horror. The secrecy of my disability was suddenly out in the open, on display for a group of teenagers, for the first time in my life. Ellen Samuels would likely classify this discussion as a "coming out *to*" friends (237) rather than "coming out," which is more nuanced: "When we look at narratives of disabled people about their own coming-out processes, we see that the language of coming out is used liberally but often carries very different meanings" (238). For me, coming out has been a lifelong process of understanding my own identity as a person living with diabetes while fostering understanding and advocacy with other nondisabled communities. *Panic Room,* and other depictions of disabilities in the media, enable these "coming out *to*" moments for persons with nonvisible disabilities. The filmmakers reflect this through the storytelling: the need for viewers to monitor Sarah throughout the film is a clever design choice that shows a character who "passes by default" to the audience until she cannot.

Panic Room also accurately demonstrates the vexed parent-child relationship typical with disabilities. When Sarah's glucose level dips into the 40s, she becomes too weak to self-manage her diabetes. It is a scene that comes intimately familiar to diabetics who have had severe hypoglycemic episodes, and perfectly demonstrates suspense caused by a desire-frustration gap. Sarah's mother takes dramatic action by leaving the panic room to obtain her daughter's glucagon kit across the hall, and in turn, literally and figuratively entering the den of thieves. Kevin L. Ferguson notes that the paternalistic theme of *Panic Room* is common to diabetic narratives: "Cinema tends to place diabetics under others' protection" (195). Ferguson suggests that this storytelling pattern of parental overseers can be offensive to a diabetic viewer and is in line with Carrie Sandahl's assessment of the "nondisabled guide" troupe. As Sandahl argues in "It's All the Same Movie: Making Code of the Freaks," "In Hollywood movies, audiences are often asked to identify with what I call the 'nondisabled' guide. This guide appears as a character in the film—typically a non-disabled white, cisgender, heterosexual man—who keys audience members to the appropriate emotional responses to the disabled character" (2019, 148). While Meg fits the bill to some extent, as a non-disabled, white, cisgender, heterosexual female guide, I would argue that her role is more complex. Meg also operates as a caregiver for Sarah, guiding the audience practically and emotionally. During a severe episode of hypoglycemia, when the brain is operating on low levels of glucose, self-management becomes difficult or impossible, as it was for me on the side of the road. While I was able to survive without assistance, the episode and experience would have been less frightening and less panic-laden if I had help. I wished I had a Meg to bring me food when my logic was compromised, and the notion of self-control became illusive. In retrospect, I can see that my reluctance to reach out for help only exacerbated the problem.

Fear can be a great motivator, but so too can shame. Here, suspense is generated by Meg's desire to save her daughter from a severe low, and her frustration is paired with entrapment in the panic room. As a caregiver she, too, experiences "panic," and the desire-frustration model of suspense mirrors the lived experience of diabetics and caregivers who may be unable to treat a low during a severe episode of hypoglycemia.

Crucially, Meg's role as caregiver is only situational. Take, for example, Sarah's autonomy throughout the rest of the film. In an early scene, it is Sarah who suggests that the two hide in the panic room. She then shows her mother how to reset the elevator to trick the intruders and avoid capture. Sarah is also more knowledgeable about her symptom presentation and hides the hypoglycemia from Meg for as long as possible. Whereas Ferguson argues that "*Panic Room*'s point seems, more simply, to be that mother knows best" (196), I would argue that mother only knows best when Sarah's knowledge is compromised by her episodic impairment. In fact, Sarah's defeatist attitude toward her mother—"I'm sorry. I was trying not to tell you… I'm dizzy and hungry"—reverberates with surrender and shame. It is not until the glucagon injection that Sarah sheds the need for a caregiver and re-emerges with convalescent strength and renewed autonomy. The scene acknowledges that sometimes we have needs that require assistance. Disability studies scholars who write about disability justice approach this shared panic through the lens of interdependence (Ashby et al. 2015). They describe care and dependence as a false dichotomy often portrayed at odds with one another (Walmsley 1993), which is what we see challenged in Meg and Sarah's relationship.

At Meg's behest, Sarah is given the glucagon injection by the more compassionate intruder, Burnham, played by Forest Whitaker, after she emerges from the seizure. At the film's climax, Sarah's conscious thought is restored as the burglars try to escape the brownstone with their stolen bonds. In a thrilling confrontation, the deranged burglar, Raoul, portrayed by Dwight David Yoakam, tries to strangle Meg with bloody hands, and Sarah suddenly becomes the caregiver of Meg in a significant role reversal. She leaps onto Raoul and stabs him repeatedly with her insulin hypodermics. It is a cathartic moment where Sarah weaponizes her diabetes, the very disease that has fostered her resilience, empathy, and courage. Absent "frustration," Sarah is motivated solely by the desire to save her mother. They mutually care for and protect each other.

Flawed Representations of Lived Experience

While *Panic Room* gets much about Type 1 diabetes right, it would be remiss not to mention its flaws when viewed through the lens of my own lived experience. The most glaring issue: under no circumstances would Sarah be able to talk a stranger through a glucagon injection while midway through a seizure, a flaw noted by Tracey Neithercott in her "Guide to Diabetes in Fiction" (Neithercott 2013). This is absolutely a blemish in an otherwise resonant film. My own experience with a hypoglycemic seizure consisted of blacking out followed by memory loss followed by a fairly lengthy recovery. I also could not have attempted to subdue an intruder shortly after the seizure.

Additionally, critics note that it is unlikely stress would cause hypoglycemia, and that Meg's offer of bottled water is a meaningless gesture for a hypoglycemic episode (Editor 2018). I disagree with these assertions, in particular, as instances of physical and emotional stress have expedited the onset of hypoglycemia in my own life; the days when I am running around to complete errands, work assignments, and frantic phone calls tend to be accompanied by a low. Similarly, while a bottle of water would not resolve hypoglycemia, the gesture suits the circumstances as keeping hydrated could keep Sarah calm and focused on the present.

Tackling these individual examples one-by-one is less productive than looking at the big picture. Largely, I find overly-technical analyses of disabilities in media to be problematic. Understandably, the stakes are high and nobody wants to propagate a stereotype; however, a critic should not hold a microscope to a work of fiction and expect all the details to perfectly match the experiences of a person living with diabetes. As Sandahl notes, "Disabled characters in mainstream movies reflect little of the interesting complexities of our actual lives … Authenticity is never achievable in any case, and attempts at it can be, frankly, pretty boring" (145). *Panic Room,* too, fudges a few of the rules, but I would argue that filmmakers must be afforded these creative liberties, especially in a genre that relies upon suspensions of disbelief, plot holes, and highly improbable events.

For instance, when Meg lights the propane gas being pipped into the room, the ignition would not cause the gas cylinder to shoot around the room like a deflating balloon; the explosion would have likely killed Meg and left the burglars unscathed. Yet, we accept this logical goof in service of suspense, and we should allow for similar storytelling shortcuts in representations of disabilities. Being overly critical of flawed representations can lead filmmakers to shy away from inclusiveness, and I'd rather a marginally flawed representation of Type 1 diabetes than none at all, so long as the representation is not considered wildly inaccurate by the diabetic community (as in the unfortunate case of *Con Air*). After all, inclusion allows for more "coming out *to*" moments with friends and family, where honest, accurate information can be shared.

Concluding Thoughts

Panic Room's representation of diabetes becomes significant not necessarily for what the film gets right or wrong, but for how both the movie and the disability conform to Aaron Smuts's desire-frustration theory of suspense. While, in reality, the climax of a hypoglycemic episode may not have the same dramatic flair of a high stakes burglary in a Manhattan brownstone, a Whopper in a Burger King parking lot can offer competing sentiments of panic and suspense. And, like the falling action and denouement of a blockbuster thriller, the convalescence is filled with relief, optimism, and a renewed appreciation for the ordinary. By applying this lens to *Panic Room* and exposing the realities of suspense in the day-to-day lives of people with diabetes, we can deepen a dialogue around the perception of banality of diabetic life. In doing so we foster greater intimacy, compassion, love, and support for the whole cast of characters in our lives.

References

Ashby, Christine, Eunyoung Jung, Casey Woodfield, Katherine Vroman, and Fernanda Orsati. 2015. 'Wishing to Go It Alone': The Complicated Interplay of Independence, Interdependence and Agency. *Disability & Society* 30 (10): 1474–1489.

Editor, DH. 2018. Diabetes Health Type 1: Diabetes in the Movies. *Diabetes Health*, January 18. Accessed August 1, 2020. https://www.diabeteshealth.com/diabetes-in-the-movies/.

Ferguson, Kevin L. 2010. The Cinema of Control: On Diabetic Excess and Illness in Film. *Journal of Medical Humanities* 31 (3): 183–204. https://doi.org/10.1007/s10912-010-9110-8.

Fralick, Michael, and Aaron S. Kesselheim. 2019. The U.S. Insulin Crisis—Rationing a Lifesaving Medication Discovered in the 1920s. *The New England Journal of Medicine* 381 (19): 1793–1795.

Neithercott, Tracey. 2013. Your Guide to Diabetes in Fiction. July. http://www.diabetesforecast.org/2013/jul/your-guide-to-diabetes-in-fiction.html.

Samuels, Ellen. 2003. My Body, My Closet: Invisible Disability and the Limits of Coming-Out Discourse. *GLQ* 9 (1–2): 233–255.
Sandahl, Carrie. 2019. It's All the Same Movie: Making Code of the Freaks. *JCMS: Journal of Cinema and Media Studies* 58 (4): 145–150. https://doi.org/10.1353/cj.2019.0044.
Smuts, Aaron. 2008. The Desire-Frustration Theory of Suspense. *The Journal of Aesthetics and Art Criticism* 66 (3): 281–290. Accessed August 1, 2020. http://www.jstor.org/stable/40206345.
Walmsley, Jan. 1993. Contradictions in Caring: Reciprocity and Interdependence. *Disability, Handicap & Society* 8 (2): 129–141.

My Tale Told by a Woman: *Lucille* and The Dramaturgy of Diabetes

G. William Zorn

In September of 2007, I was commissioned by the School of Nursing at Ohio University to write a play about diabetes. Sharon Denham of the School of Nursing wanted to utilize the play as part of an educational campaign to combat the rising number of diabetes diagnoses throughout the Appalachian region, known as "Diabetes: A Family Matter." For several weeks, I tried and failed to come up with an overarching story that would be both entertaining and educational. The primary reason for this failure was that I didn't have any direct experience with diabetes. I had no relatives with the condition, no friends or acquaintances. No one who could provide any first-hand knowledge in which to springboard my imagination. Oh, sure, I did my due diligence with research, but each description was scientific and lacked any human connection.

In December of that year, I started to have bouts of blurred vision. After going to the doctor, she could not determine a cause for the abnormality. I chalked it up to a fluke and viewed it more as an annoyance than

G. W. Zorn (✉)
Millikin University, Decatur, IL, USA

B. C. Frazer, H. R. Walker (eds.), *(Un)doing Diabetes: Representation, Disability, Culture*, Palgrave Studies in Science and Popular Culture, https://doi.org/10.1007/978-3-030-83110-3_10

anything too terribly threatening. A few days later, the furnace in my apartment stopped working efficiently and I called my landlord to have it repaired. The technician who came to fix the furnace informed me that it had been spewing carbon monoxide for what could have been months.

For the uninitiated, carbon monoxide may cause headaches and blurred vision at levels of 35 and above. My furnace was reading 80. By now, it was winter break and the student health center was closed, so I took a trip to the emergency room to confirm my exposure—and subsequent blurry vision—to carbon monoxide. There, just on a hunch, the ER doc decided to test my blood sugar as well. I'm glad he did.

As many of you reading this already know, a glucose reading of 140 and above is considered high. My glucose was at 982. I was basically in pancreatic failure. So, while I was exposed to carbon monoxide, my blurry vision was most likely caused by my blood sugar level. This was puzzling to me as I had an A1C ordered and completed in April of 2007 and was at a 6.0 reading (well within normal range). Despite the puzzling nature of this number, I didn't have much time to ponder as I was admitted immediately to the hospital for a week.

If I was struggling before to overcome my lack of experience with diabetes, I was certainly going to get an education now. My semi-private room was typical of what you would see in a hospital: a bed, television, over-bed table and a chair. The staff started almost immediately with educating me about diabetes management. Finger-sticks, glucose monitoring and the correct way to inject insulin were all on the menu. Next was the lecture and demonstration on carb-monitoring, delivered with the suitable seriousness and aplomb that a nurse named Candy should give. While I thought it was particularly cruel to give a new diabetes patient a nurse named Candy, my mind began taking notes for the future draft of my diabetes play.

The Playwriting Process Begins Again

Lucille began as any good play should, with a conflict. Drawing on my newfound experience, the conflict would be that of character versus self. Indeed, a medical model of disability understands diabetes as the body in conflict with normative endocrine function. However, in my play, Lucille's conflict stems from her having to integrate a diabetes identity and new behaviors into her established way of being in the world. Only, there was an inherent problem: Who was the audience for this play? Thirty-nine-year olds? No. Studies have shown that the main audience for theatre is an aging population. In 2009, regional theatres reported that the average theatregoer was a white retiree in their 60s (Beckhusen 2017).

I had to find the best way to tell my story but through "older" eyes. I knew it would also be helpful to enable race-flexible casting, as a key demographic in diabetes education is the African American community. Thus, the character of Lucille was born. I would tell the story of my experience through the eyes of a non-racially specific woman in her 60s. This would be accomplished by making her whole: a whole person with values and experiences and no patience for foolishness like being talked down-to. Readers and audiences, and certainly performers, can infer their own ethnicity on Lucille. As Sarah Baird tells us in her article, "Stereotypes Of Appalachia Obscure A Diverse Picture": "There's no one story of Appalachia, no one voice. It's time for everyone to feel like they can speak up, like their story is important" (Baird 2014). This would target both the demographics of a typical theatregoer and a typical Appalachian diabetes patient.

As a playwright, I have written characters from all aspects of life. Male, female, old, young, fat, thin, outgoing or introverted. I was—at the time—a 39-year-old, white, homosexual male in graduate school. I realize that it could be dangerous, inherently so, to write an educational play centered on a character whom I have very little in common. But here's the thing: My mother was in her seventies at the time I wrote the play and I had been her caretaker for a few years. I witnessed as my mother struggled with what was being taken away from her because of aging. I observed her good-natured, yet somewhat real animosity toward in-laws. And, perhaps most importantly, my mother demonstrated for me what it meant to show positivity and perseverance in the face of medical adversities. It was easy to see my experience through my mother's eyes.

Scene Analysis: Choices That Reflect the Lived Experience

Lived experience now informed the development process for *Lucille*. While I was recovering from my initial hospital visit, I began my work on a draft of the script (Zorn 2000). It began with Lucille, alone in her hospital room, and Candy, meeting for the first time:

CANDY:	Hello. Mrs. Myers?
LUCILLE:	If you've come for more blood, I'm all out. Empty. Caput. The tank is on E and I'm runnin' on fumes.
CANDY:	I'm Candy, your transition nurse.
LUCILLE:	Transition to what?
CANDY:	Well, I hear you're going home tomorrow.
LUCILLE:	News to me.
CANDY:	Oh. Well, you're going home tomorrow. Ta-da!

It was important to give Lucille a sparring partner—someone to whom she could outwardly "wrestle" with her inner demons. Transplanting the experiences of a thirty-nine-year-old diabetic playwright into the mouth of a sixty-something woman makes her particularly feisty, principally when confronting stereotypes concerning Appalachian people. There is a prevailing stereotype that Appalachian folks are "poor, backward and white" (Baird 2014). One aspect of my own experience fueled this belief, though it's hardly prone to only this region.

When dealing with diabetes education—or any medically-necessary education for that matter—the educators tend to talk down to the patient. In *The Birth of the Clinic*, French philosopher Michel Foucault went so far as to say that "doctors are doctor-oriented, not patient-oriented, and thus medicine creates an abusive power structure" (Misselbrook 2013). Though not going so far to call the dynamic abusive, several scholars writing about the stigma towards "lifestyle" diseases have noted that doctors tend to view patients with diabetes as "foolish" or "ignorant" (Boero 2007; Bock 2012).

Diabetes educators infantilize adult patients when the word choice and concepts are simplified to be something even a child could understand. Therefore, it became vital to me that Lucille be an active, educated character who would not tolerate this kind of belittling behavior. In this scene, both Lucille and Candy show off their extensive knowledge of English literature:

CANDY:	That's right. You used to be an English teacher.
LUCILLE:	Retired now, yes. How do you know—?
CANDY:	Let's see. (Reciting.) "A wise man should consider that health is the greatest of human blessings and learn how, by his own thought, to derive benefit from his illnesses."
LUCILLE:	Well now. That was one o' those Greeks. If I was the bettin' sort, I'd say Hippocrates.
CANDY:	Very good.

LUCILLE:	(Reciting.) "The only way to keep your health is to eat what you don't want, drink what you don't like, and do what you'd druther not."
CANDY:	Mark Twain. (Reciting.) "Medicine to produce health must examine disease; as music, to create harmony must investigate discord."
LUCILLE:	Plutarch. Gimme a hard one at least. (Reciting.) "Attention to health is life's greatest hindrance."
BOTH:	Plato.
	(They laugh.)
CANDY:	Say, am I going to have trouble with you, Lucille?
LUCILLE:	Prob'ly. You want trouble?
CANDY:	Honestly? Yes.
LUCILLE:	Brave girl.
CANDY:	If you've got something to fight about, you've got something to fight for.

It was important to me to give Lucille a foil, someone who she could banter with outside of the hospital setting. This would let the audience know that she was going to be all right once she left the monitoring that a hospital necessitates, as the source of her "spunk" lies in her ability to argue. She is very much a woman who would only argue with you if she cared about you. Her experience in age was her credibility, her cache in any argument. She is a tough woman with a lifetime of skills and practices, and she will not be outcredentialed.

In the following scene, Lucille again pushes back against being treated like a child. In fact, Lucille interrupts Candy to set her straight regarding how Lucille wants to be treated:

LUCILLE:	What was your name again?
CANDY:	It's Candace, but everyone calls me Candy.
LUCILLE:	Candy, I love my family.
CANDY:	I am very happy to hear that. It is so import—
LUCILLE:	Let me finish. I love my family, but I am not a child. I was born in the middle of the depression, number seven of fourteen kids. I've lived to see a half dozen wars. I was a riveter in dubya-dubya two. A damn good one, too. The Japanese never sank one of my ships. I married my Alvin in forty-seven, ran a household, raised two boys, taught English to children who would rather read comic books and I've been president of the Elks Club Lady's Auxiliary twice. Does that sound like somebody you can run roughshod over?

CANDY:	No—
LUCILLE:	Does that sound like someone who doesn't deserve to be addressed directly?
CANDY:	No—
LUCILLE:	Does that sound like someone who can't take care of herself?
CANDY:	No, ma'am.

I cannot stand being talked down to or infantilized, yet I have experienced this treatment throughout my journey with diabetes. This, along with what I have witnessed in hospital care with my mother, made it clear that Candy, while well-meaning, should not be the primary antagonist in the play. Lucille was too formidable a foe. I gave her a daughter-in-law whom she loves but doesn't particularly like—Judy (affectionally referred to as "Bony-butt").

Judy was a tough character to write since she isn't heard from until the end of the play, so much of her had to be built from the discovery of Candy. The character had to come from Lucille's storytelling. Since she wasn't physically present in the play, I decided to use an old psychology trick: role-playing. In this scene, Candy role-plays as Judy in order for Lucille to practice telling a family member about her diabetes. The audience learns about Judy through Lucille's description and Candy's guesswork:

CANDY:	Now, it's Tuesday morning and your doorbell rings.
LUCILLE:	Don't have a doorbell.
CANDY:	Then there's a knock at the door.
LUCILLE:	She's never knocked on a door a day in her life. Usually she just—
CANDY:	(As LUCILLE.) Come in!
LUCILLE:	(As JUDY.) Morning, mother Myers. Sorry I'm late.
CANDY:	(As LUCILLE.) Well, hello there, Judy.
LUCILLE:	(As JUDY.) Oh good. You've got coffee on. I just didn't have the time before I left. Rush rush rush. That's all I do these days. My nails. My hair. I simply must spend your son's money before he gets smart and divorces me. Are you outta sugar? Oh that's right. I'm sorry. Well, Equal will just have to do, I guess. How are you feeling?
CANDY:	I'm feeling fine, Judy. Just fine.
LUCILLE:	I'm glad. You know you gave us quite a scare the other night. How you could have let yourself get that sick I'll never know, bless yer heart. At death's door—

CANDY:	I wasn't at—
LUCILLE:	And you arguing with that poor nurse in the emergency room.
CANDY:	I told her my veins roll—
LUCILLE:	She was only trying to help you.
CANDY:	Well, she wasn't—
LUCILLE:	Honestly, you just have to be a little nicer to people and they'll do whatever you want them to. I should know. But, you scared us half to death, bless yer heart. I came this close to singin' it.
CANDY:	(As CANDY.) Singing what?
LUCILLE:	Your song, of course. You know. Kenny Rogers. Yer favorite. I told you I'd be singing it at your funeral. (Singing.) *Ya picked a fine time to leave me, Lucille.*
CANDY:	(As CANDY.) Oh, Lucille, that's awful.

It seems that all of Candy's training in how to deal with difficult patients is worthless in the face of adversarial Lucille. Also, she cannot believe that a person such as Judy really exists. For her to succeed in getting through to Lucille, Candy must try another tactic: Thanksgiving.

When deciding on the time of year the play was set in, I choose Thanksgiving because I couldn't imagine a more heightened time of year for a mother. For many mothers, so much time, preparation and love are wrapped up in one holiday when you are the one who determines its success. For Lucille, it was all about the meal itself and the love she could offer to those who ate her Thanksgiving feast. Once again, her background with English literature serves to illustrate her true feelings about the insulin she needs, literally the poisoning of her expression of love. Would she rather die than give up the love of providing a meal to her loved ones? In this exchange, Lucille makes the connection explicit:

(LUCILLE	picks up the insulin syringe.)
LUCILLE:	(Reciting.) "I sell thee poison; thou hast sold me none. Farewell. Buy food and get thyself in flesh."
CANDY:	(Reciting.) "Come, Cordial and not poison, go with me to Juliet's grave; for there I must use thee." I know what you're doing, Lucille. That is not poison and this is not the end of your life.
LUCILLE:	Maybe not. But it's the beginning of the end, isn't it? I was about five, I think, when my grandmother called me into the kitchen to teach me how to make her stuffing. *This* was

> important. This was the equivalent to a state secret. The entire county clamored to get their hands on that recipe. Including my mother. And here I was, my precocious, little five-year-old self, learning about soaking the celery in bacon grease overnight and using biscuits instead of croutons and never letting a utensil get anywhere near that stuffing. Your hands, she said. Your lovin' hands are what make people envious. People think there's some mysterious ingredient, and there is, but not what they think. No herb or spice or temperature can replace your own hands, baby girl. That's where the love comes from. But Candy, I ain't makin' Thanksgiving this year. It's bein' brought in by people I don't even know. In big foil pans kept warm with Sterno. Touched by plastic and metal. And strangers' hands. Where's the love in that? It's the beginning of the end.

What is "the beginning of the end"? For Lucille, it's about her vitality, her ability to provide food (love) to her family. Here, I drew on my own fears around food and change. Not the fear of making the meal or its success, but what I would no longer be able to enjoy at that time of year. Christmas and Thanksgiving come with quite a lot of baggage in terms of eating and enjoying the comradery of loved ones. For a person newly diagnosed with diabetes, I wondered what I could no longer enjoy.

In order for Lucille to transition from thinking about the end of her vitality as a mother and provider, Candy suggests that Lucille see herself as the teacher once again. As they discuss in this interaction, perhaps it's okay to "pass the torch" of tradition to the next generation (Judy):

CANDY:	Maybe it's time to pass it along.
LUCILLE:	What?
CANDY:	Your grandmother's stuffing. Maybe Miss Bony-Butt never had that kind of relationship. She doesn't know that a caterer can never live up to her mother-in-law.
LUCILLE:	And maybe Sean Connery will ask me to marry him.
CANDY:	I can't imagine that someone who has as much fight, as much pure, unfiltered, unfettered orneriness would—could—ever go gently into that good night. You've taken everything I've thrown at you today and sent it back to me twice as fast. I'll bet you match ol' Bony-Butt toe to toe, too. You don't love that girl because you have to. You love her because she's a good sparring partner. But, she can't

read your mind. Sparring is good. Keeps your mind sharp, but talk to her. Have a real conversation and see where that takes you.

LUCILLE: Well, not to toot my own horn, but I can give as good as I get.

CANDY: I'll bet you do. And something tells me as long as you can hold your own against somebody like that, you're gonna be just fine, Lucille.

In terms of the "education" part of the commission, Lucille learned to check her glucose level, grasped how to count carbohydrates, the correct way to inject her insulin and that moderation is the key to controlling blood sugar, not abstinence. For the most part, the audience's educational portion of the commission happened virtually on its own. Audiences saw Lucille's struggle and ultimate mastery of these tasks. Yes, it was a part of my experience that I wanted to include, but it was also a necessary part of Lucille's experience.

Lucille in Production and Concluding Thoughts

For me, theatre has always been a transformative medium. Transformative in the way that you can key into what you (the playwright) and your target audience have in common, your audience's attitudes and beliefs as well as their struggles. In telling my story, through identities that differ from my own, depending on casting, *Lucille* has allowed my story to go beyond myself. Lucille and I share many aspects of our personality and belief, but more than that, being a diabetic and a scholar and someone who does not suffer fools gladly makes me my own subject matter. Making her a female made use of my own observations regarding my mother's struggles with aging and fear of being useless.

I reflect on both my commission as a playwright and my subsequent diagnosis and I feel grateful. After the live feedback and many letters and emails I have received, I know that *Lucille* and "Lucille" touch a nerve. There is something relatable in both her experience as a newly diagnosed diabetic and her reaction to that diagnosis. Audiences connect with her bewilderment, her denial and her ultimate acceptance and refusal to let this disease disrupt her belief system.

Lucille will forever be a part of me, after all. She is the embodiment of my own experience both as a diabetic, as a playwright and even as an actor.

For, yes, I have played Lucille (the character) a couple of times when needed. Having lived this experience is a bit unsettling, to say the least, when performing parts of your own life.

At one certain performance in 2008, the actress who was to play Lucille was ill and I was asked to stand-in for her. It wasn't the first time I was asked to play a woman and it certainly wasn't the first time I was asked to read my own work. The experience was both enlightening and a bit uncomfortable. After all, I was reliving my experience. One thing it proved to me, though, was that even a man playing the title character still resonated with an audience. It was still funny and poignant and free from comment or judgment.

All in all, my experience creating *Lucille* has informed my own writing since. My plays have almost always centered around family and underserved populations, but through the power of the spoken word, *Lucille* goes beyond these aesthetics. It helps its audience by presenting a strong, vital woman who does not suffer fools gladly, someone to both identify and to emulate. It entertains and it never talks down to them.

References

Baird, Sarah. 2014. *Stereotypes Of Appalachia Obscure A Diverse Picture*. National Public Radio, April 6. https://www.npr.org/sections/codeswitch/2014/04/03/298892382/stereotypes-of-appalachia-obscure-a-diverse-picture. Accessed 6 Mar 2021.

Beckhusen, Theresa. 2017. Priority Report: Theatre Facts 2016. *American Theatre*, November 21. https://www.americantheatre.org/2017/11/21/priority-report-theatre-facts-2016/. Accessed 22 Feb 2020.

Bock, Sheila. 2012. Contextualization, Reflexivity, and the Study of Diabetes-Related Stigma. *Journal of Folklore Research* 49 (2): 153–178. https://doi.org/10.2979/jfolkrese.49.2.153.

Boero, Natalie. 2007. All the News that's Fat to Print: The American 'Obesity Episdemic' and the Media. *Qualitative Sociology* 30 (1): 41–60.

Misselbrook, David. 2013. Foucault. *British Journal of General Practice* 63 (611): 312. https://doi.org/10.3399/bjgp13X668249.; https://www.ncbi.nlm.nih.gov/pubmed/23735390.

Zorn, G. William. 2000. *Lucille*. Athens, Ohio: Ohio University.

PART III

Staring, Coding, and Reading the Diabetic Body

The essays in Part III take up markers of race, class, and gender to address how these categories shape representations of the diabetic body. While diabetes may be a non-apparent disability, the intersection of these categories complicate the hidden and visible elements of the body. In a playful nod to how medicine *codes* diabetes in medical records, we refer to *coding* as a cultural practice of reading meaning in visible signs of a social group.

By looking at race, class, and gender, these essays enter into in the extensive history of disability scholarship on the social practice of *staring*. Disability studies scholar and bioethicist Rosemarie Garland-Thomson discusses staring as an expression of human curiosity with the modern impulse to "observe and seek our own proof." Garland-Thomson notes that *staring* and gathering visual information to reconcile "the curious with the common" asserts a power dynamic that the staree must manage. Authors in this section take up different categories of visibility, staring, and power dynamics to examine their objects of inquiry.

Additionally, theories of *intersectionality* inform these authors' arguments. A term first coined by lawyer and civil rights advocate Kimberlé Crenshaw; *intersectionality* describes the diversity of experiences with a social category. Crenshaw explains that experiences of oppression differ based on overlapping identities. In the case of diabetes, authors ask how bodies are read and coded differently when race, class, gender, age, culture, and citizenship status are considered. With an intersectional analysis at the forefront, each author pays particular attention to resource distribution based on category. Our authors point to the material effects of such readings and trouble entrenched beliefs about intersectional diabetes experiences.

In her chapter, "Waking Up Metaphors of Diabetes," Sheila Bock draws our attention to the use of "contagion" and "contamination" as root metaphors for how diabetes spreads. Bock examines pop culture, news media, and her own interpersonal encounters to "wake up" these metaphors. Through tracing the eugenics movement of the 1950s and the COVID-19 pandemic, Bock argues that "implications of these metaphors differ significantly depending on the social meanings attached to different types of racialized and classed bodies." To conclude her chapter, Bock urges readers to consider how broader hierarchies of power shape concepts of communicability.

In Taylor Johnson's essay, "Please Don't Pet: Reflections on Life with My Diabetes Alert Dog," Johnson recounts the way social groups read and code her body as a Black diabetic with a service dog. Johnson brings readers attention to the staring, racism and ableism she manages from strangers and from within diabetic communities. In a culminating argument, Johnson calls attention to how "the non-disabled world prioritizes their convenience and profits over our access to an equitable life."

In "How To Wear (And Hide) Your Insulin Pump: Managing Device Connectedness With Gendered Bodies Online," Stephen Horrocks presents a narrative and visual analysis of Andrea Deck's video "How I Hide My Insulin Pump." Horrocks analyses Deck's video as an example of YouTube videos devoted explicitly to "wearing" and "hiding" the insulin pump. In his analysis, Horrocks argues that gendered cultural practices with insulin pumps simultaneously reinforce and resist "problematic visions of embodied normalcy." He goes on to question how social standards of normalcy are reinforced through "biomedical intervention and US cultural representations of gender."

These essays collectively address three central questions:

- How do the social categories of race, gender, and class shape readings of the diabetic body?

- How do visibility and coding cultural practices shape the "coming out" experience and social awareness of the diabetic body in public spaces?
- How might metaphor in the cultural imagination inform intersectional representations of diabetes and their subsequent material effects?

Waking Up Metaphors of Diabetes

Sheila Bock

Introduction

One afternoon, I walked into a new optometrist's office for my annual eye exam. Filling out the new patient paperwork while sitting in the lobby, I checked various boxes to address different questions about myself: Gender: Female. Race/Ethnicity: White/Non-Hispanic. Profession: University Professor. Under the section that included a long list of health conditions, I checked the box indicating that I had Type 1 diabetes. Indeed, this was the primary reason I made this appointment in the first place—so that the doctor could dilate my eyes and check to see if my diabetes, which I have had since I was 13 years old, a little less than 20 years at that point, had started to cause damage to my eyes. When it was time to see the doctor, she looked over the paperwork I had just filled out, and she began to ask me questions about my diabetes, questions I was used to answering in doctor's offices at this point: How long have I had diabetes? ["Since 1995."] Do I see an endocrinologist? ["Yes."] Do I take insulin? ["Yes,

S. Bock (✉)
University of Nevada, Las Vegas, Las Vegas, NV, USA
e-mail: sheila.bock@unlv.edu

B. C. Frazer, H. R. Walker (eds.), *(Un)doing Diabetes: Representation, Disability, Culture*, Palgrave Studies in Science and Popular Culture, https://doi.org/10.1007/978-3-030-83110-3_11

Humalog."] How much? ["I have an insulin pump, so it depends"]. Do I check my blood sugar? ["Yes."] How many times a day? ["Around 6 times a day."] When I test my blood sugar, what levels do I have? ["It varies by day, of course, but my last A1C test a couple of months ago was 6.7"].

She then turned away from me, rummaged through a desk drawer in the exam room, and turned back around carrying a handout that offered some basic information about diabetes. I expected her to use this handout as a way to enter into a conversation about my own experiences and things I should be aware of moving forward. I was expecting her to bring my attention to the section of the handout that listed some of the negative effects of uncontrolled diabetes on the body, including heart disease, stroke, kidney damage, and nerve damage, which in turn could lead to amputation and (most relevant to the purpose of my visit) blindness. Instead, she began reading to me the section of the handout that listed the risk factors for diabetes (weight, age, family history, being a member of particularly "high risk" groups including African Americans, Alaska Natives, American Indians, Asian Americans, Hispanics/Latinos, Native Hawaiians, or Pacific Islanders.) At this point, I began to think that the handout seemed primarily geared toward people with (or who were at risk for) Type 2 diabetes, a form of diabetes that manifests differently than mine. Once she started reading through the section on how to prevent diabetes (eating more healthfully, getting more physical exercise), I quipped, "Well, I have it already, so that ship has sailed!" She seemed a little bit taken aback by my interruption. I hoped at this point that she would bring the focus of the appointment back to my eyes. After a short pause, she switched gears, though still remained focused on the handout she was holding, pointing to the text that identified family history as a significant risk factor. "Yes, but if you have kids, they will be more likely to get it because you have it. If you have kids, you will have to be very careful."

I didn't ask her to clarify what she meant by this rather vague admonition to "be very careful." I did recognize (both in that moment and now several years and two children later) what David Hufford terms the "bloating of cultural authority," referring to the ways in which "professional authorities have set the boundaries of their expertise far beyond the limits that can be rationally defended" (1991: 13). As this optometrist talked to me not about the potential effects of diabetes on my eyes, but rather the potential effects of diabetes on hypothetical children in the future, I recognized her "presenting authoritative statements that [were] actually intensely moralistic and doctrinal but that [were] nonetheless presented *as expertise*" (Goldstein 2004: 170, italics in original). I also recognized in her words the representation of diabetes as a lurking threat that spreads, that transmits from one person to another, that contaminates. A condition that is not just a danger to the person who has it, but a danger to others as well.

I had spent several years at that point researching the stigma associated with Type 2 diabetes, specifically how it was discursively naturalized and the ways in which individuals and communities used storytelling to reframe and resist some these stigmatizing discourses. This experience with the optometrist was jarring to me not so much because of the connections she was drawing between contamination and diabetes, but rather because I found *myself* positioned in the category of "already contaminated," as a potential threat to others. In most of my experience, references to my own (white, Type 1 diabetic) body in conversations about diabetes are typically made in terms of familiar (and often racialized) binaries structuring prevalent and problematic understandings of diabetes: control vs. chaos, innocence vs. blame, victimhood vs criminality. As one surgeon expressed to me during a casual conversation at a social gathering, upon hearing that I had Type 1 diabetes: "I tend to have more sympathy for the Type 1 diabetics I get than the Type 2 … A Type 1 diabetic is just walking down the street and gets shot. A Type 2 diabetic is in a gang, robs a liquor store, pulls a gun, and then gets shot."

I have unpacked this surgeon's metaphoric framing of the different types of diabetes elsewhere (Bock 2012), highlighting how the focus on *bad choices* works in highly problematic ways to "spoil" the identity (Goffman 1963) of individuals with Type 2 diabetes. Though within the logic of this metaphor, the blame does not lie solely in the poor choices of the individual. Notably, the Type 2 diabetic's "gang" affiliation serves as a primary factor contributing to those choices. In other words, group membership is understood to be a source of contamination that the individual must resist or be overtaken by.

My aim in this chapter is to help "wake up the sleeping metaphors" (Martin 1991: 501) of diabetes, particularly the prevalent root metaphors of contamination and contagion, while also recognizing that the implications of these metaphors differ significantly depending on the social meanings attached to different types of racialized and classed bodies. My own surprise at being positioned as already contaminated, for example, illustrates quite clearly that the stigma so often attached to diabetes has *not* been a significant part of my own experiences with the condition. Just as disability studies scholars have recognized the importance of rhetoric in reinforcing the devaluation of certain bodies and minds—and even constructing these bodies and minds as a threat to others (cf O'Brien 2011; Yergeau 2020)—it is important to turn our critical attention to the rhetorical framings of diabetes and their consequences.

Envisioning a "Threat" that Spreads Beyond the Individual

Looking back historically, the responses of eugenicists after the introduction of insulin therapy in the early twentieth century transformed diabetes from an acute, lethal condition to "a disease of chronic complications" (Foy 2013: 35). This transformation led to great concern among eugenicists who bemoaned the newfound abilities of people with diabetes to pass on their "defective" genes. In a 1954 issue of *Eugenics Quarterly*, for example, Alan F. Guttmacher, vice president of the American Eugenics Society and Chief of Obstetrics and Gynecology at Mount Sinai Hospital, characterized "diabetics' pursuit of motherhood [as] 'illogical' and against the 'welfare of the community'" (Farley 2019: np). As people with diabetes began to live longer, this perceived threat to the community was envisioned not only in terms of the biological transmission of "flawed" genetic material from one generation to the next, but in terms of the economic costs to society at large (a vision, notably, that extended well beyond diabetes and has had tragic consequences for people with disabilities who underwent forced sterilizations [O'Brien 1999, 2003, 2011; see also "History of Eugenics Resource Guide"]. As historian Marjorie Elvin Foy explains, "From lost workdays due to illness to the need for charity or government-subsidized care for lower-income patients, chronic diseases like diabetes replaced contagions like yellow fever and tuberculosis as the biggest [perceived] impending threats to the health of the nation's workforce" (Foy 2013:37).

In the midst of these concerns about how individual choices to have children could have negative consequences for the community at large, diabetes's early associations with upper- and middle-class whiteness saved people with diabetes from being subjected the coercive eugenic practices inflicted most often on indigenous, immigrant, and African American women. As Arleen Marcia Tuchman tells us, while diabetics were seen as passing along "defective" genes [i.e., contaminating the bodies of others], "'Good' diabetics fit the eugenicists' ideal: white, affluent, intelligent, and above all capable of exercising self-control" (2013: 28). Despite the "threat" to future generations lurking in their bodies, their *social* attributes were understood to be assets to society and thus outweighed the potential harm. Their "good" choices—bolstered by the noble qualities ascribed to their group affiliations—protected them from being cast in the role of the dangerous infector of the collective gene pool, as the villain that must be stopped by any means necessary.

In contrast, as rates of Type 2 diabetes have increased drastically in recent decades, particularly among marginalized communities, so, too, have the rhetorics of contamination and transmission in relation to this condition. While diabetes is not a communicable disease, contagion is a dominant metaphor structuring how many people think and communicate about it, as in phrases like "I have to avoid diabetes like the plague" or "Stop! you'll give me diabetes ..." (Sinnenberg et al. 2018). Articles and blog posts abound online with titles like "Are Healthy (And Unhealthy) Habits Contagious?" (Hamilton 2011), at times even explicitly likening "bad" habits to viruses (cf. drake 2017). One most vivid illustration of the rhetorics of contamination and contagion is the imagery invoked in "Bad Blood," a 2006 series of articles in the *New York Times* introduced as "a series about Type 2 diabetes and how it has become an epidemic in New York" (Olsen 2006). Knowing the content of the articles, the title itself, "Bad Blood," then situates diabetes as a bodily contamination through the adjective "bad," while also echoing language used to reference syphilis, an infectious sexually transmitted disease, during the now infamous Tuskegee Syphilis Experiment. The articles' framing of diabetes as not just *contaminating* but *contagious* are furthered reinforced by the description of the high rates of diabetes as "an epidemic," offering support of Lorenzo Servitje and Kari Nixon's argument that "Epidemic discourse so thoroughly structures our world that it is endemic to our processes of social construction. That is, our current social constructions rely on paradigms that represent nearly everything as communicable" (2016: 3).

Contagion and Culture

Bringing critical attention to how contagion discourses shape widespread understandings of queerness and disability, Margaret F. Gibson explains how "Discourses of contagion call up affect-saturated histories where certain people, traits, ideas, or substances have been understood as producing undesirable—perhaps even irreversible or life threatening—effects for those with whom they come into contact" (2018: 118). The structuring metaphors of contagion bring with them a strong sense of urgency, as well as a call for surveillance and action to help minimize the "threat." Gibson observes that the responsibility for this surveillance falls heavily on mothers, the locus of social and cultural reproduction, an observation that resonates with the call to action embedded in my optometrist's warning to "be very careful." Sociologist Natalie Boero offers valuable insights into what she terms "mother blame" in common sense and professional understandings of childhood health issues, focusing in particular on the so-called "epidemic of childhood obesity" (2009) (offering yet another illustration of Servitje and Nixon's argument about epidemic discourse). In addition to their discursive links with nature, "women's association with culture and the socialization of children often holds them implicitly accountable for the spread of the 'epidemic'" (Boero 2007: 53). Mothers, as the perceived stewards of culture, are tasked with filtering out the "bad" and passing along the "good" to the next generation.

We can see these ideas dramatized within one episode (Season 13, Episode 1) of the popular animated television show *King of the Hill.* In this episode, the character Bill Dauterive—who is characterized as slovenly and childlike throughout the series—is diagnosed with diabetes. From the moment Bill is first diagnosed, he fails to take personal responsibility for his health and change his eating habits, placing the blame (at least in part) on his mother's actions. For example, when Bill's more responsible friend Hank Hill takes him shopping for healthful foods and scolds him for selecting cookies, Bill exclaims, "It's my mom's fault. When I was sad, she'd give me cookies. But when I was happy, she'd give me cookies. All of my emotions demand cookies, Hank!" This "failure" to take responsibility constitutes a classic example of a "spoiled identity," one made visible here by what Goffman terms "blemishes of individual character" (1963: 4).

This equation between diabetes and character flaws, however, is destabilized as a second storyline develops in which the female character Peggy Hill decides that she will not let diabetes happen in her own family. She begins to serve her son, Bobby, *only* healthful foods, including alfalfa sprouts, carrots, onions, seaweed, and wheat grass. At first Bobby is repulsed, but by the end of the episode his tastes transform as he finds candy to be too sweet, and he describes wheat grass as "not that bad." The replacement of "junk" food diets with foods that fall within the category of "clean" eating invoke binaries of filth and cleanliness, indulgence and discipline, contamination and purity. Through this secondary storyline, we see Peggy actually instilling a taste for healthful foods into her son, introducing the possibility that Bill's mother could have, should have, done the same. Through her surveillance of her son's eating habits, Peggy not only recognizes the lurking threat of diabetes (within a larger discursive context proclaiming an emerging diabetes "epidemic") but acts on it. Bill's choices and its consequences are presented as the result of failed parenting; Peggy's actions are presented as the better alternative, and her son Bobby's pathway toward adulthood shifts from a future that looks like Bill's to one that is more socially desirable.

Ultimately, though, self-control, discipline, and personal responsibility are presented as the central tenets to living a good life. Indeed, personal responsibility is a key ideal in the neoliberal landscape we are living in, an ideal that calls on people to take control over their health while also using poor health as evidence of "failure" and, by extension, socially undesirable character traits. In public framings of the larger consequences of this kind of "failure" at the individual level, though, metaphors of contagion creep in to highlight the danger these individuals pose to the people they come in contact with.

This dynamic is clearly evident in the 2006 *New York Times* article "Medicaid Plan Prods Patients Toward Health," which was published right when I was embarking on my research on the discursive framings of diabetes. The article describes a pilot program in West Virginia which aimed to reward people on Medicaid with "enhanced benefits" if they signed a pledge "to do my best to stay healthy" and attend health improvement programs (for weight loss and anti-smoking). The purpose of this incentive program was to reward "responsible" behavior. Those who did not sign the pledge would have their health benefits restricted significantly. Those who did sign it would receive additional benefits.

The first thing the reader encounters in this article is a picture of an older man sitting in an easy chair, smoking a cigarette, and looking not at the camera but off to the side. On the table next to him lies an ashtray filled with cigarette butts. The caption below this picture reads, "John Johnson has lost a leg to diabetes but eats 'what I want' and continues smoking. He says he will not participate in the enhanced-benefit plan" (Eckholm 2006). The article begins with the sentence, "No question, John Johnson is a doctor's nightmare" (Eckholm 2006). It then goes on to describe Mr. Johnson in more detail, framing him as the representative target of the incentive program: "Speaking from the easy chair where he spends his days in a small wooden house near this small

Appalachian town, his left trouser leg folded by a safety pin where a limb was lost to diabetes, he lighted another cigarette" (Eckholm 2006). From this brief description, the reader understands that Mr. Johnson is 1) not working since he spends his days sitting in an easy chair at home, and 2) not healthy, since he smokes and has already suffered complications from diabetes ("abominations of the body," to borrow language from Erving Goffman classification of different types of stigma). The description of Mr. Johnson continues: While "taxpayers foot the bill" of his medical treatments, he has no intention of quitting smoking: "'I've been smoking for 50 years—why should I stop now?' he added for good measure. 'This is supposed to be a free world'" (Eckholm 2006). In reference to his diabetes, he says, "I told [my doctors] I eat what I want to eat and the hell with them" (Eckholm 2006). Situating his purported lack of control (Broom and Whittaker 2004) within his invocation of freedom, the article presents Mr. Johnson as a man who has failed to manage his responsibilities for his health. Such a "failure" at the individual level affects him negatively, as well as the taxpayers who have to pay for his indulgences and indiscretions. Individual health choices become intertwined with morality and social responsibility (or its perceived lack). As we see with the fictional Bill Dauterive, Mr. Johnson's diabetes is constructed as a marker of his "blemishes of individual character" (Goffman 1963: 4), a marker that in turn "spoils" his identity.

Foundational to this set of representations is the ideology of ability, an ideology which, at its most radical, "defines the baseline by which humanness is determined, setting the measure of body and mind that gives or denies human status to individual persons" (Siebers 2013: 273). Bringing an intersectional approach to his consideration of this ideology, Tobin Siebers further explains that "the ideology of ability uses the language of pathology to justify labeling some identities as inferior to others" (2013: 285). And this process is clearly apparent in how the article connects Johnson's poor lifestyle choices to another type of stigma identified by Goffman: "the tribal stigma of race, nation, and religion" (1963: 4), where the contaminating "attribute" extends beyond the individual to all members of a group, in this case those who are part of Appalachian culture. In other words, culture becomes a pathology, a mechanism embodied within individuals and passed along through social contact that facilitates the contagion of diabetes. For example, within the article, the state commissioner of medical services, a voice of medical authority, offers *culture* as an explanation for why West Virginia has such high rates of obesity, smoking, heart disease, and diabetes when she says, "We're in an Appalachian culture where there's a fatalism, and many people don't go in for checkups or preventive services" (Eckholm 2006). Explaining individual choice in terms of cultural fatalism, culture is constructed here as a contaminating force that stands in the way of making responsible choices, thus creating a way for diabetes to spread.

The article does acknowledge briefly the poverty in the area, noting that some people cannot afford the transportation to go to the health programs, and writing that "[n]o one questions that West Virginia, more than most other states, needs more healthful lifestyles and better primary and preventive care" (Eckholm 2006). Its focus on Mr. Johnson, "the cantankerous diabetic," however, diverts attention away from the material conditions affecting health care, focusing instead on how this man, and presumably the others whom he represents, the others who purportedly have inherited (or been infected by) the fatalism of Appalachian culture, willfully refuse to take advantage of the resources available. The metaphor of contagion is foundational to this representation of diabetes.

Contamination, Contagion, and the Construction of Undesirable/Expendable Citizens

Whether implicit or explicit, the recurring metaphors of contamination and contagion in relation to diabetes (and the "bad" health behaviors that are discursively linked to it) is quite striking, especially when viewed through the lens of existing scholarship on the social meanings of contagion and its metaphors (cf. Kitta 2019; Mitchell 2014; Sontag 1989; Wald 2008). Alan Kraut (1994) introduced the term "medicalized nativism" to help explain how contagious diseases are used to validate anti-immigrant sentiments. Building on this idea, Priscilla Wald, Nancy Tomes, and Lisa Lync assert that "Cultural margins and national borders are often summoned, if not articulated, through the figure of specific contagious diseases" (2002: 619). In other words, the imagery of contagion invokes binaries of self and other, stability and disruption, purity and contamination, which in turn map onto and naturalize discourses of nationhood. What is at stake in these processes of drawing boundaries, of course, is the designation of who is entitled to the benefits of citizenship and who, by extension, is not. Importantly, these designations extend well beyond legal status and work to justify various forms of social inequality within national borders.

And when metaphors of contagion are employed to make sense of the high rates of non-infectious conditions like diabetes within certain communities, similar processes are at play. For example, the fatalism that spreads within the Appalachian community, the *New York Times* article addressed above seems to indicate, transforms members of the community (like the "cantankerous diabetic" John Johnson) into exemplars who fail to take responsibility for their own health—and thus do not deserve governmental help. Well-documented in contexts of communicable diseases, the idea extends also to contexts of diabetes and other so-called lifestyle diseases that "cultural beliefs and practices [transform] individual bodies into natural bearers of disease" (Briggs and Mantini-Briggs 2003: 9). Human value comes to be articulated in terms of economic costs. "Failure" to live up to what has been termed "sanitary citizenship" (Briggs 2003; Briggs and Mantini-Briggs 2003) transforms the carriers of a disease into entities that cost more than they are worth, that come to be seen as expendable, as not deserving the benefits of citizenship. And once "contaminating" forces are understood to be *contagious*, it becomes easier to justify engaging with "contaminated" individuals, cultures, and communities as tangible threats to the greater good, as things that needs to be defended against, as things that will not be missed when they are gone.

Sadly, the COVID-19 pandemic that has served as significant backdrop while I have written this essay reveals some of the logical consequences that play out when discourses of contamination converge with discourses of contagion. Given that the root metaphor of contamination has become so naturalized in how diabetes is currently characterized, it is perhaps not at all surprising how it has manifested itself in the wake of the devastation wrought by the highly infectious SARS-CoV-2. I have encountered people asserting that the virus is not dangerous to young, healthy people, that the virus is only dangerous to the elderly and to those with pre-existing conditions like asthma, heart disease, and diabetes (with the implication that people who fall within these categories are somehow expendable). Once again, human value comes to be articulated in terms of economic costs.

I have seen people calling into question the validity of the mounting death count for COVID-19, referring to the prevalence of pre-existing conditions like diabetes as evidence that these bodies were already contaminated, already "spoiled," so to speak, on a trajectory toward death that preceded their encounters with the novel coronavirus. And as it has become clear that there are disproportionate rates of infection, hospitalization, and death among people of color due to the novel coronavirus (among populations that also experience disproportionate rates of diabetes and its complications), these discourses of contamination (as we so often witness in both the past and the present) converge with discourses of race that similarly work to naturalize boundaries between those who *do* and *do not* deserve the full benefits of citizenship and the recognition of one's value and dignity. In short, marking the bodies of the dead as already contaminated—even before they were infected with the virus—has worked to mark some COVID-19 deaths as less tragic than others, and to downplay the scale of the tragedy as a whole. Though, of course, the tragedy of these deaths is in fact exacerbated by the insidious intertwining of the widespread contagion of the novel coronavirus and the "contagion of stigma" (Goldstein and Shuman 2016: 4) always already attached to bodies deemed not only expendable, but threatening to the greater good.

As Emily Martin tells us, it is important to wake up sleeping metaphors in order not only to become "aware of their implications" but also "to rob them of their power to naturalize our social conventions" (1991: 501). Attending to their different implications for different types of racialized and classed bodies, I would add that looking closely at these metaphors also helps us understand the broader hierarchies of power shaping the consequences of the various forms of communicability (Briggs 2005) we encounter in our lives at the individual level, the community level, and where these two domains inevitably intersect.

References

Bock, Sheila. 2012. Contextualization, Reflexivity, and the Study of Diabetes-Related Stigma. *Journal of Folklore Research* 49 (2): 153–178.

Boero, Natalie. 2007. All the News That's Fat to Print: The American "Obesity Epidemic" and the Media. *Qualitative sociology* 30 (1): 41–60.

———. 2009. Fat Kids, Working Moms, and the Epidemic of Obesity Race, Class, and Mother-Blame. *The Fat Studies Reader*: 113–119. https://doi.org/10.18574/9780814777435-015.

Briggs, Charles L. 2003. Why Nation-States and Journalists Can't Teach People to Be Healthy: Power and Pragmatic Miscalculation in Public Discourses on Health. *Medical Anthropology Quarterly* 17 (3): 287–321.

———. 2005. Communicability, Racial Discourse, and Disease. *Annual Review of Anthropology* 34: 269–291.

Briggs, Charles L., and Clara Mantini-Briggs. 2003. *Stories in the Time of Cholera: Racial Profiling during a Medical Nightmare*. Berkeley and Los Angeles: University of California Press.

Broom, Dorothy, and Andrea Whittaker. 2004. Controlling Diabetes, Controlling Diabetics: Moral Language in the Management of Diabetes Type 2. *Social Science & Medicine* 58 (11): 2371–2382.

drake. 2017. Bad Behavior and Other Viruses: Bad Habits are Contagious. *Flashionista*, September 18. http://flashionista.com/bad-behavior-and-other-viruses/.

Eckholm, Erik. 2006. Medicaid Plan Prods Patients Toward Health. *New York Times*, December 1.

Farley, Audrey. 2019. Against Medical Advice: Priscilla White and Diabetic Pregnancy. *Lady Science*. https://www.ladyscience.com/features/priscilla-white-diabetic-pregnancy.

Foy, Marjorie Elvin. 2013. *"Our Objective Wasn't to Belittle People's Behavior": The History of Gestational Diabetes, 1921–1991*. PhD Diss: The University of North Carolina at Greensboro.

Gibson, Margaret F. 2018. Subtle Neglect and Yuckiness: Queerness, Disability, and Contagion in Mother Narratives. *Feminist Formations* 30 (1): 117–140.

Goffman, Erving. 1963. *Stigma: Notes on the Management of Spoiled Identity*. New York: Simon & Schuster, Inc.

Goldstein, Diane E. 2004. *Once Upon a Virus: AIDS Legends and Vernacular Risk Perception*. Logan: Utah State University Press.

Goldstein, Diane E. and Amy Shuman. "Introduction: The Stigmatized Vernacular: Where Reflexivity Meets Untellability." In The Stigmatized Vernacular: Where Reflexivity Meets Untellability, eds. Goldstein, Diane E. and Amy Shuman. Bloomington: Indiana University Press, 2016, 1-11.

Hamilton, David R. 2011. Are Healthy (And Unhealthy) Habits Contagious? *HuffPost Life*, May 29. https://www.huffpost.com/entry/health-social-networks_b_867433.

"History of Eugenics Resource Guide". *Disability Studies—University of Washington*. https://disabilitystudies.washington.edu/history-eugenics-resource-guide. Accessed 1 April 2021.

Hufford, David. 1991. AIDS, Culture, and Authority. In *Talking AIDS: Interdisciplinary Perspectives on Acquired Immune Deficiency Syndrome*, ed. Diane E. Goldstein, 7–22. ISER Research and Policy Papers. St. John's, Nfld.: Institute for Social and Economic Research.

Kitta, Andrea. 2019. *The Kiss of Death: Contagion, Contamination, and Folklore*. Logan: Utah State University Press.

Kraut, Alan M. 1994. *Silent Travelers: Germs, Genes, and the "Immigrant Menace"*. Baltimore, MD: Johns Hopkins University Press.

Martin, Emily. 1991. The Egg and the Sperm: How Science has Constructed a Romance Based on Stereotypical Male-Female Roles. *Signs: Journal of Women in Culture and Society* 16 (3): 485–501.

Mitchell, Peta. 2014. *Contagious Metaphor*. London: Bloomsbury.

O'Brien, Gerald. 1999. Protecting the Social Body: The Use of the Organism Metaphor in Fighting the 'Menace of the Feeble-Minded'. *Mental Retardation* 37: 188–200.

———. 2003. People with Cognitive Disabilities: The Argument from Marginal Cases and Social Work Ethics. *Social Work* 48: 331–337.

———. 2011. Anchors on the Ship of Progress and Weeds in the Human Garden: Objectivist Rhetoric in American Eugenic Writings. *Disability Studies Quarterly* 31 (3). https://dsq-sds.org/article/view/1668/1603.

Olsen, Erik. 2006. Bad Blood: The Diabetes Problem. *New York Times*, January 5. https://www.nytimes.com/video/nyregion/1194817098447/bad-blood-the-diabetes-problem.html.

Servitje, Lorenzo, and Kari Nixon. 2016. The Making of a Modern Endemic: An Introduction. In *Endemic*, ed. K. Nixon and L. Servitje, 1–17. London: Palgrave Macmillan.

Siebers, Tobin. 2013. Disability and the Theory of Complex Embodiment—For Identity Politics in a New Register. *The Disability Studies Reader* 4: 278–297.

Sontag, Susan. 1989. *AIDS and Its Metaphors*. New York: Farrar, Straus and Giroux.

Sinnenberg, Lauren, Christina Mancheno, Frances K. Barg, David A. Asch, Christy Lee Rivard, Emma Horst-Martz, Alison Buttenheim, Lyle Ungar, and Raina Merchant. 2018. Content Analysis of Metaphors about Hypertension and Diabetes on Twitter: Exploratory Mixed-Methods Study. *JMIR Diabetes* 3 (4): e11177.

Wald, Patricia. 2008. *Contagious: Cultures, Carriers, and the Outbreak Narrative*. Durham, NC: Duke University Press.

Wald, Priscilla, Nancy Tomes, and Lisa Lync. 2002. Introduction: Contagion and Culture. *American Literary History* 14 (4): 617–624.

Yergeau, M. Remi. 2020. Cassandra Isn't Doing the Robot: On Risky Rhetorics and Contagious Autism. *Rhetoric Society Quarterly* 50 (3): 212–221.

Please Don't Pet: Reflections on Life with My Diabetes Alert Dog

Taylor Johnson

The Incident at the San Angelo Hotel

I noticed the hotel desk attendant frowning at me as soon as I walked in the door. After making the long drive from Austin to San Angelo, I didn't have the energy to think about what may have been bothering her. I needed to check-in into my room so I could try to relax and double check that I was ready for graduation tomorrow. "Hi! My name is Taylor Johnson and I just need to check in.," I said, forcing a cheerful tone. "You can't have a dog in the hotel," the attendant—and hotel manager, I later found out—spat out. "I'm sorry ma'am I should've explained that she's a service dog who performs medical alerts as soon as I walked in," I explained, hopeful that the information with a touch of humility would diffuse the situation. Unfortunately, my explanation didn't suffice as the woman continued shaking her head "No" and loudly exclaiming that animals were not allowed in her hotel for any reason. This back and forth lasted over an hour and ended with me, my mom, and my sister frustratedly crying angry

T. Johnson (✉)
Austin, TX, USA

B. C. Frazer, H. R. Walker (eds.), *(Un)doing Diabetes: Representation, Disability, Culture*, Palgrave Studies in Science and Popular Culture, https://doi.org/10.1007/978-3-030-83110-3_12

tears. There were no other hotel rooms available in San Angelo. So, it seemed as if I was going to spend the night before graduating with my Master's degree sleeping in our car. This treatment was infuriating, and I was trying everything I could. In a last-ditch effort I called the owner, Kim, of the service dog company, Lonestar Diabetic Alert Dogs, that trained my service dog, Claire. I was hopeful that, on my behalf, she could clarify that what the hotel manager was doing was illegal in a way that would be understood. I was also hoping Kim would be willing to ask questions about how to file a complaint in this particular unfolding situation. Kim had mediated situations like this in the past with business owners who don't quite understand the protections afforded by the American Disabilities Act. And she did call and try to ensure I was not being discriminated against on the basis of disability. That was four years ago. I still do not know exactly what was said on that phone call, but another hotel employee came outside to give us our room key and we were able to stay for the night. Kim later shared with me that the hotel manager told her that she wasn't to blame for me being "too stupid to manage my diabetes"—an ableist slur that took me back to being a scared teenager in my endocrinologist's office and years of struggling to manage my diabetes without support.

Contextualizing the Incident

As much as I would like to believe that the hotel manager was just having a bad day and that she would have had the same reaction to anyone who walked into the hotel, I am not naive. I am a larger bodied Black woman who has lived in rural Texas most of my life. I often reflect on how that conversation would have gone if I had been lighter skinned and or skinnier. It's also not lost on me that the hotel manager only listened after speaking with another White woman, who to the manager's knowledge, was also non-disabled. My word wasn't enough. I wasn't trusted to represent myself and the accommodations I needed.

It is impossible to separate race from any discussion of ableism, othering, or diabetes. "Too stupid to manage my diabetes" is a statement loaded with stereotypes diabetics are constantly pushing back against. In my experience, most people don't have sympathy for diabetics especially Black ones because they assume that diabetes is something we have done to ourselves. Some people will claim that stigma is common to all diabetics but I would argue, and there is a good amount of evidence, not only that the history of diabetes is racialized, but also that the vast majority of negative stereotypes about diabetics are connected with race (Bock 2012; Hatch 2016; Keval 2016; Tuchman 2020). Fat, lazy, uneducated, poor, and eating "bad foods" are all things unequivocally associated with Black people. I mention these associations because they help to conceptualize the experiences I've had with my service dog.

"But You Don't Look Sick": Ableism, Accessibility, and Othering

"Invisible illness" is the umbrella that diabetes is often described as falling under. Invisibility is a misleading descriptor, though, because the episodic nature and available technologies of diabetes means invisibility is a choice, often informed by privilege (Samuels 2003). Diabetes can be hidden, but only by those who have not developed apparent complications like blindness and amputations. And small wearable diabetes devices like insulin pumps and continuous glucose monitors. These devices, on the market only for those who can afford them, can be easily hidden in or by clothing. While I have never made any efforts to hide my diabetes, because it is a safety hazard to be a Black person in America and have an illness that can occasionally look like being intoxicated, it was never as visible as it is now that I have Claire. Claire is a small Golden Retriever. She attracts attention wherever we go. She is trained to alert me to high or low blood sugars outside of a specific range, by sitting and putting her paw on me. Claire's coming with me everywhere I go has been a constant test of my self-advocacy skills as well as my tolerance for being visibly disabled.

Every time I enter a public place with Claire, I silently brace myself for the stares and questions. I almost always wear headphones while out because it's the easiest to avoid, what can only be described as, harassment. Headphones, however, do not stop people from getting in my personal space without my consent. The worst offenders are the men who refuse to take "No" for an answer, try to pet Claire, whistle or even make kissy noises at us. All of these behaviors are distracting and scary for Claire, and create a dangerous situation for me. I try to explain this to people who approach us unabashedly. Usually I say something like "*I am an insulin dependent diabetic. Claire's job is to monitor my blood sugar. When you distract her, that puts me in very real danger.*" That explanation is often met, though, with sheepish looks and even protests about how diabetes is not something service dogs are for. I also get a decent amount of unsolicited diet and workout advice given with the intention of getting me to see that Claire can "just be a puppy" and I can "cure" my diabetes. Again, stigma and stereotypes are baked into all of these interactions. The "fat, lazy diabetic" archetype looms over most conversations about Claire. For example, I've even been asked, "You need a dog to tell you eat less?" No, I need a service animal because I have hypoglycemia unawareness and don't want to die in my sleep. I need a service animal because glucose monitors have an acceptable margin error and my blood sugar often drops faster than they can read. I need a service animal because she makes diabetes a little more bearable. It's exhausting to defend this justification to people over and over again.

In the years since the San Angelo hotel incident, I have had short term rental listings cancelled, been denied ride-sharing services, and lost job opportunities because I have a service dog. It is demoralizing, and resonates to me as a testament to just how much society has little interest in making things accessible for people with disabilities if it inconveniences non-disabled folks at all...even if the inconvenience is mostly imagined. For example, the most common accessibility pushback that I get from non-disabled people is that they will have to clean up after Claire or think that she will behave like their household pets and be disruptive. Both assumptions are completely untrue. As a service dog handler, it is my responsibility to ensure Claire is always groomed and is as unobtrusive as possible and if I don't—it is well within someone's right to deny access. Furthermore, when we are accommodated, it often comes at the expense of our privacy or dignity. It is almost as if we are compelled to exaggerate our pain and suffering to justify every specific need we have. Surprisingly, outsiders are not the only ones who demand such justifications, but also my fellow diabetics.

Diabetics and Diabetic Alert Dogs

When another insulin dependent diabetic at a coffee shop said to me, "Oh, you just wanted a fancy dog." after noticing Claire and my insulin pump, I was taken aback. I had only interacted with other diabetic service dog owners since I had gotten Claire so it never occurred to me that other diabetics would see having a service dog for diabetes as extravagant or odd. Or worse, that it is an unnecessary luxury given the amount of technology available to manage diabetes. It was truly a jarring experience.

Truth be told, I already feel like an outsider in diabetes spaces due to my race and being misdiagnosed with Type 2 diabetes as a teenager. Based on the representations of diabetes I see on social media and in-person Type 1-specific events I don't share many of the typical Type 1/insulin dependent diabetic experiences. For example, a part of the normal "getting to know each other" conversation between Type 1 diabetics is sharing diagnosis stories and how long they have lived with diabetes. I have a three yearlong diagnosis saga and no real answer for how long I have been diabetic—it differs by 2–3 years depending on which diagnosis we're talking about. I have also never been in DKA, gone to diabetes camp, and didn't see an insulin pump until I had been diagnosed for over a decade. And it doesn't help that I am Black and diabetes communities, online and off, are predominantly White. My interactions with other diabetics with service dogs has always been very affirming and one of the few places I really felt like I fit in the diabetes world. However, it can be difficult with diabetics who do not have service animals because it feels as if they are constantly testing me and Claire. It's no secret that diabetes is expensive so people will ask questions like "Well how did YOU afford a service dog if you think diabetes supplies are expensive?" Or they'll question why Claire isn't alerting them or saying that her range is too high and that they prefer to keep their blood sugar much lower than I do. It's at best a not-so-subtle way of telling me that they don't approve of how I'm managing my diabetes, and at worst semi-intentional exclusion based on assumptions. So, even from within the community, I face the stereotype that being a larger bodied black woman with diabetes must mean I am uneducated and unwilling to manage my diabetes without Claire's assistance. That is, even members of my own community read the accommodation that Claire provides me as legitimizing the racist stereotypes ascribed to my physical body by society.

The Stigma Is Everywhere

I work in mental health education. Specifically, I teach classes that teach strategies for wellness and promote awareness of mental health resources, especially for those experiencing mental health challenges. I enjoy the work, but find within it contradictions. One of the phrases my colleagues throw around a lot is that "We should treat mental health the way we do physical illnesses." To my understanding, they mean that there should be no stigma around struggling with, seeking support for, and having conversations about mental health. As a person with a chronic incurable physical illness, I don't have the heart to tell them that the support systems for physical illnesses are not a great point of comparison. From my experience and point of view, there is a lot of stigma attached to most chronic illnesses. Ableism, racism, and the capitalist structures that support them permeate every part of how we define and experience health. They dictate who we, as a society, offer support to and the quality of that support.

I am incredibly privileged. I have an insulin pump, a continuous glucose monitor, and a service dog. I know how to systematically research treatment options and seek out diabetes education and support. However, I also have experienced discrimination from non-disabled people, other diabetic/disabled people, and medical providers. To non-disabled people, the most basic of accommodations for people with disabilities outlined in the American Disabilities Act (ADA) probably seem like enough. From where I stand, they must not know or care that these basic protections are often ignored or violated and then ignored. Even when the media highlights instances of ADA violations (e.g. by institutions of higher education, businesses and organizations, public entities, etc.), the general public often brush off as individual bad people doing unkind things. To use a colloquialism, rather than seeing ADA violations as systemic repetitions of ableist structures, they see it as "a few bad apples".

In reality, the non-disabled world prioritizes their convenience and profits over our access to an equitable life, over and over again because disabled people aren't considered as important as non-disabled folks. On, what I would consider a small scale, deprioritization and discrimination looks like distracting a service animal or denying a rideshare to a disabled person with an assistance animal. On a larger scale, it looks like telling those of us with disabilities to stay home during a pandemic or die so that the economy and non-disabled folks can carry on business as usual. It is in this environment that Claire and I carry on, challenging "business as usual" when we can, and surviving when we can't.

References

Bock, S. 2012. Contextualization, Reflexivity, and the Study of Diabetes-Related Stigma. *Journal of Folklore Research: An International Journal of Folklore and Ethnomusicology* 49 (2): 153–178.

Hatch, A.R. 2016. *Blood Sugar: Racial Pharmacology and Food Justice in Black America*. U of Minnesota Press.

Keval, Harshad (2016). *Health, Ethnicity and Diabetes: Racialised Constructions of "Risky" South Asian Bodies*. Palgrave Macmillan. https://doi.org/10.1057/978-1-137-45703-5.

Samuels, E.J. 2003. My Body, My Closet: Invisible Disability and the Limits of Coming-Out Discourse. *GLQ: A Journal of Lesbian and Gay Studies* 9 (1): 233–255.

Tuchman, A.M. 2020. *Diabetes: A History of Race and Disease*. Yale University Press.

How To Wear (And Hide) Your Insulin Pump: Managing Device Connectedness With Gendered Bodies Online

Stephen Horrocks

In July 2020, actress Andrea Deck—owner and content producer for the YouTube channel She's Diabetic—uploaded a video titled, "How I Hide My Insulin Pump." As one of a handful of influential YouTubers producing explicitly Type 1 Diabetes-oriented content, Andrea reached out to her followers earlier that summer to gauge their interest in topics for discussion in future videos. She received many responses, "mainly women," she notes, asking her to detail "where I sort of store, and kind of hide my insulin pump with different outfits." Though she says up-front that in most cases she just clips it to her waist band where it is "out and about," she acknowledges her followers' desire to conceal the device depending on the context. "I totally know what you mean," she affirms, "when you are wearing a nice outfit, or maybe you're going on a date or something like

S. Horrocks (✉)
Purdue University, West Lafayette, IN, USA
e-mail: stephenhorrocks.amst@gmail.com

B. C. Frazer, H. R. Walker (eds.), *(Un)doing Diabetes: Representation, Disability, Culture*, Palgrave Studies in Science and Popular Culture, https://doi.org/10.1007/978-3-030-83110-3_13

that, and you don't want your pump to be front and center—TOTALLY get it" (She's Diabetic 2020b).

Discussions of fashion decision-making and insulin pump placement have been playing out on YouTube for nearly a decade. Even if in limited numbers, they serve as a visual/virtual sounding board for people attempting to navigate various cultural practices alongside the constraints of their chronic illness. For people with Type 1 diabetes, and some with other forms of Diabetes as well, insulin injection is a regularized (and medically necessary) aspect of daily life. Enacting those therapies multiple times per day can be exhausting and overwhelming, and over the past two decades insulin pumps have been established as the standard of care among prescribing endocrinologists to aid in making injections take less time- and attention-consuming (though it should be noted that insulin pumps' significant up-front and disposable supply costs make access to their use structurally unequal, often barring poor and some middle-class patient-users due to insurance-related hurdles). Because they must be connected to the body—usually somewhere on the abdomen, and often near the belly button—insulin pumps are physically front-and-center in ways that must be negotiated all day, every day.

Perhaps even more significant in the context of both YouTube and social constructions of gender, however, insulin pumps make diabetes technologically visible in new ways as well. Though the embodied realities of living with Type 1 diabetes frame nearly every aspect of one's life to varying degrees, Diabetes itself is not outwardly visible to those who are unfamiliar with its nuances. As individuals switch to treatment regimens such as insulin pump therapy and continuous glucose monitoring, however, the medical devices at the center of those systems remain on and near the body at all times—a presence that visually and materially signifies their health status in unprecedented ways. This new techno-visibility requires navigation through dominant/dominating systems of what Robert McRuer (2006) calls compulsory able-bodiedness, a process that weighs disproportionately upon the bodies of women, who must also navigate visual and material cultures of patriarchy.

In this chapter I perform a narrative and visual analysis of Andrea Deck's video "How I Hide My Insulin Pump" as an example of the several-dozen YouTube videos devoted explicitly to representing the practice of "wearing" and "hiding" the insulin pump.[1] By examining this video through the

[1] Between 2014 and 2020 I compiled an archive of approximately sixty YouTube videos produced for the purpose of demonstrating how to "wear" and/or "hide" an insulin pump.

lens of Crip Theory and Feminist Technoscience, I situate these gendered Type 1 diabetes cultural practices as simultaneously reinforcing and resisting problematic visions of embodied normalcy—gendered, racialized, and (dis)abled—social standards that are regulated through both biomedical intervention and US cultural representations of gender. For Deck and the thousands of people interacting through her various social media accounts, YouTube functions as a hub for negotiating cultural decision-making among the constraints placed on women with Type 1 diabetes, particularly

The earliest of these, as far as I can identify, was uploaded in 2008 by the user 1HappyDiabetic. Titled "How to wear your insulin pump in a Cell phone case," this video (and the channel more generally, which was active until 2014) is one of a proportionally small number of Type 1 diabetes how-to videos produced by and rhetorically oriented toward a masculine-presenting man (https://www.youtube.com/watch?v=prGeTZcC78Y).

The majority of these videos, however, were made by feminine-presenting women and detailed a variety of tips and products that would aid the viewer in securing an insulin pump on their person while wearing culturally stereotypical feminine clothing items. Over the past two-to-three years there has been an increase in the number of content creators specifically devoted to the life and needs of people with Type 1 diabetes, a small number of whom have built their YouTube presence around an "influencer" aesthetic that carries particular gendered/racialized/sexualized/classed/able-bodied connotations on its own. Some of these videos include:

"Where to Wear the Insulin Pump!" by DiabeticDanica (2012, https://www.youtube.com/watch?v=WYc-NBnkviQ);

"EASIEST WAY to HIDE and WEAR your insulin pump w/ dresses" by ukikawasaki (2013, https://www.youtube.com/watch?v=FGh99Oshs8s);

"Places to Put Your Insulin Pump" by TypeOneTeen (2014, video removed);

"The Reason my insulin pump died….and where to put your pump" by imtype.01 (2015, https://www.youtube.com/watch?v=rwrjVIhYZVI);

"HOW TO WEAR AN INSULIN PUMP WITH A DRESS!" by Michelle Lord (2017, https://www.youtube.com/watch?v=adsFSEUF74I);

"Pump cases and boy shorts: ways to wear your t:slim (and other insulin pumps)" by nicky ghaleb (2019, https://www.youtube.com/watch?v=wDjoqRfTi_I);

"SUMMER OUTFITS 2019 // How I wear my t:slim insulin pump!" by Michelle Lord, (2019, https://www.youtube.com/watch?v=5KFCCT49Lcc);

"WAYS TO WEAR A DIABETIC PUMP WITH DRESSES" by Megan Dang (2020, https://www.youtube.com/watch?v=xFO5brJKDG0);

"Top 3 Best Places to Hide Your Insulin Pump!" by Really REL with Ariel (2020, https://www.youtube.com/watch?v=R_g5AL07O6I);

"How to hide an insulin pump| Come nascondere il microinfusore é le varie zone di infusione" by Laura and Sabina (2020, https://www.youtube.com/watch?v=oVhqYhoB28Y).

in the United States. "Wearing" and "hiding" the pump are socially compulsory in part because the visuality/visibility of disability and chronic illness places people and bodies outside the bounds of hegemonic normalcy, and thereby outside the bounds of desirability. As I will show, fashion(ing) emerges as a central practice in managing insulin therapy and reconstructing its social invisibility, thereby allowing individuals such as Deck discursively back into the relative social safety of the visible normal. In a Goffmanian sense, fashion(ing) conceals Deck's medical devices that signal a stigmatized Diabetic/chronically ill body (to her and potentially to others, whether others decode that in practice or not), and thereby functions as a vessel for her to pass as able-bodied and not-chronically-ill. Through this process, Deck can inhabit the privileged social position she otherwise enjoys on account of her race, class, size, otherwise able-bodiedness, and conformity with cultural standards of beauty. And as I will demonstrate herein, as Deck's creative digital media practices attempt to normalize the social visibility of Type 1 diabetes in public, those very practices often rely on the continued stigmatization of the *optical* visibility of Type 1 diabetes and chronic illness more broadly.

Framing Pump-Wearing with Type 1 Diabetes Expertise[2]

"Hello, guys!" With this medium-defining sign-on phrase, Andrea Deck welcomes new and returning YouTube viewers to her video titled, "How I Hide My Insulin Pump" (She's Diabetic 2020b). According to the video's description, it is one she has "wanted to make for a while," and that subscribers have requested "quite frequently": a demonstration of where she puts her insulin pump while wearing different types of outfits. Deck began producing video content during the summer of 2018, describing the channel in her first video as a forum for "[her] documentation of what

[2] Though I do not have the same embodied expertise as Deck and others diagnosed with Type 1 diabetes, it was established as an ever-present aspect of my life long before I started thinking about it academically. My partner of over fifteen years was diagnosed with Type 1 diabetes at age 9, and I have been as devoted to the needs/realities associated that chronic illness (as well as the devices involved in its treatment) as I have to my partner's needs/realities more broadly. Over the past six years I have devoted my professional energies to understanding the social and cultural life and worlds of Type 1 diabetes and its networks of treatment devices, and both of these play a significant role in how I conduct the analysis here in this chapter.

it's like being a Type 1 Diabetic," and detailing successful (and often unsuccessful) practices she has enacted since her diagnosis in 2001. Alongside the mashup of vlog/how-to content that function as the primary focus of her videos, she aims to manage the comments section as a virtual commons for interaction among fellow Type 1 diabetes YouTube users on the subject of "being Diabetics, and also just being human beings" (She's Diabetic 2018). Having a virtual community space where people with Type 1 diabetes can relate with and support one another is important for many in the United States and globally. Though in-person diabetes communities and support spaces can be effective resources for a variety of social and medical needs, utilizing them relies heavily on individuals' ability to access the physical locations where meetings are held. Virtual spaces, on the other hand, offer asynchronicity and increased accessibility in terms of location and cost—though internet access is layered with its own problems of unequal access as well—providing alternate means for producing human connections with others to whom they can relate. The drive behind Deck's pivot toward broader connections as "human beings," however, is a bit opaquer and deploys universalizing language that does much less rhetorical work than the words make it appear.

Classically trained in acting at the London Academy of Music and Dramatic Arts, Deck boasts a number of high-profile film, television, and video game credits including Showtime's *Homeland*, Netflix's *The Crown*, and Creative Assembly's *Alien Isolation*—a side of her professional persona rarely discussed throughout her forty-five videos on the channel to date (She's Diabetic 2020a). That training does, however, appear to influence her online presence in the form of clear enunciation and effective oration written into most videos, as well as her delivery with a believable, conversational tone oriented to an imagined audience.

Deck enters the discussion at the nexus of device placement and clothing decisions by introducing herself. "My name is Andrea," she begins, "and I have been a Type 1 Diabetic for over nineteen years." Her personal introduction is her hook, a YouTube-standard rhetorical move intended to connect with viewers and keep them watching ("10 Fundamentals of a Creative Strategy" 2020). What is particularly interesting about Andrea's hook, however, is the type of information she leans on to do so, which demonstrates her authority to speak to the issues surrounding insulin pump placement in the process. Rather than leading with a clothing-related content teaser (or even the insulin pump), Andrea immediately deploys her Type 1 diabetes diagnosis and her personal connection to the illness. At least in this context, Deck makes the decision to position herself directly within the stigmatizing "discrediting information of self," to use Erving Goffman's term, rather than concealing its "shameful differentness" (Goffman 1963, 42, 10). Foregrounding Type 1 diabetes in this way complicates assumptions about both the function of its related stigma and its relative invisibility; the fluctuations of blood glucose levels typical of Type 1 diabetes experiences and insulin regimens are only expressed outwardly through their symptoms and/or the devices used to track and treat them. Thus, by centering Diabetes in this video and her channel more broadly, Deck makes it *discursively* visible in the process of making it optically visible online.

To add gravity to the deployment of her Type 1 diabetes, Deck constructs credibility by calling attention to the amount of time she has lived in diagnosis. Nineteen years of experience in any endeavor can glean much in the way of tacit knowledge, but especially so in activities requiring focused and deliberate repetition (Duckworth et al. 2011). In the context of a chronic illness such as Type 1 diabetes—requiring almost constant attention, decision-making, and therapeutic acts all day, every day—the repetition of processes and practices spanning two decades produces radically unique sets of expertise. As Deck and others enact those processes upon the body, expertise and embodiment become inextricably intertwined. Though largely unintentional and limited by some factors discussed later in this chapter, Deck orates a key aspect of Critical Disability Studies by invoking this time-expertise matrix.

Time, Alison Kafer (2013) argues, frames not only medical/cultural definitions of disability, but how people are oriented in relation to it. The confluence of Deck's time in diagnosis and her Type 1 diabetes expertise produces a space for negotiating what Kafer calls "crip time," a radical reconfiguring of disabled people's relationships to the dominant imaginaries that deny their worthiness for existence, past, present, and future (26–28). Whereas dominant normative cultural understandings of disability and chronic illness code those years following diagnosis in opposition to the still-desired, "lost" able-bodiedness of pre-diagnosis, this subtle deployment of Type 1 diabetes crip time casts those years as inherently productive. Deck does not engage her therapeutic technologies solely on the basis of medical need, though it certainly remains the central compelling force in their use. Here too she acts as an agent negotiating the constraints of device use from a position of embodied knowledges and expertise, a position only constructed/able because use is medically and socially compelled. To paraphrase Kafer's complication of "the cyborg," Deck is not an expert simply due to her proximity to the technology; her expertise is political. Her expertise is rooted in the ways she navigates structures of health, gender, disability, class, and race among others (104–106).

And here I return to Deck's language that began this chapter, as it gestures toward many of the intersecting systems of social inequality demarcated by the "tips," "tricks," and "hacks" she outlines throughout the video. A majority of requests for this guide to wearing and hiding her insulin pump were made by women asking for insights into practical concerns of using an insulin pump while dressed in culturally conforming women's clothing. Given the significant differences in how gender is inscribed in/on articles of clothing using markers of size, shape, drape, style, and material, this may not come as a surprise to many. These gendered cultural norms associated with fashion and clothing make the use and placement of medical devices such as insulin pumps more complicated for gender-conforming women and feminine-expressing people than men and masculine-expressing people. The device, as a material object, must be placed somewhere, and storage space among articles of clothing is inconsistent. Pockets on women's pants are considerably smaller than those designed into men's pants (when they are sewn in at all), too small to fit any of the most widely used smartphones in the US (Diehm and Thomas 2018). Dresses usually lack pocket space as well, and each design's cut, drape, and flow restrict access to different alternative locations such as waistbands and bra straps. Jumpers and rompers often introduce combinations of these and related issues. The silhouette and profile of feminine-gendered clothing are frequently constructed around an external (coded-male) perspective of the clothed body that often cannot account for "other" objects such as medical devices connected to the body.

Deck hints at her own desire and/or preference to avoid the device's visible presence among her clothing. She doesn't want the pump "front and center" during social situations where certain cultural performances are being enacted (like going on a date, as she suggests). These moments of her video provide an entry point to explore the ways in which her technical expertise—like that of other pump users—does not exist in a vacuum. Not only is she an insulin pump and Diabetes expert, but a tacit expert in navigating the social realities of gender (and, importantly, of middle-class whiteness) as well. It is within this framework, where practical need meets cultural influence, that Andrea Deck outlines her tips for how to best hide one's insulin pump.

Repurposing the Waistband as Device Storage

In organizing her ideas about how to hide her insulin pump, Deck explains that she decided it would be advantageous to display some variety of clothing style and form, and to conduct an informal compare/contrast discussion thereof. In that pursuit, she cut together five video sequences while wearing five different outfits to provide a visual guide to her most common storage/concealment practices. Before cutting to those video segments, however, Deck notes that in a vast majority of cases, her pump is clipped to the waistband of her pants, "and it's out and about, pretty much" (She's Diabetic 2020b). With the exception of outfits that do not have them, Deck describes and displays a preference for waistbands as accessible and comfortable locations to place the pump device throughout the course of a routine day.

After detailing a well-hidden accessory with her first outfit (discussed later in this chapter), Deck demonstrates her waistband-clipping technique on a black, flowing, strappy jumpsuit with a triangular cutout in the midsection. In lauding this jumpsuit, Deck refers to it as "my most Diabetes-friendly jumpsuit," and the cutout is the key feature. By cutting out the front, designers put together a jumpsuit with an accessible waistband where Deck clips her pump, an act she excitedly describes as "very, very convenient." Part of the reason why the waistband works so well in the context of device use requires a return to the intended purpose of the pump object itself: to inject insulin as needed. Bolus injections, made manually to balance carbohydrate consumption any time an individual eats food, must be performed by interfacing with the pump. If the device was tucked beneath a jumpsuit without a front cutout, for example, accessing the controls when it is needed could be quite difficult and even obstruct its use altogether. By wearing a piece with an open waistband, Deck applies her experiential knowledge related to clothing and device access directly to her clothing choice, making room for similar modes of disrupting the constraints of broader fashion trends. "I pretty much live in this in the summer. [laughs] Let's be honest."

Much of the convenience of this jumpsuit, however, is wrapped up in the financial and social factors that allow individuals to obtain and publicly wear it in the first place. The primary reason this piece serves Deck's purpose so effectively is the strategically placed cutout in the midsection. Though a wide range of jumpers could provide the type of comfort she describes, they serve no pump-related purpose if they do not provide easy access to the waistband (i.e. if they do not also feature an abdomen cutout—which the vast majority do not). The limits of fashionable and exclusive clothing such as this (which is no longer for sale at the time of this publication) call into question the efficacy of this type of display for the purposes of advising viewers at all. What is more, as Deck outlines in the video's description, this outfit combines pieces from Urban Outfitters, American Apparel, Lululemon, and Birkenstock, again raising question about who Deck envisions the audience will be.

Following her discussion of waistband storage in/on her jumpsuit, Deck cuts to a segment on pump placement while wearing workout gear. Comprised of black Lycra leggings, a black loose-fitting tank top, and a sports bra, the storage capacity of Deck's third outfit is once again limited by its lack of pockets and tight profile—a material reality of gender's social imprint on clothing in most cases in the U.S. And yet, as with her last combination, the pants' waistband functions as the most stable and accessible location to clip her pump—two features particularly important during typical exercise activities where people and bodies move constantly and somewhat sporadically. Equally significant, however, is the extent to which this particular style can effectively hide the device—and by connection, the technological marker of embodied otherness that forces her to negotiate what Rosemarie Garland-Thomson refers to as the instability of her social normalcy (from "Roadkill Truths," in Brune et al. 2014, para. 8). "If you're the type of person that wants to, kind of, conceal more," she begins, "... I mean, you're in all black, and your pump's black... It all kind of washes into one" (She's Diabetic 2020b).

In this moment, as the discussion of accessibility and storing the insulin pump morphs into a focused discussion of concealing it, Deck enacts the type of flexibility required of disabled and chronically ill people to conform to culturally dominant conceptions of the body. In his widely influential book *Crip Theory: Cultural Signs of Queerness and Disability*, Robert McRuer (2006) analyzes the power structures involved in the normalizing discourses related sexuality and disability in the twenty-first century. Key to these embodied cultural standards today—systems of domination that he calls compulsory able-bodiedness—is their flexibility. "According to the flexible logic of neoliberalism," he argues, "all varieties of queerness—and, for that matter, all disabilities—are essentially temporary, appearing only when, and as long as, they are necessary." Which means those with disabilities and chronic diseases can be made visible when they are palatable ***enough*** to maintain comfort among the able-bodied, yet can be easily moved off of center stage when systemic discomfort arises (29). Whereas Goffman's (1963) notion of passing is hyper-specified to individual interactions and decision-making, McRuer's framing here makes it clear how largescale social systems are invested in compelling disabled people/bodies in and out of states of passing for the benefit of the unmarked normal (16).

Deck's ability to perform the fashioned process of her pump and clothing "wash[ing] into one," as she says, is highly dependent on the extent to which her body matches the intended silhouette of the exercise clothing she is demonstrating. Since bodies differ dramatically, and therefore the ways they match and/or contrast with the designed ideals of the clothing designers, that ability to blur her medical device among her clothing is not shared by all. Deck is thin, white, cisgender, and conforms to a number of embodied attributes culturally constructed within traditional standards of beauty. Her performance of those standards on-screen in the context of both medical device use and fashion(ing) further normalizes both those cultural standards themselves and their barriers-to-entry. In this moment the contingent boundaries of able-bodied normalcy for chronically ill people and bodies become increasingly visible and discriminating.

With her fourth pump-wearing outfit example, Deck dons a button-down denim shirt with black jeans, and as she alluded to at the beginning of the video, she once again claims the waistband as a primary storage space. "Because the shirt is long enough," she explains, as she tugs at the bottom of her shirt tails, "it kind of covers it. You can't really see it, so I feel pretty darn comfortable with it there." Though in context this statement seems to be a straightforward expression of physical comfort obtained by getting the always-on device out-of-the-way, "comfort" in the context of social and cultural practices that express aspects of one's identity can carry many different connotations. As McRuer (2006) outlined in the quoted text above, the comfortability of able-bodiedness is rooted in the ability to move out of sight that which does not fit social standards of normalcy. In a more colloquial sense: for the able-bodied, ignorance is bliss; passing as able-bodied can provide (brief) respite from the exhaustion of living with and treating chronic illness. But read at the intersection of gender and systemic sexism, that which produces comfortability in fashion and clothing often polices non-normative bodies, beauties, and practices at the same time. Finding comfort in "covering up" has some roots in Puritan and Victorian conceptions of gendered bodies as "dirty" or "fallen" in need of obscuring as not to sully the purity of others (i.e. men) (Reis 1995; Welter 1966). On the other hand, in the context of large-scale objectification and sexualization practices that put the bodies and lives of women disproportionately at risk of violence, the comfort of covering up can be a radical claim to one's own agency in resistance to those systems (Strelan and Hargreaves 2005; Tiggemann and Lynch 2001).

Lest we forget, however, the "covering up" that plays out in this video has to do with covering the medical device that simultaneously keeps Deck alive and outwardly signals to others that she lives with a major chronic illness (especially those who are already familiar with Type 1 diabetes and/or the pump itself). She not only covers the device from the view of others, but from her own. By hiding it she demonstrates her desire to pass as non-diabetic, as non-disabled, an act that highlights some of the larger implications of "desiring." As Kelly Fritsch (2015) has argued, desirability has always been reserved for the able-bodied, and gendered constructions of those boundaries overlay able-bodiedness with white middle-class heteronormativity (44, 48). Breaking away from those limits of desirability is complicated, in part because that conceptualized opposite of desiring disability entails a fear and disdain for the disability itself and the coding of the body/person as inherently undesirable (Kafer 2013, 28; Fritsch 2016, 11–12). As an upper/upper-middle class, thin, cis-het, white woman, Deck inhabits a position deeply invested in normativity and privilege—of desirability—and her desire to outwardly present as able-bodied is an attempt to quell the Type 1 diabetes threat thereto.

Pump Visibility and Techno-Medically Disrupted Fashion

Appropriately, in her efforts to cover the technological marker of medicalized difference attached to her body, Deck turns to other technologies of the body. Clothing, as a complex fabric of cultural practice itself, functions as a "technological fix" for the social fallout of medical device use (Rosner 2004). In the end, as Deck turns to one last outfit to demonstrate her wearing/hiding technique—a t-shirt and jeans—she once again mentions her use of the waistband. This time, however, she follows that by donning an extra clothing accessory to aid in securing the pump on her body and keeping it out of sight. “Here I’ve just thrown on a jacket,” she shrugs. “This is just something I will throw on often times because I’m just generally a cold person, but,” she says while putting up one finger, “it’s an excellent way to hide your pump.” After opening the jacket and showing her pump-free waistband, Deck reveals that her pump is stored in the outer pocket of her jacket.

Though this move seems like a small departure from the waistband-focused discussion that dominates most of the video, her decision to use a pocket on another item of clothing—one that drapes open and fits quite loosely on the abdomen—requires some irreversible modification that aid in the act of hiding the pump’s tubing. “Within my jacket, I’ve actually cut a little hole,” she says as she lightly touches the spot on the back of her pocket through which she has fed the tubing. The need and/or desire to create a material situation around the body that can obscure her technological markers of illness is powerful enough to all but require her to keep not only the pump, but the tubing out of her outfit’s silhouette. Tucking the tubing serves many purposes, most notably the desire to avoid having the tubing snagged on objects such as doorknobs, tearing infusion sets out of the abdomen. But Deck mentions no purpose for modifying her jacket other than keeping the device out of sight.

In deploying this and other objects as part of a broader effort to hide the insulin pump, she (possibly subconsciously) compiles and displays a tool kit which she uses to disrupt the optical visibility of her insulin pump through a discursive social visibility of Type 1 diabetes online. In her depictions of each of the five outfits in this video, Deck offers an alternative method for hiding the pump through the use of fanny packs and—in the case of outfit number one—an athletic ankle-strap pouch she used to conceal microphones on-sets. Each of these, like the jacket, are relatively minor additive accessories, but in each case visually replaces the insulin pump, a socially stigmatized on-body object, with a more socially acceptable on-body object. Though not a uniquely Type 1 diabetes aesthetic in and of itself, when understood as part of the larger system of the medicalization and material cultures of Type 1 diabetes, they take on new meanings specific to that space and experience.

As Aimi Hamraie and Kelly Fritsch (2019) argue in their “Crip Technoscience Manifesto,” “Disabled people are experts and designers of everyday life,” making and utilizing things to stake a claim in the inherent desirability of disabled life (2–3). Though, as I have just argued, Deck is invested in breaking down certain taboos related to displays of chronic illness in public, she relies on reinforcing others as a means of escaping some of the difficulties of having to be chronically "out" all the time. So while these wear-and-hide videos do attempt to normalize the *discussion* about Type 1 diabetes, the *visible materialities* remain stigmatized without the kind of "commitment to disability culture and aesthetics" typical of crip practices and movements (Sheppard 2019).

What remains transformative about her performance in this video is her reliance on managing both her health practices and device visibility through material practices and online visual media simultaneously. As she physically enacts these material cultures of Type 1 diabetes on-screen, it provides a counter-narrative to challenge the dominant discourses surrounding medical devices and chronic illness in public. Her performance is as much about normalizing the lived experience of Type 1 diabetes as it is about the practical issue of where to put the object itself. In that discursive sense, Deck stands on-screen as a kind of digital media liberator, signing off at the end of the video with a hope that viewers will garner some practical tips to hide their pump and "enjoy the freedom of not having something around your waistband 24/7."

And yet, much surrounding Type 1 diabetes and the platform (YouTube) remain as entrenched in discourses of inequality and normativity as ever before. Disability and chronic illness in public remain socially unacceptable due to the discomfort they evoke among the able-bodied. Evidence of that can be seen in the Type 1 diabetes YouTube content in 2020. It, today, remains a primarily white, middle-class, thin, cisgender woman's space, as it has been for a decade or more. Deck's descriptions here, and in many ways her own physical and visual presence in the video, demonstrate the gendered and able-bodied identity politics that define YouTube more broadly. But as medical technologies continue to disrupt normative body frames through the act of use—necessary for the survival of the people with Type 1 diabetes who use them—YouTube channels such as She's Diabetic may continue to disrupt the platform's normative digital frames, and push those boundaries to a place that can encompass the complexities of embodied difference more generally.

References

"10 Fundamentals of a Creative Strategy". 2020. YouTube Creator Academy. https://creatoracademy.youtube.com/page/lesson/creative-fundamentals-bootcamp#strategies-zippy-link-3.

Brune, Jeffrey, Rosemarie Garland-Thomson, Susan Schweik, Tanya Titchkosky, and Heather Love. 2014. Forum Introduction: Reflections on the Fiftieth Anniversary of Erving Goffman's Stigma. *Disability Studies Quarterly* 34 (1) https://doi.org/10.18061/dsq.v34i1.4014.

Diehm, Jan, and Amber Thomas. 2018. Pockets. *The Pudding*. August. https://pudding.cool/2018/08/pockets/.

Duckworth, Angela Lee, Teri A. Kirby, Eli Tsukayama, Heather Berstein, and K. Anders Ericsson. 2011. Deliberate Practice Spells Success: Why Grittier Competitors Triumph at the National Spelling Bee. *Social Psychological and Personality Science* 2 (2): 174–181. https://doi.org/10.1177/1948550610385872.

Fritsch, Kelly. 2015. Desiring Disability Differently: Neoliberalism, Heterotopic Imagination and Intra-Corporeal Reconfigurations. *Foucault Studies* 0 (19): 43–66. https://doi.org/10.22439/fs.v0i19.4824.

———. 2016. Cripping Neoliberal Futurity: Marking the Elsewhere and Elsewhen of Desiring Otherwise. *Feral Feminisms* 5 (2016): 11–26.

Goffman, Erving. 1963. *Stigma: Notes on The Management of Spoiled Identity*. Prentice-Hall.

Hamraie, Aimi, and Kelly Fritsch. 2019. Crip Technoscience Manifesto. *Catalyst: Feminism, Theory, Technoscience* 5 (1): 1–33. https://doi.org/10.28968/cftt.v5i1.29607.

Kafer, Alison. 2013. *Feminist, Queer, Crip*. Indiana University Press. http://www.jstor.org/stable/j.ctt16gz79x.

McRuer, Robert. 2006. *Crip Theory: Cultural Signs of Queerness and Disability*. New York: NYU Press.

Reis, Elizabeth. 1995. The Devil, the Body, and the Feminine Soul in Puritan New England. *The Journal of American History* 82 (1): 15–36. https://doi.org/10.2307/2081913.

Rosner, Lisa, ed. 2004. *The Technological Fix: How People Use Technology to Create and Solve Problems*. New York: Routledge.

She's Diabetic. 2018. *WELCOME TO MY CHANNEL*. YouTube video. https://www.youtube.com/watch?v=5Jg5zhkmjv0.

———. 2020a. She's Diabetic. YouTube. https://www.youtube.com/c/ShesDiabetic.

———. 2020b. *How I Hide My Insulin Pump*. YouTube video. https://www.youtube.com/watch?v=-csDveXqR_c.

Sheppard, Alice. 2019. Staging Bodies, Performing Ramps: Cultural-Aesthetic Disability Technoscience. *Catalyst: Feminism, Theory, Technoscience* 5 (1): 1–12. https://doi.org/10.28968/cftt.v5i1.30459.

Strelan, Peter, and Duane Hargreaves. 2005. Women Who Objectify Other Women: The Vicious Circle of Objectification? *Sex Roles* 52 (9–10): 707–712.

Tiggemann, Marika, and Jessica E. Lynch. 2001. Body Image across the Life Span in Adult Women: The Role of Self-Objectification. *Developmental Psychology* 37 (2): 243–253. https://doi.org/10.1037/0012-1649.37.2.243.

Welter, Barbara. 1966. The Cult of True Womanhood: 1820–1860. *American Quarterly* 18 (2): 151–174. https://doi.org/10.2307/2711179.

PART IV

Re-scripting and Resisting Spoiled Identities

In 1963, sociologist Erving Goffman famously presented his theories on the nature of *stigma*. Goffman argued that the modern experience of stigma constitutes social information, which depending on the context, results in a *spoiled identity*. Stigma occurs when a person has attributes that make them different and those differences are thought of as "bad, or dangerous, or weak." In a social group, stigma makes an individual seem less than human. As such, stigma can have devasting consequences including discrimination, dehumanization, and reduced life chances.

Part IV features writers who contest representations of diabetes that use stigma and shame as strategies to impose normalcy on diabetic bodies. In these representations, diabetes often functions as a discrediting attribute. Here, our authors point out that outsiders frequently use shame and stigma as strategies to "help" people with diabetes. These authors pay particular attention to stigmatizing representations of diabetes and food, social gatherings and medical contexts, fear-tactics as motivation to change behavior, and stigma in romantic relationships. Writers here point to the decisions that diabetic people make to resist stigma. They also raise provocative questions about the limitations and consequences of resisting stigmatizing representations.

In "Desiring Decay: The Power of Unwellness and the Dynamics of Cure in Lina Meruane's *Fruta podrida* (2007)," Elizabeth Jan Jones analyzes this dystopian Chilean novel. In Meruane's novel, the main character Zoila is diagnosed with diabetes and resists compliance with medical treatment. Zoila rejects cure and embraces the unwellness that comes from diabetes, even though such a stance will ultimately lead to her death by decay. Jones argues that Zoila's "desiring of unwellness and diabetic decay" presents a radical form of female agency, but "forces the reader to reckon with how far liberal society is willing to go in embracing female bodily autonomy."

Mila Clarke Buckley reflects on the stigma and medical racism she experienced in her piece, "The Blame and Shame Game: Transforming Medical and Social Interactions." Using the story of her misdiagnosis, Buckley brings other stigmatized elements of her identity, including Blackness and fatness, into conversation with diabetes stigma. Buckley offers a cogent argument that "shame in the social and medical contexts do not work as motivational strategies for managing any type of diabetes." To conclude, Buckley draws a parallel between how shame and stigma are deployed in social media memes and the way the medical community treats people with Type 2 diabetes.

Cynthia Martin takes on the stigma entrenched in public service announcements (PSAs) intended to reduce diabetes incidence. In her essay, "The Monstering of Diabetes: The Failure of Fear and Sarcasm in Public Health PSAs," Martin accounts for rhetorical strategies in international PSA campaigns that use "appeals to fear and sarcastic humor" in their advertisements. Martin argues that such strategies are not only unsuccessful at changing behavior, but they also reproduce diabetes stigma.

In the chapter, "Hurt, Comfort and Intimacy: Representations of Diabetes in Fan Fiction," Justine Debelius approaches the realm of fan fiction. In Debelius' analysis of the subgenre of "Hurt/Comfort," she explores the depiction of the diabetic character's emotional vulnerability. According to Debelius, Hurt/Comfort fan fiction stories depict diabetic characters as reacting to stigma in two primary ways: receiving caretaking and taking control. Debelius argues that the diversity of perspectives in this genre speak to different aspects of the lived diabetic experience, and what "one diabetic considers comforting may in fact, be another's fear."

Taken together, these essays speak to the questions:

- Why do some believe stigma and shame work as a strategy to change the behavior of diabetic people?
- How can diabetic people resist and re-script the stigmatizing stories written about them?
- What are the limitations or consequences of an empowered diabetic character?

Desiring Decay: The Power of Unwellness and the Dynamics of Cure in Lina Meruane's *Fruta Podrida* (2007)

Elizabeth Jan Jones

In 2008, global pharmaceutical company Eli Lilly's Mexico branch won the Aspid publicity award for their diabetes ad campaign ("Eli Lilly México" 2008). The campaign featured four photos, including one example with a middle-aged man eating an innocuous snack, but with the shadow of a wheelchair—what Susan Antebi (2014) refers to as the universal symbol of disability (226)—haunting the background of the image. All four images in the campaign include text that states: "Si tienes diabetes evita que la sombra de las complicaciones te alcance" [If you have diabetes don't let the shadow of complications get you].[1] Not long before the

[1] English translations will be included in brackets after all Spanish quotes. All translations are my own.

E. J. Jones (✉)
The University of North Carolina at Chapel Hill, Chapel Hill, NC, USA
e-mail: eljjones@unc.edu

B. C. Frazer, H. R. Walker (eds.), *(Un)doing Diabetes: Representation, Disability, Culture*, Palgrave Studies in Science and Popular Culture, https://doi.org/10.1007/978-3-030-83110-3_14

creation of this campaign, Eli Lilly found themselves embroiled in scandal when they were accused of manufacturing a drug that caused diabetes as a side effect (Antebi 2014, 226), and the Mexican government also sued the company for price collusion in its sales of insulin between 2003 to 2006 (Randewich 2010, n.p.).

The ad campaign, and the scandals surrounding Eli Lilly, sum up the complications and contradictions of diabetes in Mexico in particular and the Global South in general. While diabetes is ubiquitous enough to warrant major publicity ads and to be a public health concern,[2] the ultimate party responsible for achieving health is the individual. If a person does not use diabetes treatment, then the consequences are their fault. Diabetes is both an illness and a disability. Diabetes is a problem, but also an example of modern scientific and medical progress, even as it demonstrates the costs of medical care. Diabetes has been treatable since of the advent of insulin and other pharmaceutical and technological therapies. However, those treatments are not universally accessible, thus creating systems of inclusion and exclusion, particularly in neoliberal markets consisting of what James Cypher (2004) calls an "experiment in unregulated capitalism" (30).[3] For profit-health care systems demonstrate the power of the medical industry and how certain customers are collateral damage in the name of profit.

Chilean writer and literary scholar Lina Meruane (1970–) incorporates, exaggerates, and goes beyond these quandaries and contradictions as she examines the complex reality of diabetes in a medicalized world in her 2007 novel *Fruta podrida* [Rotten Fruit]. Meruane is recognized for her frequent inclusion of disability, illness, and the corporeal in her novels and this work is no exception. In the novel, which features two half-sisters named Zoila and María, Meruane pushes the limits of conventional

[2]While it is difficult to find statistics on diabetes in Latin America as a whole, the rate is certainly increasing, as can be demonstrated in recent statistics on Chile—Lina Meruane's home country. In a 2017 press release by Chile's Ministry of Health, one in ten Chileans had diabetes ("Día Mundial de la Diabetes, n.p.).

[3]As Cypher (2004) states, neoliberalism in Chile has complex domestic and international consequences. Augusto Pinochet's horrendous military dictatorship was responsible for the country's transition to neoliberalism with its unregulated capitalist framework. Though the dictatorship is most famous for its terrible abuses of human rights, the country did experience an economic boom, partially due to Chilean economists under Pinochet who were trained in the United States. While Chile's economy eventually plateaued and stagnated, those who followed Pinochet were still hesitant to disrupt to the "ultra-free-market" economy (30).

narrative in the book's unusual structure and its often-disturbing plot points. The novel's leading characters eat flies, drink urine, and utilize their bodies in abnormal ways: Zoila rejects her diabetes treatment while María purposefully gets pregnant in order to sell the babies on the black market.

This analysis will focus on the character of Zoila. Paradoxically, as Zoila's bodily health declines due to the progression of diabetes complications, her individual autonomy and power increases. Beyond former interpretations of the novel, this chapter examines the dynamics of treatment and the power of unwellness, demonstrating the empowering and transgressive in Zoila's unconventional and dangerous actions as she misuses and appropriates medical care. By applying critical disability studies theory and a close reading approach to Meruane's unique narrative, the protagonist's actions can be understood as a radical form of female agency and empowerment as she seeks, to borrow Robert McRuer's (2006) phrasing, "to welcome the disability to come, to desire it" (207). This chapter will first review the novel and its connections to disability studies theory. It then will continue to an analysis of its overarching themes, such as the meaning of the body in *Fruta podrida*, followed by a close reading of key scenes. The analysis will conclude with a meditation on the meaning of cure and how Zoila's rejection of cure is ultimately an act of self-love and a vindication of life, even as it leads to her ultimate death.

Overview of the Novel

While Meruane is one of the better-known authors in contemporary Latin American literature, *Fruta podrida* is less studied and less read than her work *Sangre en el ojo* (2012), which was translated into English under the title *Seeing Red* (2016b). For this reason, a summary of the book's contents and structure is helpful for readers who may be unfamiliar with the unique and disturbing novel that is *Fruta podrida*. The book is divided into four parts, which alternate voice and style. The first section "plan fruta" [plan: fruit] is narrated by an extratextual speaker, which then transitions to Zoila's voice in the longest, second section "moscas de la fruta" [fruit flies]. The last two parts incorporate more unusual narrative techniques, with "fruta de exportación" [exported fruit] being narrated in the "tú" [you, informal] form and the last, very brief, part being narrated from the perspective of a nurse who uses a stream of consciousness style in all italics.

While Zoila only narrates "moscas de la fruta" in her own voice, she is the character around whom the novel rotates. Over the course of the novel, Zoila is diagnosed with diabetes, subsequently misuses treatment for her own means, including choosing to exacerbate her symptoms via an overuse of insulin or consumption of forbidden foods. Rather than record her symptoms as she is supposed to, she writes poems in what she calls her "cuaderno de deScomposición," [deComposition notebook], which can be found interspersed between the parts. Eventually Zoila absconds to the North, where her father is from, in order to cut off terminally ill patients from their IVs and life support—an act she sees as liberating them.[4] As Lina Meruane (2016a) states of the character, she is "[t]he girl with sweet blood, native of Ojo Seco, a blind alley in the middle of Chile's industrial fruit belt, [who] chooses to travel and die in front of a foreign hospital, in a performance of critical resistance against a system that discarded her as useless" (35). Around Zoila's physical decline operates María, the agricultural chemist who gets pregnant in order to sell the babies and pay for Zoila's medical care. She, too, after years of being taken advantage of by her neoliberal employer engages in her own acts of terrorism by poisoning a shipment of fruit with cyanide. These two principal characters and the novel's unique style weave together to create a narrative that is critical, strange, and fascinating in its combination of the disturbing and the different alongside illness and disability.

Diabetes and Disability

Before embarking on a textual analysis of the novel and Zoila's strange brand of resistance, a discussion of how diabetes and diabetes-induced physical decay fits into the realm of disability studies is crucial. Disability studies has long engaged in debates on the defining line between disability

[4] Beth E. Jörgensen (2019) points to the dangerous nature of Zoila's choice: "Zoila 'frees' them into death, in a highly problematical move that fails to grant or even acknowledge their potential agency, albeit a move carried out in response to perceived injustices. The novel sidesteps the fraught and controversial topic of assisted suicide for 'terminal' patients, itself a controversial medical status, by portraying Zoila's solitary and unbidden acts of medical terrorism without making reference to that debate. The narrative resists passing judgment on Zoila's actions or labeling her a criminal" (1635). I bring this plot point up not to celebrate or condone Zoila's troubling actions, but Zoila's killing of these patients does fit in with the character's overall worldview that characterizes being stuck in a medicalized system as a fate worse than death.

and illness, with scholars often getting stuck in the analytical weeds that split these two, often socially constructed and certainly mutually influential, categories.[5] The desire to define disability as separate from the experience of illness stems from the activist roots that created disability studies. As Susan Wendell (2001) states, "modern movements for the rights of people with disabilities have fought the identification of disability with illness and for good reason" (17). In the fight to demedicalize disability and call out its social construction, disability activists rejected the notion that they were sick and should be constantly seeking out cures, medicine, or the diminishment of their difference. Nonetheless, like Wendell (2001) further argues, "some people with disabilities *are* sick, diseased, and ill" and these bodies are the ones that were often ignored by the influential social model (18, emphasis in original).

In the realm of literary analysis and cultural studies, much can be gained from applying a disability studies lens to conditions that may have been considered diseases or illnesses. Disability—in its signaling of social construction, dynamics of power, critique of medical perspectives and considerations of what is considered normal and why—provides an approximation to deconstruct the supposed givens of health, illness, and cure. Such an approximation falls in line with Alison Kafer's (2013) political-relational model of disability, which also addresses chronic pain and illness and their connections to disability. As Kafer states, "the problem of disability is located in inaccessible buildings, discriminatory attitudes, and ideological systems that attribute normalcy and deviance to particular minds and bodies" and asserts that disability allyship and desires for medical care are not mutually exclusive (23). Disability thus creates a nexus where personal desires and societal norms meet, allowing for an examination of both individual ideas of the body and social ideals undergirding a preference for the normative.

In the intersection between disability and illness, diabetes presents an exceptional case that demonstrates the fruitful points of applying a disability approach to the condition. As Antebi (2014) argues, diabetes is a condition that lends itself to analysis of the various components of disability as it contains "un núcleo de representaciones de la discapacidad: de cuerpos y poblaciones, de diagnosis y prognosis, de salud pública y prácticas

[5] See Wendell (2001) for a discussion of how chronic illnesses can be viewed as disabilities and Price Herndl (2005) for an attempted splitting of disease and disability into two separate categories.

individuales en las cuales se imponen y se intercalan, implícitamente, las imperativas del mercado farmacéutico y la mirada médica" [a nucleus of disability representations: bodies and populations, diagnoses and prognoses, public health and private practice wherein the motives of the pharmaceutical market and medical gaze are implicitly linked] (230). Within Antebi's discussion of disability, I would like to signal two components that are especially relevant for an analysis of *Fruta podrida*: public health and individual practice. Type 1 diabetes, which is the type Zoila is diagnosed with, is a salient condition for examining the tension between these two components because of its status as a treatable, though not curable, condition. In the frame of *Fruta podrida,* Zoila questions the sincerity of public health goals via her individual practice of self-destruction. Rather than use medical interventions, such as insulin, to treat her diabetes, Zoila employs them to highlight and exacerbate her condition. *Fruta podrida* also presents a future in which a transplant would be able to completely cure the disease–a cure that Zoila is determined not to see (26–7). Thus, the novel lends itself to an examination of cure and treatment and the dynamics of power in the rejection of life-prolonging—if not life-saving—medicine.

I, like Zoila, have a long history with medical systems that have viewed my body as being a problem to be fixed. After a multi-trauma accident in my early twenties that resulted in a dozen broken bones and a variable level of permanent disability, I have spent the better part of a decade being treated by surgeons, physical therapists, orthopedists, and other medical professionals. At first, this level of care was necessary to save my life. Without the blood transfusions and emergency surgeries, I would not be here to write this essay. Now, it remains as I seek to mitigate my level of chronic pain and preserve my joints. Nonetheless, I have a complicated relationship to care and treatment. I appreciate the benefits it gives me—I recognize and appreciate the debt I owe to modern medicine—and I also resent my body being constantly framed as nothing more than an amalgamation of issues to be eliminated. Though I have no intention of using and misusing medicine in the way Zoila does, I understand the motivations behind her actions and feel a sense of liberty in reading her path to self-destruction. Zoila's ownership and celebration of her problematic and rebellious body is as freeing as it is disconcerting.

With this in mind, *Fruta podrida* raises complicated questions for both myself as a reader and disability studies as a field. As Tobin Siebers (2008) states: "The medical model defines disability as an individual defect lodged in the person, a defect that must be cured or eliminated if the person is to achieve full capacity as a human being." Disability studies scholars often reject medical model approaches to disability and focus on analysis of "the social meanings, symbols, and stigmas attached to disability identity" (3). *Fruta podrida* creates a distorted reflection back on the idea of cure and medicalization of the body. The book affirms fundamental tenets of disability studies, such disability being a positive identity, yet signals their limit points. Is our society willing to accept bodily agency when cure or treatment are viable and relatively accessible options? The remainder of this analysis will explore this question to demonstrate the way *Fruta podrida*'s unusual narrative highlights how Zoila's desiring of unwellness and diabetic decay forces the reader to reckon with how far supposedly progressive society is willing to go in embracing female bodily autonomy and radical agency.

The Body and Rebellion in Fruta Podrida

Within Zoila's world, two qualities define bodies, and especially women's bodies: medicalization and commodification. Bodies are kept alive, even if the individuals would prefer otherwise, and healthy bodies are expected to be productive and docile. As one doctor states at the beginning of the novel, after María asks him if Zoila will die: "¿morirse? repitió el Médico palidecido aún más y balbuceó: morirse nadie. Sobre mi cadáver se morirá alguien en este hospital" ["Die?" repeated the Doctor, growing even paler and stammering. "No one dies. Over my dead body will someone die in this hospital"] (23). Thus, the doctor and María decide for Zoila's body without consulting Zoila the person: she is placed on a transplant list and given a strict regimen to follow.

Commodification, like medicalization, privileges health at all costs. As Mónica Barrientos (2015) argues, bodies and fruit are linked throughout the novel, "ya que el cuerpo y la fruta son tratados de la misma forma, son uno solo" [given that body and fruit are treated in the same way, they are one entity] (96). This means that bodies, and particularly women's bodies, like the fruit produced in Chile's agricultural belt, should be aesthetically pleasing and economically productive. They should also participate in the systems that surround them willingly, or at least quietly. María represents the hyper-realization of this ideal. Not only does she dress in her uniform every day and report to work, but she also convinces the women who work as seasonal workers to give up their strike. María encourages other bodies to maintain their economic productivity and sells the infants she creates for economic and scientific gain.

However, even she eventually reaches her limit in how she participates in these systems when she poisons fruit meant for exportation. Zoila, on the other hand, is the antithesis of the commodified ideals that surround her from beginning to end. While María works endlessly, Zoila states: "Mientras ella produce fruta perfecta en el campo yo produzco azúcar en mi cuerpo: en esta casa yo soy la encargada de mí, pero no como mi madre abnegada ni como una laboriosa hermana rodeada de venenos. Mi empresa es la del descuido" [While she makes perfect fruit in the fields I make sugar in my body: in this house I am in charge of myself, but not like my abnegated mother or my industrious sister surrounded by poisons. My business is neglect] (42). Even when Zoila's body is producing something—in this case an overflow of sugar—it is not for sale or productivity, but rather to make a body that is collapsing, disintegrating, and refusing to be controlled.

Several scholars have stated, in their analyses of the novel, that Zoila's body is rebelling against her, a clear reference to the diagnosis given to her in the first part of the book:

> como le decía, dijo el Médico, no es una enfermedad contagiosa pero sí transmisible, porque, posiblemente, muy probablemente, es una condición latente, hereditaria, que de pronto se detona, estalla sin aviso, y a partir de ese momento el sistema defensivo empieza a recibir órdenes contradictorias, resoluciones suicidas. El propio cuerpo se rebela contra sí, el cuerpo hace de sí mismo su propio enemigo. (24–5)
>
> [As I told you, says the Doctor, it's not a contagious illness, but it is transmissible because, possibly, very probably, it's a latent condition, hereditary, that eventually detonates, explodes without warning, and after that moment the immune system starts to receive contradictory orders, suicidal decisions. The body rebels against itself, the body makes itself its own enemy.]

As Barrientos (2015) argues, affirming the doctor's statements, "el cuerpo de Zoila se rebela contra sí como símbolo de la resistencia a las tecnologías médicas que intentan mantenerla sana" [Zoila's body rebels against her as a symbol of resistance against the medical technologies that attempt to keep her healthy] (100). In this assertion, it is Zoila's physical body that is rebellious, not her actual self. Rather than view Zoila's decisions as merely symbolic or separate from her autonomy, I view her decisions to hasten her diabetic decline as personal and as a decision to rebel *with* her body rather than *against* her body. As the young woman leans into her chronic condition, assuming it as her own, she engages in a radical, transgressive, and dystopic form of bodily acceptance. Instead of engaging in cures or treatments meant to manage her diabetes, she claims decay in a way that simultaneously establishes control over her body and recognizes diabetes as a fundamental component of her bodily identity, even if this level of recognition also leads to her inevitable decline.

This understanding of Zoila's rebellious and atypical actions as her own and focusing on her relationship with her body is the focus this analysis will use in its remaining pages to understand and frame specific decisions the character makes throughout the novel. While Zoila's decisions are undoubtedly made in concert with the world that surrounds her—including large systems, like medicine and neoliberal economics—the following section of analysis will focus on the character's relationship with her own body, rather than examine that body as a metonym or metaphor for other political concerns.[6] In other words, the systems around Zoila may influence how the character views her body and thus frame her actions as especially transgressive, but it will be the body and the self that take the center. This attention gives value to the character in and of herself, rather than as an illustrating tool for extratextual systems, and allows the analysis to focus more deeply on the value of her autonomy and agency.

With this in mind, a scene at the beginning of "moscas de la fruta" illustrates how Zoila rebels with her body and takes a position of agency in determining the condition of that body. Zoila is overcome with an insatiable hunger, stating "tengo más hambre que posibilidades de saciarla. Hambre de todo lo prohibido, hambre de lo que quedó pegado en las ollas, de lo que sobra y se despacha en las bolsas de basura" [I have more hunger than ways to satiate it. Hunger for everything forbidden, hunger for what's left stuck at the bottom of pots, for what is left over and thrown in the trash] (35). In order to eat sweets and satisfy her intense hunger, Zoila gives herself insulin; however, she accidentally gives herself an overdose when she discovers that María has hidden the "compotas, el dulce de membrillo, los chocolates, el pan fresco en una bolsa y las galletas y las mermeladas" [preserves, quince jelly, chocolates, fresh bread in a bag and the cookies and the marmalade], thus keeping Zoila from satisfying her

[6] See, for example, César Zamorano (2016) and his discussion of capitalism in the novel and Jörgensen's (2019) examination of global systems, such as neoliberal markets and the Global North's subjugation of the Global South.

intense desire for "azúcar" [sugar], which appears written many times in increasingly small font to the end of the page as Zoila loses consciousness (37).

Zoila's use of medicine to exacerbate her symptoms instead of minimize them, as is the standard use of insulin, is one of the most striking components of this scene. Rather than using the insulin to regulate blood sugar levels and consume a standard diet, Zoila employs it for her own purposes—in this case, to eat with abandon. Her plan is only thwarted by her sister's hiding of the sweets Zoila craves and needs to counteract the excessive use of insulin. The fact that Zoila's desire is to eat without repercussion is especially transgressive when viewed with a long history of women being encouraged to suppress their desires. As Susan Bordo (2004) argues, women are expected to suppress their appetites to maintain a sense of control over their bodies and, as she provocatively claims, "[a]lmost all of us who can afford to be eating well are dieting" (103). Advertisements praise the hungry woman who successfully controls her desires, but outwardly maintains a cool and easy relationship with food (102–3).

For the dieting woman in the Global North, bodily control results in an aesthetically pleasing corporeal self that satisfies the gaze of others. The body is a consumable object, rather than a consuming being. Zoila's rebellion with her body gives her a degree of control—it is an active decision on her part to not minimize her symptoms in a way that would give her a normative body—but it is not a state that makes her societally appropriate or beautiful when taken to the lengths Zolia takes them. As Zoila's uncontrolled diabetes continues, she has an exchange with her sister:

Estás pálida, ojerosa, me dice sin energía. Estás demasiado flaca.

> Estoy perfectamente, le digo aunque sé que no es cierto. Mi cuerpo empezará a capitular, más temprano que tarde. Debo apurarme: mi vista siempre borrosa, los cada vez más frecuentes calambres en los pies me anuncian la ya inevitable disolución. Pero no tengo miedo, no siento angustia. Nunca me he sentido más dueña de mi cuerpo. (101)
>
> [You're pale, haggard, she tells me without energy. You're too thin.
>
> I'm perfect, I tell her even though I know it's not true. My body will start to give up, sooner than later. I need to hurry: my sight always blurry, the increasingly frequent shocks in my feet are announcing their already inevitable dissolution. But I'm not scared, I don't feel anguished. I've never felt more in charge of my own body.]

First, María signals that Zoila's body does not have positive aesthetic value. She is pale, thin, and haggard. As Zoila has allowed, and even hastened, the process of developing diabetes complications, she has also chosen to become ugly, or at least very different from the dominant aesthetic standards placed upon the female body.

Additionally, the fact that Zoila's "ya inevitable disolución" [already inevitable dissolution] is from diabetes, and not a different, possibly more aesthetically pleasing ailment, raises questions regarding meaning and gender norms (101).[7] While many have connected the appearance of diabetes to the fact that Lina Meruane herself has diabetes, it undoubtedly possesses a unique literary significance within the novel as it fosters in Zoila qualities that run both parallel and counter to the feminine norm. Very literally, diabetes creates sweetness as it creates an overproduction of sugar in the bloodstream and tell-tale symptoms, such as sweet breath. In another sense, humans generally seek out and desire sweetness. In the metaphorical sense, women are also expected to be sweet and subservient. Nonetheless, Zoila's bodily sweetness is far from pleasing or palatable and her personality far from sweetly submissive. She unleashes vomiting, frequent urination, and a sweetness that eventually turns into diabetes-related complications, or the sweetness of decay. These repulsive and corporeal qualities make Zoila's body uncontrollable to others—and especially to her sister and the medical establishment—but, paradoxically, results in the protagonist's feeling completely at home in her decaying body. Her proclamation of "Nunca me he sentido más dueña de mi cuerpo" [I've never felt more in charge of my own body] represents the personal agency and autonomy Zoila finds in her creation of an uncontrollable body via her rejection of normative blood sugar control. (101).

[7] Susan Sontag (1990) in *Illness as Metaphor; and, AIDS and Its Metaphors* discusses how diseases are (or are not) able to be romanticized. For example, as she claims, "[t]he dying tubercular is pictured as made more beautiful and more soulful; the person dying of cancer is portrayed as robbed of all capacities of self-transcendence, humiliated by fear and agony" (17). This contrasts with AIDS, which Sontag argues resists such romantic characterizations (111–2). While Sontag does not speak to diabetes specifically, it is nonetheless possible to speculate the metaphorical significance the stereotypes of this condition have in our world, which seem to range from a tragedy to the innocent, in the case of children with Type 1 diabetes, to a condition of sloth and gluttony, in the case of Type 2. While both of these metaphorical stereotypes are far too simplistic, Zoila manipulates both of them. It is implied that she has Type 1 diabetes, but she uses that diagnosis as an excuse to engage in the self-indulgent behaviors, often incorrectly and harmfully, associated with Type 2.

This embracing of the ugly and the unappealing comes with its own power. As Zoila choses to operate outside of the society that surrounds her, she is able to frame her body as a construction with benefits only for herself. By rejecting beauty standards of the Global North and behavior, she is beholden to no one. Though self-destructive, Zoila's diabetic decline is also representative of a normally unachievable level of freedom for the woman's body. Her excessive consumption of food continues by taking an autoerotic twist throughout the novel. At one point, left home alone, Zoila loses track of time and fills the house with "[c]ucharas con mermelada diseminadas por el suelo," [spoons with marmalade thrown on the floor] artifacts of her time spent "comiendo sin pausa" [eating without pause] (89).

Zoila's autoerotic eating serves the contradictory function of giving primacy to the physical self—the need and desire for sweetness and food—while also taking control over one's own body in the act of desiring it for what it is and exacerbating that state. Food and diabetes are inextricably linked. For Zoila, rather than serving as a form of nourishment or cultural significance, food without tightly controlled insulin dosing serves as a catalyst to declining ability and increasing impairment. This is confirmed in María's chastisement of her sister, as she reprimands: "Apestas a mermelada. A pan con mucha mantequilla y demasiada mermelada. ¿Crees que me engañas porque estás en los huesos? ¿Crees que no sé que toda esa azúcar te desnutre, que acorta tus posibilidades y apura tu muerte?" [You reek of marmalade. Like bread with a lot of butter and too much marmalade. Do you think you're fooling me because you're skin and bones? Do you think that I don't know that all this sugar malnourishes you, that it shrinks your possibilities and pushes you closer to death?] (70). In this way, Zoila's decision to indulge her gastronomic desires is also an indulgence of her desire for disability. By consuming all the sugar and carbohydrates she craves, Zoila allows—and even welcomes—disability to consume her as it becomes the primary and most apparent component of her identity.[8]

[8] Zoila's desire for diabetes has intriguing parallels to and divergences from the transable community. Bethany Stevens (2011) defines transable people as "individuals who *need* to acquire a physical impairment despite having been born or living in physically unimpaired bodies" (n.p., emphasis in original). This leads to transable people undergoing procedures, like elective amputations, in pursuit of a physical body that matches the one they feel they should possess. While Zoila certainly elects to misuse treatment, she does not communicate a feeling of being born in the wrong type of body or a sense that this was the body she was

Zoila has also been, throughout her life, the rejected one. As her father left to go north to an unnamed foreign country–which is implied to be the United States—he leaves her in the semi-unwilling care of María. María reflects on this situation, lamenting: "En qué momento dejé que su Padre se largara al extranjero. En qué momento acepté hacerme cargo. En qué momento, qué desgracia" [In what moment did I allow her Father to beat it and go abroad. In what moment did I accept taking responsibility. In what moment, what a disgrace] (15). Zoila has no friends, no other meaningful relationships, and the herculean efforts spent by her sister and the medical system to keep her alive seem to stem more from a fear of death than for a desire for Zoila herself to exist. Zoila's desiring of herself, including managing her disability on her own terns and infirmity, is an act of impossible self-love in the face of a world that has otherwise ruled her as disposable.

Difficulties of Cure and Conclusions

Zoila's decisions are doubly radical because she has treatment—if not a possible cure—at her disposal, though Zoila's economic situation in accessing that cure is ambiguous. It appears that insulin is easy to acquire and most medical care is doled out almost too willingly, as we see later in the novel where people are kept alive against their will via intensive interventions. However, access to the next level of top tier care and scientific advances, such as organ transplants, is restricted to those who can pay the high dollar entrance fee. This gatekeeping is what leads María to sell the babies she creates on the black market and clearly reflects a coercive environment, but this coercion is also obviously predicated on a narrow definition of health and worth. Only bodies that are capable of capitalist productivity, which then allows them to engage in a capitalist medical environment, belong in the narrative world of *Fruta podrida*.

Additionally, Zoila's rejection of cure—the experimental and fictional organ transplant—and treatment—the use of insulin and a controlled diet—reflects the uneasy home that medical treatment has in the realm of disability studies. While the general idea that disability must be cured is

always meant to have. Rather, the misuse of insulin serves as a vehicle for a particular type of rebellion in her quest for total freedom. It is not so much that Zoila felt the need to be diabetic, but that her diagnosis functions as a catalyst to get closer to complete autonomy in the rigid world in which she lives.

rejected, many disabled people rely on medical care and would be hesitant to increase their levels of impairment or pain without these treatments. Wendell (2001) writes of the difficult place chronic illness has in disability studies, stating that "it is striking that everyone, including disability scholars and activists, tends to assume that prevention is desirable when the cause of disability is war, famine, poor medical care, accident, or illness, and that cure is desirable when the cause is illness" (31). Kafer (2013) similarly speaks to the allure of what she calls the "curative imaginary," or "an understanding of disability that not only *expects* and *assumes* intervention but also cannot imagine or comprehend anything other than intervention" (27, emphasis in original). The desire for a future where this curative imaginary comes to fruition is even more present in the world of diabetes where much money and advocacy is spent in the quest for a cure.[9] Even as disability studies seeks to value difference and undo ableism, you would be hard pressed to find someone who would tell an individual with diabetes to reject treatment in the way that Zoila does.

Eli Clare (2017) succinctly sums up the contradictions of cure: "I landed inside a knot of contradictions. Cure saves lives; cure manipulates lives; cure prioritizes some lives over others; cure makes profits; cure justifies violence; cure promises resolution to body-mind loss" (xvi). In the case of *Fruta podrida*, cure represents a lack of options for our protagonist because worthy bodies are so narrowly defined and the path of the curative imaginary so strongly sought for any and all non-normative bodies. Zoila's rejection of treatment is, in its paradoxical way, a celebration of life and freedom even as it shortens her actual life span. The protagonist is aware of the suicidal nature of her actions and what her rejection of cure will ultimately lead to, but she still choses to continue down this path because it allows her to be exactly who she wants to be and have a body that only she desires. Kafer (2013) speculates, "how might we begin to read [...] practices of self-care not as preserving one's body for productive work but as refusing such regimes in order to make room for pleasure?" (39). While it might be difficult to read Zoila's actions under the traditional rubric of self-care—her decline would be incredibly painful, though descriptions of

[9]JDRF is one such advocacy organization seeking a cure above all else. The organization seeks a cure for Type 1 diabetes, clearly stating "Our focus is on finding a cure" and other ways to minimize the impact of Type 1 diabetes on the lives of those who have it ("Research"). This desire for a cure for a condition that causes pain and necessitates uncomfortable treatment is incredibly valid, but it is also worth recognizing the equally valid desire of people with diabetes to band together in community and celebrate their lives as they currently are.

pain are notably missing in the work—we can still recognize the pleasure and desire she has for her own body, even if it is not a pleasure most would seek.

Though it is not specifically about disability, ray(nise) cange's (2016) discussion of the death, and speculated suicide, of Sandra Bland is salient here. Bland, a Black woman, died in police custody in Texas after a troubling arrest that received criticism for its unjust and racist nature. Though many refused to believe it so, Bland's death in her jail cell was ruled a suicide. Cange writes:

> The shifting of suicide from a position of weakness is why I want us to not take suicide off the table and to recognize the power within that action, if she did commit suicide. Sandra, from the beginning, refused to give up her power. And in that jail cell suicide may have been a form of resistance and an astounding statement of self-love. A statement saying[:] I will not give you the power to kill me and I love myself enough to not endure you killing me slowly. (n.p.)

Though the fictional situation of Zoila is clearly different from Bland's in crucial ways—I do not wish to compare Zoila's quest for autonomy with the presence of systemic racism in the United States—the idea that suicide can come from a position of power and even love in the face of unjust systems certainly connects to *Fruta podrida*.

To many literary critics, Zoila is the novel's most compelling and most off-putting character because she is the only person—and certainly only woman—who gets to be exactly who she wants to be. As Jörgensen (2019) writes of the novel:

> Zoila's extreme actions [...] and the graphic descriptions of her physical state are shocking in their 'abnormality' and criminality, but they encourage the reader to draw a connection between the character's very limited options for freedom, and the limited options for all vulnerable people who live under the regime of neoliberal economics and medical research". (1635)

That level of freedom is as appealing as it is dangerous, which is where Zoila's actions reveal themselves as ultimately impossible. It is impossible to be truly autonomous in a world that is so guided by systems, hierarchies, and structure in its goal to restrict individual agency in the name of a supposed societal good. Since the novel's beginning, the protagonist has been given one choice: use treatment as directed and seek an eventual cure. As Zoila rejects this dictum and opts for a different path, the rigid world of *Fruta podrida* cannot allow her to continue to exist. Zoila's implied death—we never actually see the character die, but instead only get a strange stream of consciousness description from a possibly hallucinated nurse—is the only reasonable option for the character in the literary world she inhabits. Instead of viewing Zoila's quest for inevitable death as a fruitless suicide mission, it can perhaps be better understood as a radical quest for desiring disability and freedom in the shadow of a medicalized world.

It is easy to dismiss the lessons from *Fruta podrida* because of its transgressive and hyperbolic narrative, but the novel also has lessons for the extratextual world and the novel's readers. In both our current moment and in an easy to envision future, more medical technologies will be at our disposal. The lightning speed development of a vaccine for the, at the time of writing this essay, ongoing COVID-19 pandemic is just one example. The debate among citizens over refusing a future vaccine—whether that be due to ideology or legitimate scientific concerns—demonstrates the delicate place choice has in our world. Though the most progressive among us believe in individual autonomy and choice, how far are we willing to let that go? When is a decision for independence, like those we see in Zoila, a thing to be celebrated and when is it to be squashed? How does society feel about the quest for freedom when it poses a threat—both to our values and to our physical safety? These are questions I do not have the answer for, but I believe there is the beginning of an answer in Maren Tova Linett's (2020) statement that "[l]iterary texts serve as thought experiments that help us envision the ramifications of given values" (loc. 85). *Fruta podrida* demonstrates both the cost of freedom and the cost of "health"—an equation that more of us will struggle to balance in a neoliberal and medicalized world.

References

Antebi, Susan. 2014. El haplotipo cósmico: discapacidad, mestizaje y el mapa del genoma mexicano. In *Heridas abiertas: Biopolítica y representación en América Latina*, ed. Mabel Moraña and Ignacio M. Sánchez Prado, 225–246. Madrid and Frankfurt: Iberoamericana and Vervuert.

Barrientos, Mónica. 2015. La fisura del espacio y la toxicidad de los cuerpos: *El contagio* de Guadalupe Santa Cruz y *Fruta podrida* de Lina Meruane. *Chasqui* 44 (1): 91–103.

Bordo, Susan. 2004. *Unbearable Weight: Feminism, Western Culture, and the Body.* Berkeley: University of California Press.

cange, ray(nise). 2016. Why I'm Not Ready to Rule Out Suicide in the Case of Sandra Bland. *Black Girl Dangerous*, July 8. www.bgdblog.org/2015/07/why-not-ready-rule-out-suicide-in-the-case-of-sandra-bland/.

Clare, Eli. 2017. *Brilliant Imperfection: Grappling with Cure.* Durham: Duke University Press.

Cypher, James. 2004. Is Chile a Neoliberal Success? *Dollars and Sense* 255: 30–35.

"Día Mundial de la Diabetes". 2017. *Ministerio de Salud*, November 14. https://www.minsal.cl/dia-mundial-de-la-diabetes/#:~:text=DIABETES%20EN%20CHILE,y%20chilenas%20padece%20esta%20enfermedad.

"Eli Lilly México se lleva el oro en los premios Aspid 2008". 2008. Merca2.0, September 11, https://www.merca20.com/eli-lilly-mexico-se-lleva-el-oro-en-los-premios-aspid-2008/.

Jörgensen, Beth E. 2019. Globalized Food and Pharma: The South Bites Back in Lina Meruane's *Fruta podrida. Disability in the Global South* 6 (1): 1622–1639.

Kafer, Alison. 2013. *Feminist, Queer, Crip.* Bloomington: Indiana University Press.

Linett, Maren Tova. 2020. *Literary Bioethics: Animality, Disability, and the Human.* New York: NYU Press. Kindle.

McRuer, Robert. 2006. *Crip Theory: Cultural Signs of Queerness and Disability.* New York: NYU Press.

Meruane, Lina. 2007. *Fruta podrida.* Santiago: Fondo de Cultura Económica Chile.

———. 2012. *Sangre en el ojo.* Santiago: Mondadori.

———. 2016a. Blind Spot. Trans. Beth Jörgensen. In *Libre Acceso: Latin American Literature and Film through Disability Studies,* edited by Susan Antebi and Beth Jörgensen, 29–46, Albany: SUNY Press.

———. 2016b. *Seeing Red.* Trans. Megan McDowell. Dallas: Deep Vellum.

Price Herndl, Diane. 2005. Disease versus Disability: The Medical Humanities and Disability Studies. *PMLA* 120 (2): 593–598.

Randewich, Noel. 2010. Mexico Fines Eli Lilly, Others for Collusion. *Reuters,* February 23. https://www.reuters.com/article/mexico-pharmaceutical/mexico-fines-eli-lilly-others-for-collusion-idUSN2310744920100223.

"Research". n.d. *JDRF,* https://www.jdrf.org/impact/research/.

Siebers, Tobin. 2008. *Disability Theory.* Ann Arbor: University of Michigan Press.

Sontag, Susan. 1990. *Illness as Metaphor; and, AIDS and its Metaphors.* New York: Doubleday.

Stevens, Bethany. 2011. Interrogating Transability: A Catalyst to View Disability as Body Art. *Disability Studies Quarterly* 31 (4).

Wendell, Susan. 2001. Unhealthy Disabled: Treating Chronic Illnesses as Disabilities. *Hypatia* 16 (4): 17–33.

Zamorano, César. 2016. Capitalismo y producción de subjetividad en *Mano de obra* y *Fruta podrida. Revista Iberoamericana* 82 (254): 27–44.

The Blame and Shame Game: Transforming Medical and Social Interactions

Mila Clarke Buckley

Every Easter, 4th of July, Halloween, Thanksgiving, Christmas, and honestly every other major holiday that centers on gathering and food, I brace myself for disappointment and frustration. It's not because I personally have a hard time with managing food and diabetes around the holidays—even though I have in the past. It's because I know there will inevitably be a disgusting diabetes joke, typically circulated online, that I have to spend my precious holiday-time debunking.

Sometimes it's jokes or memes like 'having too many Cadbury eggs will give you diabetes.' Other times it's a jab like "Man, I hope I don't get fat and get diabetes after I eat all of this turkey." Both are so inaccurate that it hurts. No, eating too much sugar will not give you diabetes. No, diabetes is not a punishment laid on anyone who enjoys a variety of foods. And in no place are diabetes jokes more prevalent than social media. No matter the year, the inevitable post comes, and I just have to take a deep breath

M. C. Buckley (✉)
Houston, TX, USA
e-mail: mila@hangrywoman.com

B. C. Frazer, H. R. Walker (eds.), *(Un)doing Diabetes: Representation, Disability, Culture*, Palgrave Studies in Science and Popular Culture, https://doi.org/10.1007/978-3-030-83110-3_15

and sigh. “Here it goes again,” I say to myself. I should have canned responses for these things to save time.

Such posts represent food as a source of shame. They circulate disturbing, widespread misconceptions about people with diabetes and how they *should* relate to food. People think we’re lazy and it’s our own fault we have diabetes. It’s widely believed that if you don’t have blood sugars in range, you simply aren’t trying your hardest to get there. If you have diabetes and you eat anything but salads and veggies, others assume that you’re actively doing a disservice to your body. Whether you have diabetes or not, if you’re fat, the stereotype says that diabetes is inevitable.

The thing is, none of those things are true, but they are perceived to be true. People with diabetes spend incredible amounts of time and energy to debunk these stigmas and misrepresentations about diabetes and food. Like other forms of disability, the outside world watches you and questions your existence. From friends to strangers, many people feel entitled to question everything about you. With diabetes, the outside world questions the choices you make with food. Unfortunately, when you embody many of the aforementioned stigmas, people will see what they want to see.

Like me, I’m not your typical person with Type 1 diabetes. I am fat and I am a Black woman. I was diagnosed in adulthood, and because of a family history of Type 2 diabetes, a high blood sugar reading at my doctor’s appointment and the way I looked, healthcare providers deemed it unnecessary for me to be tested for autoimmune antibodies. I was misdiagnosed with Type 2 diabetes in my mid-20s, but four years later I found out that I actually had Latent Autoimmune Diabetes In Adults or LADA. It’s a slow progressing form of Type 1 diabetes, where you lose beta cell function over time instead of all at once. It eventually requires complete insulin dependence.

My misdiagnosis taught me that food shame stems not only from outsiders and social media, but from medical providers as well. For years as someone diagnosed with Type 2 diabetes, my care team told me to eat fewer carbs and exercise more. I was told I couldn’t eat foods from my culture like plantains, rice and peas, and Jamaican beef patties. I can’t tell you how many times I heard “Try kale! You might like it!” (I already did, and also collards, and broccoli, and other green things). Kale is thought of as the “superfood,” when in fact only thinking of kale as a “good” food erases culture, pleasure, and complexity of how humans relate to foods.

Not only was food a threat, but insulin was too. Primary care doctors and diabetes educators presented insulin to me as a consequence of mismanagement—not as a helpful option for my body. Some would say, "I don't want to put you on insulin yet because I know you can manage this with diet and exercise." For medical experts to use my body's need for insulin as a threat goes hand in hand with food shame. They think that if only I ate better, I would not need insulin. So when I was being shamed in medical contexts, I felt like I was failing, like I was a ***bad diabetic.*** Even though I love kale, it was a long time before I realized that I wouldn't be a bad diabetic if I didn't. I also know now that I needed insulin. It would have helped me manage my blood sugars so much better, and it's a useful tool for anyone with diabetes who requires it.

When you are continually told to change your body through what you eat, or how much you exert to have optimal diabetes management, it changes your relationship with food -- for the worse. It's not just small changes either. The day you're diagnosed with Type 2 Diabetes, you're told to overhaul your life. For years, the constant thought on my mind was: eating less means I am doing better. Every time I saw my blood sugar logs, my blood sugars would reaffirm that. I honestly arrived at a point where I thought to myself "if I eat any fewer carbs, I'd probably just die." I didn't know it at the time, but I was hurting my body in pursuit of the version of "health" my medical team demanded of me.

In my story, my numbers were best when I put my body in a state of neglect. If I'd forgotten to eat, or only had a few almonds, tea and fresh clementine slices, and my blood sugars were coasting at 80 mg/dL, I felt both so happy, and so tortured. I had a sense of happiness because I knew that week was going to look really good on my blood glucose report. I felt tortured because eating that way felt like the only way I could lose weight and maintain good blood sugars. For many years, there was just no in between.

When I got my A1C down to 6.3%, it wasn't because I was healthy—it was because food restriction was the only way I knew how to keep my blood sugars from rising beyond the top of my glucose range. When I'd get praise for in range blood sugars, it was hard to accept because I knew that I wasn't achieving it in the healthiest way. I knew the harm my body was experiencing with how I related to food at this time. I had anxiety about meeting with my care team because I knew that I'd have to explain where these numbers came from, and how much I was struggling to nourish my body and maintain in range blood sugars.

Then, when I was diagnosed with LADA, the conversation shifted in a way I hadn't anticipated. Suddenly the do's and don'ts of foods weren't the conversation I was having anymore. My appointments included grace and understanding. If I had a bad blood sugar day it was less about me, or the food I ate, and more about learning the balances between food and insulin. We wouldn't start with how high my A1C was, but with how much my time in range had improved, and what I was doing well—or struggling with—from my perspective. My endocrinologist would push me to be in the figurative driver's seat of my diabetes management and to test and tinker until I found my perfect balance—something I was not encouraged to do when I was seeing healthcare providers for Type 2 diabetes.

That change was refreshing, but it made me wonder why my care teams were operating from a place of deficit and judgement when I had a different label in my chart. Why was my Type 2 treatment rooted in the shame I *should* feel for my food choices, where my LADA diagnosis was rooted in empowerment and praise for curiosity and fitting the pieces together? I still find myself in a place of confusion about it, and I find it difficult to let myself "fail" because I'm still fearful that the conversation will end in blame and shame if I don't find myself improving. Even though I'm relatively healthy, those conversations still lurk as a shadow over my diabetes management and my interactions with the healthcare system.

My updated diagnosis is still new to me, and I'm not sure when the moment of confusion will pass. Still, the one thing I firmly believe is that shame and stigma makes its way to the medical field, just as much as it does to those aggravating posts where diabetes is a punchline and used to perpetuate food and body shame. My hope is that medical experts will no longer criticize the food choices of people with diabetes of any type thinking that they are helping someone control their blood sugar. If they don't abandon this mindset, it means patients are continually set up for failure, judgement and blame. I know personally that shame in the social and medical contexts do not work as motivational strategies for managing any type of diabetes.

Until my hope is realized, I guess I'll have the internal tug-of-war over how much time I want to spend during holidays or doctor visits defending others with diabetes. In both spaces I try to make it known that living well with diabetes and isn't just about food and diabetes management isn't simple as most may think.

Hopefully, that change comes soon for patients, and it won't be too much longer.

The Monstering of Diabetes: The Failure of Fear and Sarcasm in Public Health PSAs

Cynthia Martin

A tall, shadowy apparition in a hooded cloak stalks a woman on the street. An open leg sore crafted from cake icing and sprinkles oozes pus and rotting flesh. A naïve, slovenly middle-aged male proclaims his love for bacon to his doctor. These are the images that confront viewers in various public service announcements intended to educate the public about the dangers of diabetes. But with the incidence of Type 2 diabetes increasing every year, quadrupling from 1980 to 2015 (World Health Organization 2020), one must ask how effective these ads actually are in preventing diabetes.

For the last decade, the medical and public health sectors have embarked on a public awareness campaign to educate about Type 2 diabetes in an effort to halt what was first termed an epidemic as early as 2005 (Bassett

C. Martin (✉)
James Madison University, Harrisonburg, VA, USA
e-mail: marti2cs@jmu.edu

B. C. Frazer, H. R. Walker (eds.), *(Un)doing Diabetes: Representation, Disability, Culture*, Palgrave Studies in Science and Popular Culture, https://doi.org/10.1007/978-3-030-83110-3_16

2005, 1496).[1] The public service announcements created to support these campaigns are rooted in good intentions. However, these efforts rely on representational strategies, such as fear and sarcastic humor, that are not only ineffective, but that also potentially alienate the very population they seek to reach. Instead of educating the public about diabetes in its many different forms, these PSAs, with their images of monstrosity and messages of personal responsibility, are cloaked in a rhetoric of condemnation, thereby stigmatizing the disease and those who live with it as undesirable and grotesque.

This chapter takes a rhetorical approach in its examination of recent PSAs sponsored by international public health organizations to address the global rise in incidences of diabetes. Two predominant strategies used in such campaigns are identified and examined—the use of appeals to fear and sarcastic humor. Ultimately this chapter argues that such strategies in PSAs are not only ineffective in changing behaviors, but also contribute to the growing stigma surrounding diabetes and those who live with the disease in its many different forms.

Diabetes Stigma

Few other diseases are associated with shame and blame to the extent diabetes is (Furuta 2020). Diabetes stigma refers to perceptions of exclusion, blame or judgement because one has diabetes (Major and O'Brien 2005, 394–395). An overwhelming body of research supports findings that people with diabetes often feel stigmatized for having the disease. A study conducted in association with the diaTribe Foundation and dQ&A revealed 52% of people with Type 2 diabetes and 76% with Type 1 who were surveyed perceived stigma, with the highest rates being reported by parents of children who live with Type 1 diabetes (Liu et al. 2017, 28). In

[1] In her editorial introduction to the September 2005 volume of *American Journal of Public Health,* Associate Editor Mary Bassett, MD argues with urgency that something must be done to slow the incidence of Type 2 diabetes in the US. "Diabetes is epidemic," she declares, noting "[T]he high and rapidly increasing prevalence of the disease demands this description." She also notes that identifying diabetes as an epidemic will empower medical and public health professionals to adopt "established disease control strategies" such as "surveillance, risk identification, and interventions" in their efforts to ensure patients do not develop diabetes (1496). In the fifteen years since publication, both the medical/public health communities and popular media have embraced the analogy, but without realizing the promise of the strategic control methods Bassett proposed. See Politico Staff (2018).

another study, 93% of people with diabetes (Types 1 and 2) who were surveyed believed Type 1 diabetes is stigmatized; 52% reported experiencing negative stereotyping, discrimination, and rejection associated with their disease (Browne et al. 2014). The most widely reported experience of diabetes stigma is the perception of having a character flaw/failure of personal responsibility (81%), followed by the perception of being a burden on the health care system (65%) (Liu et al. 2017, 29). Gredig and Bartelsen-Raemy (2017) found people with diabetes not only reported experiencing stigma, but nearly all participants (over 3300) also reported being discriminated against in the workplace, school, and social activities because of their condition (1627).

This stigma and discrimination are often internalized and can result in adverse effects such as poor disease management, depression, and anger. Gredig and Bartelsen-Raemy (2017) suggest perceived stigma correlates with low self-esteem, psychological distress and depressive symptoms (1628–1629). These findings are even more pronounced in youth with Type 1 diabetes, who report feeling ashamed and angry about their disease and who express a desire to feel "normal." Sanders et al. (2019) note that the transition from childhood to adulthood is particularly challenging for teens who may experience feelings of isolation or who may feel "different" as a result of the constant daily management of diabetes (1294–1295). The teens in their study often experienced biographical disruption[2] as they attempted to render their disease invisible in order to achieve a "normal self in public" (1295–1296). Jeong et al. (2018) affirm such findings in their study, focusing on how young adults perceived and respond to diabetes stigma. Study participants reported behaving in ways that can have deleterious effects on their health and management of their disease, including not checking their BGs and not dosing insulin so as not to draw attention of others and to "pass" as "normal" (47–48).[3]

[2] Michael Bury (1982) introduced the term "biographical disruption" to describe the way chronic illness threatens an individual's social and cultural identities. Those experiencing biographical disruption generally perceive social relationships and themselves differently than prior to experiences of disruption. For instance, the reciprocity of friendship starts to feel unbalanced. The resources and commitment required to maintain "normal appearances" (175) in friendships and in social environments become exhausting. Ultimately, those experiencing biographical disruption feel social participation is not worth the effort, which results in isolation (175–176).

[3] Erving Goffman (1963) suggests passing as a strategy for managing stigma associated with what he calls "spoiled bodies." Contemporary scholars working in disability studies

Liu et al. (2017) reported feelings of stigma not only affected disease management, but also prevented those who live with the disease from disclosing the disease to friends, family, and healthcare professionals (28). Gabrielle Kaplan-Mayer (2020), an author and diabetes advocate, explains:

> In my own experience, I have noticed that I always say "type 1" when telling someone I am meeting for the first time about my diabetes, and I quickly follow that with, "I was diagnosed when I was 10 years old." I haven't lost all of the weight I gained during my two pregnancies, and I know that being overweight is associated in the public mind with type 2 diabetes. I also know that many people hold the individual responsible for being overweight or for having developed type 2 diabetes.

Whether or not this attitude is fair, having lived with the challenges of type 1 diabetes for 34 years, I don't want someone to think for a minute that I am in any way responsible for having diabetes or that if I just lost some weight it would go away... considering the often inaccurate media portrayal of and public attitudes toward diabetes, this is not surprising.

Alexander Wolf and Nancy Liu (2014) suggest the media plays a role in creating diabetes stigma, citing language used by the media that portrays diabetes and those who live with it as burdens. Dickinson et al. notes that "language lies at the core of ... social perception, personal identity...and stereotyping" (2017, 551). van Huijgevoort, writing about self-identity and disability, suggests that the way social systems address disease often determines the way those living with disease are perceived by others (2002, 784). In other words, the words and images we use to portray diabetes determines how society, in general, perceives those who live with diabetes. Participants in the research noted above report terms such as "repulsive" (Jeong et al. 2018, 48), "junkies," "gluttons," (Gredig and Bartelsen-Raemy 2017, 1628), among many other labels that carry negative connotations, being used to describe diabetes. Browne et al. (2014) also

have criticized the simplicity of this concept and noted its roots in the medical model of disability, which focuses on the physical body and impairment as problems to be solved. Others who espouse a social model of disability have criticized passing as assimilation and a disavowal of impairment while Bill Hughes has suggested tropes such as the monster offer valuable sites to disrupt the normative ideal of the body. Falling somewhere in between are scholars such as Tobin Siebers, who suggests those who pass are more aware of and thus able to manipulate social organization and human perception, and Ellen Samuels, who notes the disability community doesn't necessarily make room in the community for those who live with non-visible disabilities.

implicate the media, but note other sources of stigma including family members, schoolteachers, and health care professionals. A close examination of recent ad campaigns aimed at preventing diabetes suggest another source of stigma—the public health organizations dedicated to educating about diabetes and advocating for those who live with the disease.

Appeals to Fear in Diabetes PSAs

The use of fear in messages of prevention is nothing new. Aristotle describes fear as a fundamental emotional appeal in *Rhetoric* (2011) and Walton (2000) notes its frequent use in marketing and political and health communications in modern times. Witte (1992) explains that "fear appeals are persuasive messages designed to scare people [into compliance] by describing the terrible things that will happen if they do not do what the message recommends" (329). By this definition, appeals to fear are rampant in PSAs that encourage viewers to take preventative measures to ward off prediabetes and Type 2 diabetes.

In 2013, International Diabetes Federation (IDF) launched its *Diabetes Kills* campaign. One of its televised ads to support this campaign shocked the world and the diabetic community with its representation of diabetes as a dark, cloud-like apparition similar in appearance to the life-sucking dementors of *Harry Potter* fame. In the animated advertisement, the dark, cloud-like apparition speedily makes its way along the sidewalks of a small town, encircling unsuspecting men and women, who drop to their knees under physical duress or who collapse in death. At the end of the ad, the apparition nosedives into the ground to reveal a gravestone. The words "Diabetes Kills. Learn How to Stay Healthy" flash on the screen. The backlash against this ad was so extensive, IDF removed it from airplay and scrubbed the internet of its presence with exception of only a few sites.[4]

Critics rightly took aim at this PSA for its portrayal of diabetes as monstrous and its use of fear and threat to achieve compliance. Writing for *A Sweet Life*, Michael Aviad (2013) suggests this ad misses the mark in one very detrimental way: "The 'black smoke monster as diabetes' doesn't strike me as a plausible metaphor. In fact, diabetes is not … a random monster that strikes without warning." Susan Sontag's *Illness of Metaphor* (1978) and *AIDS and Its Metaphors* (1989) argue modern metaphors of

[4] See Piemonte (2013) for the complete televised advertisement. See van Gurp (2013) for a still shot from the televised advertisement.

illness not only undermine the reality of the diseases they represent, but such metaphors lead to stigma by portraying those who live with disease as digressive and deficient in character or will. This ad, with its spectre-like representation of diabetes, not only stigmatizes diabetes as monstrous, but also stigmatizes those who live with diabetes as monstrous by extension.

Similarly, the Diabetes Association of Thailand (DAT) recently sponsored print ads for its 2016 *Sweet Kills* campaign that utilize similar fear tactics to encourage individuals to reduce their sugar intake. The campaign consists of several ads that feature graphic images of open sores on arms or legs. The pus, flesh, and vascular tissue revealed by the sores are styled from a variety of sweets—cake, cookies, brownies, chocolate, icing, ice cream and sprinkles. Despite the use of desserts, the images are grotesque and graphic. The juxtaposition of sweets with explicit anatomical illustrations are intended to shock and scare in an effort to call attention to the dangerous consequences of uncontrolled diabetes and hyperglycemia (high blood glucose). While the ads have been praised within the advertising and art worlds—art critic Justin Page (2016) refers to the campaign as "disturbingly delicious"—advocates and scholars of diabetes have again criticized this campaign for its use of fear.

Speight et al. (2020) point to the campaign and note that people are likely to react defensively when confronted with images that are intended to frighten (566). Diabetes activist and Director of the Diabetes Education program at Teachers College, Columbia University Jane Dickinson concurs. She suggests scare tactics may work initially, but if individuals are changing behaviors based on external motivators such as threats, the changes are "not likely to stick." She goes on to explain that when the threat is not immediately realized, individuals can slip into previous behaviors and then feel like failures and lose confidence in themselves (Snouffer 2018). Susan Guzman, co-founder of the Diabetes Behavioral Institute in San Diego, suggests those fear tactics and the feelings of failure can contribute to diabetes stress which could lead to individuals "disengage[ing] from diabetes management" (Snouffer 2018). In this regard, fear tactics could potentially increase negative behaviors instead of reducing them. J. Keith Simpson agrees. He notes that while it is commonly believed use of fear in health promotion can be effective with little backfire, eg. reinforcement of negative beliefs and behaviors instead of change,[5] he points out that recent research, including his own, suggests otherwise. Examining

[5] See Tannenbaum (2015).

fear appeals in health campaigns ranging from anti-smoking to chiropractic anti-subluxation, he concludes fear appeals have a negligible effect on long-term behaviors. He ultimately calls for the use of other strategies to promote behavioral change (Simpson 2017).

Humor and Sarcasm in PSAs

The American Diabetes Association has answered that call and has been praised for its use of humor in its most recent campaign (PR Newswire). But while images of monsters or grotesque wounds are absent from the PSAs, a close examination of ads such as "Bacon Lovers" and "Busy Moms" suggests these ads are just as likely to stigmatize the disease and those living with it as the ads created by IDF and DAT.

M.V. Terskikh (2017) suggests humor can be an effective alternative to the use of fear in public service announcements (155). Noting that humor is more memorable and yields positive emotions, Terskikh suggests one of the advantages of using humor is it can increase a PSA's circulation (159). However, this research is rooted in a narrow understanding of humor as relief. John C. Meyer (2000) explains that when humor is enacted to reduce stress, people laugh as a way to release nervous energy, which results in a reduction of dissonance. In theory, the relief that audiences feel makes communication less overwhelming and makes the receiver of the message more receptive (312). Accordingly, humor in PSAs could potentially make a targeted audience more receptive to the message. However, research conducted by Hye Jin Yoon (2015) suggests humor, when used in conjunction with fear or threat, has no effect on the persuasiveness of public service announcements. Iles and Xiaoli (2017), citing Sternthal and Craig (1973), notes that scholars have long been divided on the efficacy of humor in public service announcements, in large part due to the broad scope of the different types of humor (188). Focusing, in part, on the use of sarcastic humor in public service announcements, Iles and Xiaoli suggest that sarcasm can increase counterarguing (described as resistance to/arguing against the message) as well positive attitudes toward risky behaviors (197).

A recent campaign from the American Diabetes Association (ADA) titled "Do I have Prediabetes?" (2016a) eschews fear. One of the ads in this campaign, "Bacon Lovers," features a middle-aged white male patient, Thomas, in an examining room with his doctor. The patient has just been diagnosed with pre-diabetes, and the doctor is explaining that exercise and a change in diet can stop progression and potentially reverse the disease. In response to the doctor's recommendations, Thomas confesses that exercise makes him "hungry…for bacon." In what appears to be a rebuff of his duty and role, the doctor concurs: "I love bacon, too, and who likes to exercise?" The two share a laugh, seemingly about the inanity of living a healthy lifestyle. Thomas, thinking he has just been given a get out of jail free card, asks "So we're good?" The doctor returns his gaze to the patient file, shakes his head, and says with grave seriousness "No. You still have prediabetes."

A similar strategy is employed in another ad titled "Busy Mom" from the same campaign. The same examining room and doctor feature in this PSA, but the patient, Maria, is an African American female. Upon diagnosis of prediabetes, Maria exclaims, "Prediabetes? I don't have time to eat right or exercise. I am a busy mom!" The doctor responds drawing a diagram on his clipboard and exclaims, "This is great news! Busy moms never get prediabetes!" He shows Maria the diagram, which features a large circle in the middle of the page representing the public, and a smaller circle in the upper corner representing "busy moms." Unlike Thomas, Maria recognizes the sarcasm immediately, and, feeling admonished and shamed. She directs her gaze downward at her feet, rendering herself an object of spectacle—without power and without agency. The doctor's treatment of his male patient and his female patient could not be more different, though neither interaction is appropriate. Whereas the doctor shares a laugh with Thomas to call out his behavior, when treating Maria, he relies on condescension and belittlement. We cannot overlook the gender discrimination that is manifest in these two very different interactions.

That said, both ads rely on humor in the form of sarcasm to convey a message about healthy lifestyles. However, any gains in communication made initially are undermined by the use of sarcasm. Sarcasm is characterized by the rejection of an utterance (Haiman 1998, 22). In the case of "Bacon Lovers," the sarcasm rejects Thomas's love of unhealthy food. The doctor's laughter temporarily and insincerely enables the lifestyle choices perceived by the medical establishment to be unhealthy. But as Thomas realizes the moment the doctor returns to his role as gate keeper of public health, the doctor's laughter is not an expression of comradery, but rather a sarcastic condemnation of Thomas's choices. Similarly, the doctor's exclamation that busy moms never get diabetes is intended to blamefully reject Maria's defense that she doesn't have time to exercise or eat healthily. Meyer (2000) notes sarcasm is an expression of hostility that can be explained through the superiority theory of humor which, in part, allows for humor to be used as a social corrective (314). The doctor uses sarcasm in an attempt to correct Thomas's and Maria's behaviors that are perceived to be detrimental to reversing Type 2 diabetes. Instead of being inspirational or motivational, the doctor's, and by extension the ad's, message of prevention becomes discomforting because the use of sarcasm is both hostile toward and condemning of the patients.

The use of sarcasm signifies and reinscribes an unbalanced power relationship between doctor and patient. Messages of prevention that rely on sarcasm or simply imply threat (improve your lifestyle or suffer the dire consequences) are rooted in a medical model of disability that views the disability, or in this case, disease, as a personal deficiency that can only be fixed by complying with medical advice (Olkin 1999, 26). PSAs that approach diabetes from this model not only reinforce the disease as a problem to be solved, but approach those who live with the disease as aberrant. According to the medical model, people with disabilities deviate from what is "normal" (Olkin 1999, 26). In PSAs sponsored by the ADA, the patients are presented as aberrant. Whereas viewers may have identified with Thomas and Maria and their struggles to maintain healthy lifestyles, the use of sarcasm in the PSAs enwraps the viewer in the pitfalls of the medical model, othering Thomas and Maria by depicting them as deviant or abnormal in stark contrast to the doctor, who holds the power of normality and knowledge in the physician-patient relationship. The doctor empathizes momentarily, but quickly reestablishes the power-imbalance through sarcasm. Ultimately, the doctor offers correction and conventional wisdom.

Puntoni et al. (2011) suggest the construction of an undesired identity in PSAs adversely impacts their efficacy. Studying the effect of breast cancer campaigns on consumer behavior, the researchers found that when an ad posits an identity the viewer finds undesirable, the viewer tends to discard the message. In other words, when a person's positive self-conception is threatened, the viewer removes the threat by dismissing or defying the information that makes them uncomfortable. Accordingly, the ads that are part of the ADA's campaign "Do I have Pre Diabetes?" construct undesirable identities for those who are at risk for pre-diabetes. Instead of presenting Thomas and Maria as individuals with whom viewers can identify, the ads instead invite the viewer to join the doctor in mocking and judging the patients. In this respect, the use of sarcasm fails, and the aim of the ads fail. The ADA ads are no more effective in changing behavior than the ads that rely on monstrous representations of the disease.

Conclusion

These PSAs and the discourse of diabetes coming out of the public health sector suffer the same problems of representation Simi Linton noted back in 1998 in *Claiming Disability*, namely that such depictions pathologize and stigmatize disease and disability, that they objectify and oversimplify lived experience, and they silence the voices of those living with disabilities and disease. When people who live with diabetes, any type, are depicted as monstrous or are targets of the hostility associated with sarcasm, the negative feelings they experience can "contribute to an already stressful experience of living with the disease" (Dickinson et al. 2017, 551). David S. Martins, a medical rhetorician and author of "Diabetes Management, the Complexities of Embodiment, and Rhetorical Analysis," suggests that diabetes education is disembodied from real, lived experiences. The same applies to the public awareness campaigns that seek to educate. The portrayals of diabetes do not reflect the realities of the disease. It is not diabetes that kills, but the complications arising from unmanaged diabetes that kill. A love for bacon is not the sole cause of Type 2 diabetes; diet is one of many risk factors that also include age and genetics, as well as two factors the public health sector has yet to acknowledge, race and socioeconomic status.

Claudia Chaufan (2008) argues Type 2 diabetes is a good indicator of unequal and unjust distribution of social resources necessary to good health. Drawing on over a decade of research, she argues that the root causes of diabetes lie in inequality and lack of social power.[6] Auchincloss et al. (2008) found that higher diabetes rates were related to lack of access to neighborhood resources that support exercise and healthy foods. Schootman et al. (2007) noted the incidence of diabetes increases with poor housing conditions; they also noted a connection to race, as Black neighborhoods were more likely to be characterized by low quality housing than white neighborhoods. Messages of prevention that stress the importance of exercise and diet do little good if the means to exercise in a safe environment or to obtain nutritious foods is foreclosed upon because of one's race or economic situation. Until these factors are addressed, the incidence of Type 2 diabetes will continue to rise, as will the incidence of the consequences—heart disease, kidney disease, neuropathy (Rosenbloom et al. 1999).

[6] See Chaufan (2000) and Chaufan and Weitz (2009).

The public health sector has had over twenty years to get it right. And yet, still, every year the public is made to suffer through yet another campaign that relies on fear and threat, or that ridicules those who live with the disease through its use of sarcasm. PSAs that depict those who live with diabetes as undesirable, monstrous, or aberrant perpetuates an us/them dichotomy that leaves little room for understanding the causes of diabetes or the experience of living with the disease. It is time for a new model for PSAs, one that privileges lived experience and empowers those who live with the disease, one that eschews a medical model that mandates compliance without considering factors, especially those discrimination-laden socioeconomic factors, that serve as barriers to health. As Speigt et al. suggest, awareness campaigns should "create empathy among the general public" instead of stigma (567). Puntoni et al. (2011) suggest the greatest potential for success are those PSAs that elevate one's sense of self-worth (423). These findings are in line with research by Klein and Harris (2009) who found that health communications that enable self-affirmation remove defense motivations and can thus lead to behavioral change (1466). Diabetes advocate and writer for *Diabetes Self Management* Jan Chait (2014) suggests messages of hope that prescribe action instead of messages of fear only could go a long way in educating the public about the dangers of diabetes. More than anything, however, we need to public policy that enables good health, including access to sites for exercise and affordable, nutritious foods.

If the sponsors of PSAs want to impact the rate of diabetes, these organizations must first acknowledge and embrace the realities of diabetes and its causes.

References

American Diabetes Association. 2016a. Bacon Lovers. Televised Advertisement. Ad Council.

———. 2016b. Busy Moms. Televised Advertisement. Ad Council.

Aristotle. 2011. *Rhetoric*. Translated by W. Rhys Roberts. The Internet Classics Archive. http://classics.mit.edu/Aristotle/rhetoric.1.i.html. Originally written 350 BCE.

Auchincloss, A., A. Diez Roux, D.G. Brown, C. Erdmann, and A. Bertoni. 2008. Neighborhood Resources for Physical Activity and Healthy Foods and their Association with Insulin Resistance. *Epidemiology* 19 (1): 146–157.

Aviad, Michael. 2013. Diabetes as Black Smoke: Does the IDF's Scare Tactic Work? *A Sweet Life*, July 18. https://asweetlife.org/diabetes-as-black-smoke-does-the-idfs-scare-tactic-work/.

Bassett, Mary T. 2005. Diabetes Is an Epidemic. *American Journal of Public Health* 95 (9): 1496. https://doi.org/10.2105/ajph.95.9.1496.

Browne, Jessica, Adriana Ventura, Kylie Mosely, and Jane Speight. 2014. 'I'm Not a Druggie, I'm Just a Diabetic': A Qualitative Study of Stigma from the Perspective of Adults with Type 1 Diabetes. *BMJ Open* 4 (7). https://doi.org/10.1136/bmjopen-2014-005625.

Bury, Michael. 1982. Chronic Illness as Biographical Disruption. *Sociology of Health and Illness* 4 (2): 167–182. https://doi.org/10.1111/1467-9566.ep11339939.

Chait, Jan. 2014. Scared Trait: Is It Helpful? *Diabetes Self-Management*, December18. https://www.diabetesselfmanagement.com/blog/scared-trait-is-it-helpful/.

Chaufan, Claudia. 2000. To Comply or Not to Comply: In Search of the Real Question. *Clinical Diabetes* 18 (1): 46–47.

———. 2008. What Does Justice Have to Do With It? A Bioethical and Sociological Perspective on the Diabetes Epidemic. In *Bioethical Issues: Sociological Perspectives—Advances in Medical Sociology*, ed. B. Katz Rothman and E. Armstrong. New York: Elsevier.

Chaufan, Claudia, and Rose Weitz. 2009. The Elephant in the Room: The Invisibility of Poverty in Research on Type 2 Diabetes. *Humanity and Society* 33: 74–98.

Diabetes Association of Thailand. 2016. *Sweet Kills*. Print Advertisement. Ogilvy and Mather.

Dickinson, Jane, Susan J. Guzman, Melinda D. Maryniuk, Catherine A. O'Brian, Jane K. Kadohiro, Richard A. Jackson, Nancy D'Hondt, Brenda Montgomery, Kelly L. Close, and Martha M. Funnell. 2017. The Use of Language in Diabetes Care and Education. *Diabetes Educator* 43 (6): 551–564.

Furuta, Rebecca. 2020. Living 'with' Diabetes, But 'for' Something Else. *Patients Rising*. https://patientsrising.org/diabetic-stigma.

Goffman, Erving. 1963. *Stigma: Notes on the Management of a Spoiled Body*. Englewood Cliffs: Prentice Hall.

Gredig, Daniel, and A. Bartelsen-Raemy. 2017. Diabetes-related Stigma Affects the Quality of Life of People Living with Diabetes Mellitus in Switzerland: Implications for Healthcare Providers. *Health and Social Care in the Community* 25 (5): 1620–1633. https://doi.org/10.1111/hsc.12376.

van Gurp, Marc. 2013. Beautiful Animation. *Ococio*. https://osocio.org/message/beautiful-animation-diabetes-kills/.

Haiman, John. 1998. *Talk is Cheap: Sarcasm, Alienation and the Evolution of Language*. New York: Oxford University Press.

Hughes, Bill. 2009. Wounded/Monstrous/Abject: A Critique of the Disabled Body in the Sociological Imaginary. *Disability & Society* 24 (4): 399–410.

van Huijgevoort, T. 2002. Coping with a Visual Impairment Through Self-investigation. *Journal of Visual Impairment and Blindness* 96 (11): 783–795. https://doi.org/10.1177/0145482X0209601103.

Iles, Irina Alexandra and Nan Xiaoli. 2017. It's No Laughing Matter: An Exploratory Study of the Use of Ironic Versus Sarcastic Humor in Health-Related Advertising Messages. *Health Marketing Quarterly* 34 (3): 187–201. https://doi.org/10.1080/07359683.2017.1346432.

International Diabetes Federation. 2013. Diabetes Kills. Television advertisement. Kiwono Motion.

Jeong, Yoo Mi, Laurie Quinn, Nahyun Kim, and Pamela Martyn-Nemeth. 2018. Health-related Stigma in Young Adults with Type 1 Diabetes Mellitus. *Journal of Psychosocial Nursing Health* 56 (10): 44–51. https://doi.org/10.3928/02793695-20180503-01.

Kaplan-Mayer, Gabriele. 2020. Type 1 Diabetes Symptoms and Overview for Adults. *Diabetes Self Management*, March 6. https://www.diabetesselfmanagement.com/about-diabetes/types-of-diabetes/a-focus-on-adults-with-type-1-diabetes/.

Klein, William, and Peter Harris. 2009. Self-Affirmation Enhances Attentional Bias Toward Threatening Components of a Persuasive Message. *Psychological Science* 20 (12): 1463–1467. https://doi.org/10.1111/j.1467-9280.2009.02467.x.

Linton, Simi. 1998. *Claiming Disability: Knowledge and Identity*. New York: NYU Press.

Liu, Nancy F., Adam S. Brown, Alexandra E. Folias, Michael F. Younge, Susan J. Guzman, Kelly L. Close, and Richard Wood. 2017. Stigma in People with Type 1 or Type 2 Diabetes. *Clinical Diabetes* 35 (1): 27–34. https://doi.org/10.2337/cd16-0020.

Major, Brenda, and Laurie O'Brien. 2005. The Social Psychology of Stigma. *Annual Review of Psychology* 56 (Feb.): 393–421. https://doi.org/10.1146/annurev.psych.56.091103.070137.

Martins, David S. 2009. Diabetes Management, the Complexities of Embodiment and Rhetorical Analysis. In *Rhetoric of Healthcare: Essays Toward a New Disciplinary Inquiry*, ed. Barbara Heifferon and Stuart C. Brown, 75–90. Cresskill: Hampton Press.

Meyer, John C. 2000. Humor as a Doubt-Edged Sword: Four Functions of Humor in Communication. *Communication Theory* 10 (3): 310–331.https://doi.org/10.1111/j.1468-2885.2000.tb00194.x.

Olkin, R. 1999. *What Psychotherapists Should Know about Disability*. New York: Guildford Press.

Page, Justin. 2016. Sweet Kills, Deliciously Disturbing Ads Showing What Too Much Sugar Can Do to Our Bodies, March 29. https://laughingsquid.com/what-too-much-sugar-can-do-to-our-bodies/.

Piemonte, Lorenzo. 2013. Diabetes Kills—Public Service Announcement. *Dailymotion*. https://www.dailymotion.com/video/x12650g.

Politico Staff. 2018. The Diabetes Epidemic: Opportunities and Missed Opportunities. *Politico*, November 2. https://www.politico.com/story/2018/11/02/us-diabetes-epidemic-959043.

PR Newswire. 2016. First of its Kind PSA Campaign Targets the 86 Million American Adults with Prediabetes. https://www.multivu.com/players/English/7731551-ad-council-prediabetes-psa/.

Puntoni, Stephano, Steven Sweldens, and Nader Tavassoli. 2011. Gender Identity Salience and Perceived Vulnerability to Breast Cancer. *Journal of Marketing Research* 48 (June): 413–424. https://doi.org/10.1509/jmkr.48.3.413.

Rosenbloom, Arlan, Robert S. Young, Jennie R. Joe, and William E. Winter. 1999. Emerging Epidemic of Type 2 Diabetes in Youth. *Diabetes Care* 22 (2): 345–354.

Samuels, Ellen. 2003. My Body, My Closet: Invisible Disability and the Limits of Coming Out Discourse. *GLQ: A Journal of Lesbian and Gay Studies* 9 (1–2): 233–255.

Sanders, Tom, Jackie Elliot, Paul Norman, Barbara Johnson, and Simon Heller. 2019. Disruption Illness Contexts and Liminality in the Accounts of Young People with Type 1 Diabetes. *Sociology of Health and Illness* 41 (7): 1289–1304. https://doi.org/10.1111/1467-9566.12906.

Schootman, Mario, Elena M. Andresen, Fredric D. Wolinsky, Theodore K. Malmstrom, J. Philip Miller, Yan Yan, and Douglas K. Miller. 2007. The Effect of Adverse Housing and Neighborhood Conditions on the Development of Diabetes Mellitus Among Middle-Aged African Americans. *American Journal of Epidemiology* 166 (4): 379–387.

Siebers, Tobin. 2008. *Disability Theory*. Ann Arbor: University of Michigan Press.

Simpson, J. Keith. 2017. Appeal to Fear in Health Care: Appropriate or Inappropriate? *Chiropractic and Manual Therapies* 25: 27. https://doi.org/10.1186/s12998-017-0157-8.

Snouffer, Elizabeth. 2018. Ask the Experts: Why Diabetes Scare-tactics May Cause More Harm Than Good. *Diabetes Voice*, December 6. https://diabetesvoice.org/en/caring-for-diabetes/why-diabetes-scare-tactics-may-cause-more-harm-than-good/.

Sontag, Susan. 1978. *Illness and Metaphor*. New York: Farrar, Straus and Giroux.

———. 1989. *Aids and Its Metaphors*. New York: Farrar, Straus and Giroux.

Speight, Jane, Timothy C. Skinner, Kyle Jacques Rose, Renza Scibilia, and Andrew J. Boulton. 2020. Oh sugar! How Diabetes Campaigns Can Be Damaging to the Cause They Aim to Serve. *The Lancet Diabetes and Endocrinology* 8 (July): 566–567.

Sternthal, Brian, and C. Samuel Craig. 1973. Humor in Advertising. *Journal of Marketing* 37 (4): 12–18. https://doi.org/10.1177/002224297303700403.

Tannenbaum, M.B., J. Hepler, R.S. Zimmerman, L. Saul, S. Jacobs, K. Wilson, and D. Albarracin. 2015. Appealing to Fear: A Meta-Analysis of Fear Appeal Effectiveness and Theories. *Psychological Bulletin* 141 (6): 1178–1204. https://doi.org/10.1037/a0039729.

Terskikh, M.V. 2017. Humor and Fear Appeals in Public Service Announcements Discourse. *Voprosy Kognitivnoy Lingvistiki* 3: 155–161. https://doi.org/10.20916/1812-3228-2017-3-155-161.

Walton, Douglas. 2000. *Scare Tactics: Arguments that Appeal to Fear and Threats.* 2013. N.p.: Springer Science & Business Media.

Witte, Kim. 1992. Putting the Fear Back into Fear Appeals: The Extended Parallel Process Model. *Communications Monographs* 59 (4): 329–349.

Wolf, Alexander, and Nancy Liu. 2014. The Numbers of Shame and Blame: How Stigma Affects Patients and Diabetes Management. *Diatribe*, August 7. https://diatribe.org/issues/67/learning-curve.

World Health Organization. 2020. Diabetes. https://www.who.int/news-room/fact-sheets/detail/diabetes.

Yoon, Hye Jin. 2015. Emotional and Cognitive Responses to Non-humorous and Humorous Threat Persuasion Public Service Advertisements. *Journal of Current Issues & Research in Advertising* 36 (1): 52–69. https://doi.org/10.1080/10641734.2014.912597.

Hurt, Comfort and Intimacy: Representations of Diabetes in Fan Fiction

Justine Debelius

I like to read, and I read a lot. I have stayed up more nights than I care to admit chasing one more chapter. I think the best stories force characters to grow, mature, and recover. I would rather read about four people in a box having a heart-to-heart than watch the same characters traipse across the galaxy and blow things up without ever talking about their emotions or changing as people. In my favorite stories, I find characters to identify with: someone whose personal or emotional journey reflects my own in some ways. After twenty years with Type 1 diabetes, I look for diabetic characters in fiction, even knowing I will sometimes I be disappointed. I find there are not enough stories about diabetics in mainstream media, and when I find them, the stories feel inauthentic. My complaints with such representations are numerous: the diabetic character may be weak and unable to manage their lives on their own; they may be diabetic only when it's convenient in the plot; the technology they use may be

J. Debelius (✉)
Department of Tumor, Microbiology, and Cell Biology, Karolinska Institutet, Stockholm, Sweden

B. C. Frazer, H. R. Walker (eds.), *(Un)doing Diabetes: Representation, Disability, Culture*, Palgrave Studies in Science and Popular Culture, https://doi.org/10.1007/978-3-030-83110-3_17

outdated; and their care based on ableist assumptions (e.g. a diagnosis of diabetes means the person ate too much sugar). I often find myself asking if it's better to have bad representation than no representation at all, or if there are ways to change the way these groups are represented.

I have a confession, though. When I say, "I read a lot," what I really mean is, "I read a lot of fan fiction." Scholars who study the genre frequently describe fan fiction as literary works derived from a common source ("canon") and produced by and for an engaged community, or "fandom" (Coppa 2017). Fan fiction falls into a broader category of "transformative works"—a legal definition that allows their continuing existence, but also a commentary on the potential power of new tellings to reshape old tales. Unfortunately, when I confess to reading fan fiction, it feels like many people are still stuck with an older, narrower view: fan fiction is a collection of poorly written stories by girls and women about cookie cutter porn. There's an undertone that fan fiction writers are people who are not creative enough to create their own worlds. And, while one can certainly find stories featuring a lot of erotica, and plenty of variations on the same plot, these are a subset of the kinds of stories that fans tell. Instead, as someone who both reads and writes fan fiction regularly, I find complex stories about found families, tired millennials, and trauma recovery. I get to see myself represented in stories and characters, even if the original creator never imagined their character sharing my experiences. Fan fiction scholar Francesca Coppa has described fan fiction as folktales for the modern age: a common narrative about current heroes and sensibilities (2017). This description ultimately rings true; my experience in fandom has been about a collaborative exploration of who we are as people, writers, and a community.

Fan Fiction and Disability

As a literary genre, fan fiction has the potential to create social change. Due to the fluidity between audience and artist, fan fiction and fandom disrupt traditional views of how media is produced and consumed (Coppa 2014). At their best, fan works can be socially disruptive by creating space to explore how non-dominant identities can change characters, stories and societies—sometimes with real world impacts (Coppa 2014, Clemons 2019, Dym et al. 2019, Fowler 2019). For example, Dym et al. describe how fandom engagement can create a safe space for content creators to explore queer identity outside explicitly queer spaces and can support trauma recovery (2019). For disability centric stories and disabled characters, fan fiction can reframe the way readers understand disability by shifting disabled bodies, voices, and experiences are presented to both disabled and non-disabled audiences (Clemons 2019: 275). However, fan works can also re-enforce privilege and dominant narratives when they knowingly or unknowingly bring in sexist, ableist, racist, or transphobic views (Clemons 2019, Newman-Stille 2019, Johnson, 2019). Fan works are still finding ways to challenge harmful views, including those that marginalize or oppress disabled characters.

Hurt/Comfort (H/C) is a major fandom subgenre that centers around disability, the perception of disability, and recovery. The core of a H/C narrative arc breaks down into four pieces (Linn 2017). First, it may optionally open with an unaddressed concern or emotional vulnerability. For instance, a varsity high school athlete might worry about what will happen in college when she is no longer on a varsity team. Second, it is followed by a "hurt": a physical injury, illness, or state of extreme physical deprivation. The hurt must be severe enough that the character cannot care for themselves on their own, although the period of dependence in and of itself may be brief. Some H/C stories only hint at the physical manifestations of "hurt." Instead, H/C focuses on emotional ramifications: in her essay on horrifying H/C Rachel Linn argues, "The danger comes from within, not without." (2017, 3.3). So, our athlete might break her arm during a game, preventing her from playing. In the third piece of the arc, the character is "comforted": aid is provided by a companion and the characters must grapple with the aftermath of their injury on both a physical and emotional level (Linn 2017, 3). For our athlete, physical comfort might include a cast, pain killers, or time away from the sport. In contrast, emotional comfort must address the character's fears and potentially challenge to her identity.

In this portion of the story, the type and consequence of the comfort depends on the H/C subgenre. Within homoerotic "slash"[1] fic, the writer

[1] As a genre, "Slash" typically refers to stories centered around non-canonical but often subtextual romantic relationships between two or more male characters; relationships between two or more female characters are sometimes described as "femslash". The name references an early fanish convention where platonic relationships were denoted using an ampersand (&; i.e. Captain Kirk & Lenard "Bones" McCoy) while romantic relationships were denoted with a slash ("/"; i.e. Kirk/Spock). Slash fics have historically relied on external events to force canonically assumed heterosexual characters to move past their inhibitions and instead find a way to be intimate in their relationships (Jenkins 1992; Russ 2014). Many

uses the hurt and the associated vulnerabilities to build intimacy within a relationship (Newman-Stille 2019). In this genre, our athlete's injury and the subsequent physical intimacy with a female friend would lead to the confession of mutual interest and the girls will likely end up dating. Linn proposes a second subgenre, "horrifying," where the arc explores the boundaries of humanity by systematically deconstructing characters by pushing them to or beyond their mental, physical, and emotional breaking points. The narrative then tries to bring them back from the brink, with the goal of exploring the limits of the human experience (2017: 7). Our basketball player would not fit into this subgenre without an additional, substantial injury, but a returning prisoner of war who has survived injury, starvation, captivity, and torture would be. A third genre exists somewhere between these spaces: an H/C story that serves to explore a character's trauma only if their trauma is not all consuming. The effect of this depiction is supposed to guide the audience to see the character emerging with more confidence (Fathallah 2011: 3).

Depending on the way in which this subgenre is written, it may fall into a trope described by disability scholars as an "overcoming narrative" where disability is presented as a failure that must be compensated for (Garland-Thompson, 2005: 1568). Less frequently, writers, especially disabled writers, can chose to avoid this trope making ultimate success and comfort the integration of their disability into their identity and relationship. If our athlete discovered that her injury permanently affected her ability to play and was thus forced to grapple with losing the sport, her process of acceptance could fall into this narrative. Arguably, this perspective of self-acceptance and an integration of the character's response to their injury into their identity moves the story closer to the ideas of newer critical disability theories. While all fan fiction stories mix together physical and emotional vulnerability and growth, the degree to which these elements are combined dictates the emotional payoff of the story. The final, optional aspect, of the arc is the establishment of a new normal or plateau. This is typically seen in longer stories. It shows the character somewhere emotionally stable. Life may not be perfect, but they have weathered the storm

scholars argue that this view focuses on the needs and desires of predominantly female slash writers through projection, rather than true representations of queer relationships between men, and indeed, there is debate about whether canonical homoerotic relationships truly quality as slash (Russ 2014; Jones 2014; Hunting, 2012: 1). The scholarship on slash and femslash is rich in its own right and beyond the scope of this work; interested readers may find works by Russ (2014), and Jenkins (1992) useful introductions.

and are either with their intended partner or have achieved a place of self-acceptance.

For creators, writing compelling H/C stories that focus on permanent disabilities (permanent injury or chronic illnesses like diabetes) requires building emotional vulnerability without painting the lived reality of the condition as horrifying. A permanently disabled character who refuses to accept their current life and instead spends their time longing for an old or able-bodied normal cannot grow. If "normal" only exists within the context of an average, nondisabled body, then disability is inherently tragic (Kafer 2013). In fan fiction, this view remains alive and well, from magical cure stories to H/C arcs that build vulnerability through ableist tropes, for example, when disabled people provide inspiration porn or portray disability as victimization (Newman-Stille 2019). Authors who wish to move their disabled characters beyond the world of self-pity projected for them by non-disabled people must therefore find new ways to engage with the idea of what it means to be disabled and what it means to be vulnerable (Kafer 2013). Reimagining disability to incorporate physical, interpersonal, environmental and political aspects actually offers more opportunities for new H/C narratives (Kafer 2013; Newman-Stille 2019). For instance, this new view might introduce social or structural barriers as a hurt. A character who cannot attend prom because it is inaccessible can be comforted by a campaign to move the venue to a place that is accessible, rather than requiring a date who is willing to carry them into the building. However, finding this new perspective depends on the disability, author, and narrative goals.

One disability that writers struggle to represent in H/C is diabetes. Moving beyond the fics that promise "comfort so sweet they will give you diabetes," readers and writers must confront an episodic disease that is non-apparent, chronic, and also marked by acute emergencies. While there is no cure, a person manages diabetes through medications like insulin and metformin, exercise, diet, and careful self-monitoring. For some people with diabetes, their self-management becomes ingrained—flowing into the background of daily life. However, to be diabetic, especially a diabetic who uses insulin, is to flirt with short term emergencies of hyper- and hypo-glycemia, also called high and low blood sugars. The onset of high or low blood sugars happens on the scale of minutes to hours and when not addressed, lead to altered consciousness, unconsciousness, and in extreme cases, death. The suspension between highs and lows makes the lived experience of diabetes to be anything but mundane or routine.

Representations must therefore find a way to encode one or both of these potential views. Film scholar Kevin L. Ferguson argues that the invisibility of diabetes necessitates a visual shorthand when it appears in media (2010, 10). This visual shorthand extends the idea that diabetes is only visible when it is poorly controlled, a representational strategy often pulled into fan fiction by authors who draw from source works (Ferguson 2010; Linn 2017: 3). This depiction parallels a medical perspective on disability: there is no cure, but with work and sacrifice, the diabetic can almost achieve normality. By its very nature, fan fiction that represents diabetes explores the way in which diabetes influences either canon diabetic characters or re-imagines established characters as diabetic. In doing so, such work opens opportunities to explore the way the dichotomy of control and crises build vulnerability.

In this essay, I look at the way in which fan fiction writers tell diabetes-centric H/C stories.[2] I do this through primarily textual analysis of three example stories by diabetic authors, gleaned from Archive of Our Own (www.ao3.org), a popular fan fiction archive with a well-documented, semi structured meta tagging system. All the stories are used with the author's consent (Kelley 2016). I approach the work from the perspective of a diabetic, hurt/comfort aficionado, and active member of multiple fandoms. From these works, two contrasting narratives emerged: stories about caretaking and stories about taking control. The stories provide multiple answers to the question of what it means to build intimate relationships in diabetes.

Comfort as Care

One diabetic-centric H/C story is what I will call a "caretaking story," designed to present intimacy between the diabetic character and a companion. All caretaking fics are told from the perspective of the non-diabetic narrator who acts as caretaker, centering the reader in a world where diabetes is an external reality, as opposed to an integral part of the character's

[2] For the purpose of this essay, "diabetes centric" H/C refers to stories where both the physical and emotional injury come specifically from diabetes. For example, a story where a diabetic character gets shot and is forced to contemplate their own mortality would not qualify, nor would a story where a diabetic character serves as the comforter for another character. In either case, diabetes may influence the diabetic's health, psychology and world view, but it would not be the core source of injury or vulnerability.

lived experience. This perspective makes it easier to gage an appropriate reaction to the disabled character's experience of "hurt."

The physical hurt in these stories can either come from an extreme in blood sugar—a severe high or low—or from the daily tasks of diabetes management. The diabetic characters are childish, a potential shorthand for their emotional vulnerability (Newman-Stille 2019). The caretaker provides physical comfort for the diabetic person by performing some daily act of diabetes care: blood sugar monitoring, giving insulin, and dietary management with little help or input from the diabetic character. The endgame for most stories is intimacy, but if any character gets to experience growth and catharsis, it is the caretaker.

When done well, caretaking H/C is about intimacy and familiarity within an existing relationship. Based on the movie, *Love Simon*, the fic titled, "it's a love that will keep me holding on," depicts Simon's boyfriend, Bram, taking care of Simon as he has high blood sugar (brooklynbis 2018). The story shows five examples of Simon's response to high blood sugar: hyperactivity; disassociation; exhaustion; frustration; and sensory overload. During each of the scenes, Bram takes care of Simon both physically and emotionally, either by helping Simon by retrieving his blood sugar meter and insulin, or by testing and dosing for Simon. Simon's degree of participation varies based on his mental state, but the author makes it clear that Simon normally performs his own self-management tasks. At the end of each scene, Simon and Bram reaffirm their love for each other and Simon makes it clear that he is grateful for the support. From a disability studies perspective, the story works have to move outside a traditional medical model of disability into a more all-encompassing one, like Kafer's political relational model (2013). We are asked to focus beyond Simon's experience, but instead on the impact of his diabetes on his family. While the story acknowledges lived medical realities of high blood sugar, it also focuses on the way in which Simon's diabetes affects Bram and their relationship. However, despite this change in perspective on disability, the story still centers Bram while denying Simon physical autonomy and narrative agency.

A second example of a caretaking story comes from "Sweet and Sour," an *Osomasu-san* anime fanfic (PastelLucio 2017). In this fic, we watch as Karamatsu cares for his twin brother, Jyushimatsu, after Jyushimatsu's diagnosis with diabetes.[3] This story uses the chronic nature of diabetes as the central conflict for the "hurt" aspect of the story, embodied by Karamatsu testing Jyushimatsu's blood sugar and performing an insulin injection for him. Jyushimatsu's emotional vulnerability comes from terror and revulsion at what he must do to stay alive. Karamatsu remains calm while Jyushimatsu throws a temper tantrum over the painful torture of blood sugar checks and insulin injections. In the caretaking story, Karamatsu mourns the pain he must cause his brother—positioning the central pain of diabetes as belonging to the loved ones of those diagnosed, rather than to the person with diabetes themselves. Though Jyushimatsu's frustration is shown while being cared for by Karamatsu, the story focuses on the emotional experiences and growth of Karamatsu while he works to keep Jyushimatsu safe.

The caretakers are the protagonists of these stories, granted control over both the other character's diabetes and the narrative. Bram and Karamatsu provide physical comfort: they are solely, in Karamatsu's case, or situationally, in Bram's case, responsible for testing the diabetic character's blood sugar and administering insulin. These actions grant them a narrative agency that both the diabetic characters are denied. Simon is sometimes able to take care for himself, but when his blood sugar is high, he reverts to a child-like state. Bram ultimately makes the complex decisions, for example, how much insulin should be dosed. In "Sweet and Sour," we see an even more extreme version of this dichotomy. Karamatsu takes action in the story, while Jyushimatsu weeps and refuses to act. The only time Jyushimatsu expresses his opinion or asks his brother to stop, he is ignored or worse, threatened. It is through such plot devices that Jyushimatsu's character is reduced to an avatar of out-of-control diabetes. Because Jyushimatsu cannot take care of himself, he arguably cannot exist in the story as anything but an extension of Karamatsu. In both caretaking stories, Karamatsu and Bram must act because they are the only capable character available.

What is more, aside from their caretaking actions, Karamatsu and Bram's narration guides the emotional response of the reader. Both serve as what Disability Studies scholar, Carrie Sandahl, describes as the

[3] I am unfamiliar with the source work, *Osomasu-san*. However, the *Osomasu-san* wiki suggests the characters were originally introduced in as children in an earlier series, *Osomasu-kun*. Based on the fandom tagged for the story and the fact that Karamatsu and Jyushimatsu are twins, I assume the characters are adults.

"non-disabled guide" (2019: 148). This character "keys audience members to the appropriate emotional responses to the disabled character" (Sandhl 2019: 148). By and large, fan fiction writers must assume their audience will be non-diabetic and is likely to not be disabled; even stories written as "gift fics" from a diabetic author to a diabetic reader, can be assumed to have a wider non-disabled audience. By selecting the non-disabled character as guide and narrator, the author can introduce diabetes-related care tasks without having to face the potential complexities of either lived experience or the physical consequences of the acute diabetes-related hurt. For instance, Simon's story would read very differently from his perspective, possibly leading the audience confused during a spiral between hyperactive to dissociated or asleep. The approach also makes it easier to leverage traditional vulnerability coding in hurt/comfort. The caretaker can depict the disabled character as vulnerable, cute, or somehow in need of support, an almost necessary cue to allow for the intimacy to come. This choice also discounts the perspective and experience of the diabetic characters: they are adorable or difficult, rather than experiencing some physical reality of diabetes. However, the way in which these two works use their guide character as emotional touchstones differs greatly.

Karamatsu paints Jyushimatsu and his emotional reaction to having diabetes as a burden that he, as a caretaker, must bear. The story depicts Jyushimatsu as a disobedient, dependent child who whimpers, whines, sniffles, and eventually escalates to "full-on bawling with tears and snot" (PastelLucio 2017). At one point, Karamatsu even threatens to spank Jyushimatsu when he says he does not want to take an insulin injection. Infantilizing imagery like we see in this fic is not uncommon to diabetes spaces.

Diabetes is often associated with infantilizing imagery. For example, a thematic analysis of interviews with adult diabetics from Australia found participants often used child-like language as they related to their diabetes (Broom and Whittaker 2004). In this study, "naughty" was a common descriptor among participants for lapses in self-care and periods when blood sugar management was difficult. While Jyushimatsu does not seem to relate to his own diabetes through conventional child-like rhetors, the descriptions of his behavior locate him squarely within that realm. In contrast, Broom and Whittaker argue that using child-like rhetors provides adults with diabetes a way to assert their moral agency by creating a dichotomy between "childlike language which diverts blame … and the requirement that they "grow up" and manage properly" (2004). Unlike the people with diabetes described in Broom and Whittaker's study, though, the character Jyushimatsu is not afforded the chance to grow up or manage diabetes tasks on his sown. Instead, he is the victim of a horrifying disease which has robbed him of his agency. Readers of this fic are led to reduce Jyushimatsu's behavior as a character deficit and as a burden to Karamatsu instead of as a complex embodiment of chronic illness. And Jyushimatsu's suffering seems to only get worse as Karamatsu forces care upon him. In this way, the plot frames diabetes almost as a fate worse than death. The insidiousness of Jyushimatsu's caretaking story, then, extends beyond locating the primary experience of disability within the growth of a non-disabled character. It also reproduces the pervasive cultural narrative that death is preferable to living a life with disability (Sandahl 2019). As a diabetic reader, there is only hurt without any chance for comfort in this representation.

In contrast, Bram's narrative perspective focuses on intimacy with Simon, guiding the reader to understand that their romantic relationship is strong in spite of the challenges disability can introduce. Henry Jenkins, an early scholar of fandom studies, observed, "Slash stories centre on the relationships between male program characters and the obstacles they must overcome to achieve intimacy" (1992, 189). Slash-centric H/C focuses on using vulnerability to build intimacy. In this genre, disabilities can easily become a natural extension for coding this vulnerability (Newman-Stille 2019). Simon and Bram's fic takes place after they have been together for several years in their shared home and we watch them move through their living room, kitchen, stairs and bedroom. The narrative indicates that even when Simon has high blood sugar, he performs self-care tasks outside their home. Only with Bram do we see Simon allow himself this vulnerability. Within this context, Bram caring for Simon becomes intimate, furthering their romantic narrative. However, one key difference between Simon and Bram's story and tradition slash fic is the canon sexuality of the characters. Traditionally, within slash, H/C has served to allow assumed heterosexual characters space to explore the possibility for an intimate homoerotic relationship (Jenkins 1992; Russ 2014). In their original canon story, Simon and Bram are explicitly written as queer; the central conflict of the source work, *Love Simon*, centers on Simon's experience of coming out in high school, leading to his relationship with Bram. The story follows the plot a typical romantic comedy, where the characters must overcome personal and societal barriers placed in the way of their relationship. Since potentials obstacles to the relationship have been fully explored in canon, the need to read them into other stories is lessened. This reading may limit the need to re-code characters as vulnerable to establish or support intimacy.

An alternative reading that does not involve trying to re-code hypermasculinity as vulnerable may be possible. The author of Simon's caretaking story notes, "again, this is mainly based off my own experience here (very heavily in fact)" and added meta-tags for "Bram is a good boyfriend" and "boyfriend goals" (brooklynbis 2018).[4] This commentary may be indicative of the author's desires for their own potential relationship. In an essay on how fan fiction taught her to write, professional author Seanan McGuire claims that storytelling starts with projecting oneself into the story (2018). In Western media, many white boys[5] learn from an early age that the hero of stories looks like them while girls were forced to find "socially acceptable avatars" as representatives to tell their stories (McGuire 2018). By placing themselves through the use of socially acceptable avatars in stories, "[women's] stories were finally judged based on what [the stories] were, and not what people thought they knew about [the writers], and them." (McGuire 2018). Using Simon as a socially acceptable avatar, the fic potentially becomes an opportunity for its diabetic author to explore what they might want to find in current or future relationships. And, in that way, this version of a caretaker story could come with a comforting promise: there is intimacy to be had with diabetes, and there are partners who will care.

Ultimately, though, the comfort as care narrative fails to live up to fan fiction's transformative potential. These stories play into a disability trope described by disability scholar Rosemary Garland-Thompson as the "sentimental narrative that sees people with disabilities abilities as occasions for narcissistic pity or lessons in suffering for those who imagine themselves as nondisabled" (2005: 1568). Although the characters are re-imagined and re-written as diabetic, they still play into dominant social views of

[4] The Archive of our Own repository uses a semi-structured meta tagging system. The tagging system identifies fandom, characters, relationships, warnings, and other content (Johnson 2014). The tags can also serve as insight into the author's view and intention: a story tagged "romance" may be approached differently by authors and readers than the same story tagged "stockholm syndrome."

[5] McGuire writes from the perspective of a queer cis-gender white woman growing up in the 80's and 90's, which she states explicitly in her essay. The choice of explicitly gendered language is not intended as a dismissal of nonbinary fans, but was intended to speak to her observations and experiences.

disability, re-enforcing an idea living with a disability like diabetes is too difficult to manage alone.

Comfort as Control

A second diabetes centric H/C narrative exists almost in response to the caretaking narrative: in these stories, the diabetic character manages their diabetes on their own. The diabetic characters are shown planning out and doing diabetes self-care tasks; making subtle calculations around food, blood sugar, and insulin; and changing insulin pump infusion sets or constant glucose monitoring (CGM) sensors. These diabetic characters are also more likely to have and rely on technology like pumps and CGMs. However, the diabetic character fears what will happen when they discuss their diabetes within their relationships; this is the central point of tension rather than any physical manifestation of the disease. Here, vulnerability is almost the anthesis of the caretaker narrative. The diabetic character is afraid of having their relationship transition from that of partners into caretaker and patient with the accompanying lack of agency. Avoiding this scenario is often worth the cost of intimacy in a relationship. For me, as a reader and writer, the conflict between intimacy and autonomy is what makes the stories so appealing and the emotional set up is key. The "hurt" portion of story can vary in severity, but it requires the diabetic character's blood sugar to be too volatile to manage without help. Comfort comes through conversation, and the diabetic character re-asserting or re-negotiating boundaries. The payout is both growth for the diabetic character and the relationship.

The fic, "True Independence" is emblematic of the comfort as control type of H/C story. The main character, a fictionalized version of YouTuber Adam Kovic, has been diabetic for several years (Orphan Work 2017b). Shortly before the beginning of the story, he entered a polyamorous relationship with his coworkers. The story, told from Adam's perspective, opens with Adam focusing on the contrast between the almost routine actions of self-care and the emotional toll of diabetes in his relationships. He performs common daily tasks like testing his blood sugar, taking insulin, and calculating the number of carbohydrates in his food without much effort. At the same time, Adam worries about the consequences of letting his lovers closer because "[he] thought [they'd] think it was too much" and leave him (Orphan Work 2017b, ch 3). Adam's thinking demonstrates an existential duality present in the comfort as control narrative—he accepts his own diabetes and wonders how non-disabled people could accept it in him.

In the story, Adam goes to the beach with his coworkers to film for their YouTube series. After strenuous exercise, Adam experiences a severe low blood sugar. His lovers come to his rescue, helping him test his blood sugar and staying with him while he recovers. This is the extent of the physical comfort Adam receives and he recovers in less than half an hour. At dinner that evening, Adam and his lovers have a discussion about his diabetes. Adam makes it clear that diabetes is his responsibility, and that it is an additional thing the group will need to navigate while they work through their romantic relationship.

Unlike caretaking fics, this archetype relies on the way disability affects interpersonal relationships to build conflict and reveal vulnerability. For instance, in "True Independence," Adam struggles with a major, interconnected fears about how his diabetes will affect his relationship: will his partners reject him, blame him, or pressure and judge him? In my own comfort as control fics, I tend to take this question a step further. My characters question whether a potential romantic interest is worthy enough of the trust needed to build an intimate relationship, rather than as a potential complication to a nascent romance. Scholarship in the area of diabetes suggests that Adam, my characters and I are not alone in concerns around the way in which diabetes will affect our relationships. For example, a study of Australian adults with Type 1 diabetes[6] found participants worried disclosing their diabetes might affect long term relationship prospects, including one individual whose mother-in-law discouraged her partner from proposing to her (Browne et al. 2014). Studies have also found that diabetic people also feared judgement and blame from close family related to their self-care. And the suspicion of judgment may not be unfounded. Some studies that are grounded in the relational side of diabetes found that partners of diabetics who had witnessed severe hypoglycemic events experienced diabetes-specific stressors like anxiety and loss of sleep, while their diabetic partners did not (Gonder-Fredrik et al. 1997; Ritholz 2014). As we see in studies, fan fic, and beyond, diabetic adults are subjected to a process of negotiation to establish healthy boundaries within relationships to address their vulnerability.

[6] "True Independence" carries the meta tags, "Type I Diabetes" and "daibetic!adam", clearly identifying Adam as type I diabetic.

Comfort and intimacy in the comfort as control narrative derive from relationship growth. In diabetes control centric stories, comfort comes in the form of negotiated boundaries. In “True Independence,” Adam establishes his boundaries, saying “I need [diabetes] to be my problem [...] I know that you guys want to help me with stuff... but the diabetes thing is my thing. My baggage to carry” (Orphaned Work 2017b, ch 3). Because the story follows an H/C narrative arc, the comfort response is reassurance from Adam’s partners. They remind him that they have known each other for years, and Adam’s diabetes never affected their friendship or acceptance before. Rather than holding Adam to an unobtainable standard of perfection, Adam’s lovers reassure him that they won’t judge him, saying that for as long as Adam had been diabetic, he’d “earned [himself] a few mistakes” (Orphaned Work 2017b: ch 3). While the language may read as somewhat ableist, the sentiment is clear: Adam’s lovers are there to support him on his terms, even when things are challenging. Subsequent works in this series reflect these boundaries: in a later story, we see Adam’s lovers working to make sure there is food available should be experience a low blood sugar, but they trust him to know when it might be necessary (Orphan Work 2017a: ch 1). This story approaches the ideals of “Crip Lit” within fan fiction by “assert new understandings of disabled bodies” (Newman-Stille 2019; 91). Adam has incorporated his disability into his lived experience and relationship, allowing the relationship to transform. As Adam creates intimacy with his partners, the character reminds readers that romantic relationships do not have to fall into the trap of caretaker and patient, but instead can exist on an equal footing of healthy boundaries and mutual respect.

Conclusions

Diabetes-centric H/C fanfiction explores what it means to be diabetic, vulnerable, and intimate. Some stories re-enforce common narratives from popular culture by building on existing ableist tropes and paint their diabetic characters as children. The representation of diabetes in these stories provides little comfort for any of their characters: the diabetic characters cannot grow, the caretakers are saddled with a burden, and the audience learns that life with diabetes is not worth living. These narratives perpetuate diabetes-related stigmas, and fail to live up to the transformative, disruptive power of fan fiction. However, readers can also find stories that reflect different perspectives on the lives and desire of characters with diabetes. Some fanfics portray characters who desire intimacy around and care for their diabetes, while at the same time demonstrating fear of the consequences of such intimacy. Together, all of these stories can create a new cultural imagination around what it means to be diabetic, whether that be a rescue by a prince charming or the complexity of navigating a multifaceted relationship.

References

brooklynbis. 2018. It's a Love That Will Keep Me Holding On. Fan Fiction. Archive of Our Own. August 3, 2018. https://archiveofourown.org/works/15554610.

Broom, Dorothy, and Andrea Whittaker. 2004. Controlling Diabetes, Controlling Diabetics: Moral Language in the Management of Diabetes Type 2. *Social Science and Medicine* 58: 2371–2382. https://doi.org/10.1016/j.socscimed.2003.09.002.

Browne, Jessica L., Adriana Ventura, Kylie Mosely, and Jane Speight. 2014. 'I'm Not a Druggie, I'm Just Diabetic': A Qualitative Study of Stigma from the Perspective of Adults with Type 1 Diabetes. *BMJ Open* 4: e005625. https://doi.org/10.1136/bmjopen-2014-005625.

Clemons, AmyLea. 2019. Enabling/Disabling: Fanfiction and Disability Discourse. *Canadian Journal of Disability Studies* 7: 247–278. https://doi.org/10.15353/cjds.v8i2.500.

Coppa, Francesca. 2014. Fuck Yeah, Fandom is Beautiful. *Journal of Fan Studies* 2 (1): 73–82. https://doi.org/10.1386/jfs.2.1.73_1.

———. 2017. Introduction: Five Things that Fanfiction Is, and One Thing It Isn't. In *The Fanfiction Reader: Folk Tales for the Digital Age*, ed. Francesca Coppa, 1–17. Ann Arbor: University of Michigan Press.

Dym, Brianna, Jed R. Brubaker, Casey Fiesler, and Bryan Semaan. 2019. 'Coming Out Okay' Community Narratives for LGBTQ Identity Recovery Work. *Proceedings of the ACM on Human-Computer Interaction* 3(CSCW): 1–28. https://doi.org/10.1145/3359256.

Fathallah, Judith May. 2011. H/C and Me: An Autoethnographic Account of a Troubled Love Affair. *Transformative Works and Cultures* 7. https://doi.org/10.3983/twc.2011.0252.

Ferguson, Kevin L. 2010. The Cinema of Control: On Diabetic Excess and Illness in Film. *Journal of Medical Humanities.* 31 (3): 183–204. https://doi.org/10.1007/s10912-010-9110-8.

Fowler, Megan Justine. 2019. Rewriting the School Story through Racebending in the Harry Potter and Raven Cycle Fandoms. In *Fans of Color, Fandoms of*

Color, ed. Abigail De Kosnik and André Carrington, special issue. *Transformative Works and Cultures*, 29. https://doi.org/10.3983/twc.2019.1492.

Garland-Thompson, Rosemary. 2005. Feminist Disability Studies. *Signs* 30: 1557–1587. https://doi.org/10.1086/423352.

Gonder-Fredrik, Linda, Daniel Cox, Boris Kovatchev, Diana Julian, and William Clark. 1997. The Psychosocial Impact of Severe Hypoglycemic Episodes on Spouses of Patients With IDDM. *Diabetes Care* 20: 1543–1546. https://doi.org/10.2337/diacare.20.10.1543.

Hunting, Kyra. 2012. *Queer as Folk* and the Trouble with Slash. *Transformative Works and Cultures* 11. https://doi.org/10.3983/twc.2012.0415.

Jenkins, Henry. 1992. *Textual Poachers: Television Fans & Participatory Culture*. London: Routledge.

Johnson, Shannon Fay. 2014. Fan Fiction Metadata Creation and Utilization within Fan Fiction Archives: Three Primary Models. *Transformative Works and Cultures* 17. https://doi.org/10.3983/twc.2014.0578.

Johnson, Poe. 2019. Transformative Racism: The Black Body in Fan Works. In *Fans of Color, Fandoms of Color*, ed. Abigail De Kosnik and andré carrington, special issue, *Transformative Works and Cultures* 29. https://doi.org/10.3983/twc.2019.1669.

Jones, Sara Gwenlian. 2014. The Sex Lives of Cult Television Characters. In *The Fan Fiction Studies Reader*, ed. Karen Hellekson and Kristina Busse, 116–129. Iowa City: University of Iowa Press.

Kafer, Alison. 2013. *Feminist Queer Crip*. Bloomington, IN: Indiana University Press.

Kelley, Brittany. 2016. Toward a Goodwill Ethics of Online Research Methods. *Transformative Works and Cultures* 22. https://doi.org/10.3983/twc.2016.0891.

Linn, Rachel. 2017. Bodies in Horrifying Hurt/Comfort Fan Fiction: Paying the Toll. *Transformative Works and Cultures* 25. https://doi.org/10.3983/twc.2017.1102.

McGuire, Seanan. 2018. The Bodies of the Girls Who Made Me: Fanfic and the Modern World. *Tor.com*, April 9. https://www.tor.com/2018/04/09/the-bodies-of-the-girls-who-made-me-fanfic-and-the-modern-world/.

Newman-Stille, Derek. 2019. From Slash Fan Fiction to Crip Fan Fiction: What Role Does Disability Have in Fandom? *Canadian Journal of Disabilities Studies* 8 (2): 73–95. https://doi.org/10.15353/cjds.v8i2.492.

Orphaned Work. 2017a. Business Trips. Fan Fiction. Archive of our Own. April 9. https://archiveofourown.org/works/10576221.

———. 2017b. True Independence. Fan Fiction. Archive of Our Own. March 6. https://archiveofourown.org/works/10124924.

PastelLucio. 2017. Sweet and Sour. Fan Fiction. Archive of Our Own. August 19. https://archiveofourown.org/works/11849889.

Ritholz, M.D., M. Beste, S.S. Edwards, E.A. Beverly, A. Atakov-Sastillo, and H.A. Wolpert. 2014. Impact of Continuous Glucose Monitoring on Diabetes Management and Marital Relationship of Adults with Type 1 Diabetes and Their Spouses: A Qualitative Study. *Diabetic Medicine* 31: 47–54. https://doi.org/10.1111/dme.12276.

Russ, Joanna. 2014. Pornography by Women, for Women, with Love. In *The Fan Fiction Studies Reader*, ed. Karen Hellekson and Kristina Busse, 82–96. Iowa City: University of Iowa Press.

Sandahl, Carrie. 2019. It's All the Same Movie: Making *Code of Fraaks*. *Journal of Cinema and Media Studies* 58: 145–150. https://doi.org/10.1353/cj.2019.0044.

PART V

Disability Identity, Crip Futures and Liberation

Chapters in the final section consider diabetes identity, futures, and liberation from internalized ableism across a variety of contexts. In each chapter, the author grapples with diabetes identity within a particular ecosystem (e.g. advocacy work, diabetes camp, online blogs). Though the authors come from different points in their own diabetic identity formation, all contend with external pressures of 'should'. For example, S.K. Sabada recalls how non-disabled adults in their life put pressure on them to meet heteronormative species-typical milestones from a young age. Such pressures gave Sabada a platform to push against in their identity development as a non-binary, queer, diabetic child. While Stephen Shaul describes how his expectation of being a diabetes advocate dictated how he 'should' appear, act, and show up. All four authors in this section contend with ontological paradoxes that make reading diabetes identity a stimulating and thought-provoking exercise.

In "Self-Exceptionism and its Counternarrative: An Autonetnography of Shifting Diabetes Identity," Heather R. Walker contemplates diabetes identity formation in a social environment that makes assumptions about what being diabetic must mean. Walker argues that bringing diabetes into her self-concept was a political act requiring unlearning and deconditioning. She describes moments of reckoning with internalized ableism, where she tried to locate herself within and apart from stereotypical formulations of diabetes. First, Walker deconstructs a representational strategy she calls *self-exceptionism*. Then, she offers an alternative framework for looking at diabetes identity which Walker terms *radical trust*.

Issues surrounding both trust and identity-building play a significant role in Kirsten E. Gardner's chapter, "'Especially Made for Them': Summer Camps for Diabetic Children." As Gardner analyzes historical documents of diabetes camp life and structure, she questions the impact of the camp funders, and researchers' good intentions. She uses the charity model of disability to upend how campers, counselors, medical specialists, and philanthropists made sense of diabetes. In contrast with the historical account Gardner shares of diabetes camp life as a "temporal accessibly built environment apart from the world that often ignores bodies disabled by chronic illness," S.K. Sabada, who attended diabetes camp in their youth, paints a more complicated picture.

S.K. Sabada's autofictive essay, "Troubling Cure and Cripping Futurity: Queering Narratives of Diabetes" positions diabetes identity against the theory of the Symbolic Child, carving out a place for diabetics to grow *sideways*. In settings like diabetes camp and charity fundraising events, Sabada identifies oppressive forces that they felt constrained their upward development as a human. They complicate diabetes identity by describing what it would look like to desire a diabetic body and diabetes embodiment. To end their chapter, Sabada calls readers from all backgrounds to "examine collective diabetic embodiment as a relatively untapped resource of knowledge and culture, [and] to fully embrace our power as disabled people capable of destabilizing ableism." Sabada's empowering concluding message sets the stage for our final chapter in the book.

We close this book with a chapter by diabetes advocate Stephen Shaul. In his hope-filled chapter "Diabetes Advocacy: Many Voices, One Message," Shaul describes and demystifies advocacy through personal narrative. Shaul questions what it means to be an advocate and represent the ever-broadening community. In this encouraging chapter, Shaul invites readers to identify as an advocate and act on their impulse to make the diabetes experience better for more people.

Four central questions guide the works in part five:

- How, and against what, do diabetic people incorporate *collective diabetes identity* into their self-concepts?
- How does collective diabetes identity shift when diabetic people deconstruct internalized ableism?

- What conundrums arise when we de-center the medical gaze from spaces like diabetes camp?
- How can we reimagine the diabetic experience, diabetes embodiment, and diabetic futures?

Self-Exceptionism and its Counternarrative: An Autonetnography of Shifting Diabetes Identity

Heather R. Walker

Until my late 20's, I was thin—or rather, thin enough to not face discrimination based on size. In those days, I was both flattered and repulsed by a common reaction I would receive after disclosing that I have diabetes. "You don't look like you have diabetes" each new acquaintance would inevitably say. I would feel flattered because their comment implicitly suggested my body met contemporary standards of beauty [coded for thinness] and I had been socialized and conditioned to understand that as a compliment. But, I would too feel repulsed because I knew that their comment subscribed to stereotypical ideas that a diabetic body *should* be "overweight." I would wonder when in my life I would stop hearing this comment. At what age? At what size? And then I would smile and respond

H. R. Walker (✉)
Medical Group Analytics, University of Utah Health, Salt Lake City, UT, USA
e-mail: Heather.Walker@hsc.utah.edu

B. C. Frazer, H. R. Walker (eds.), *(Un)doing Diabetes: Representation, Disability, Culture*, Palgrave Studies in Science and Popular Culture, https://doi.org/10.1007/978-3-030-83110-3_18

with something along the lines of "many of us don't"—believing myself to be doing the good work of education because I refuted the stereotype.

The banality of common reactions to my disclosure became numbing over time. The more I received reactions like this as a teenager and young adult, the more I internalized the stigma hidden within them. I bought into the stigmatized identity put upon diabetic people by mainstream non-diabetic society, or ***ascribed identity in diabetes.*** I believed that most diabetic bodies looked diabetic [fat embodiment], and that my diabetic body was simply an exception [thin embodiment]. In addition, I have Type 1 diabetes, which further complicates these matters. I have held back from telling anyone what type of diabetes I have for the last six or seven years—sometimes as a rejection of the way the medical establishment has categorized and sub-grouped diabetic people, and other times as a hope to not reproduce type-based diabetes stigma. The motivation behind the response I used to give (i.e. "not all diabetic bodies look diabetic") was to spark continued conversation about diabetes. At that time in my growth and development as a human and as a diabetic, I wanted the world to change its understanding of diabetes and its different types. At that time in my life, I believed I could reduce diabetes stigma by teaching people that not all types of diabetes fit the stereotypical mold. In effect, I was using myself to represent the ***ideal exception*** rather than dismantling ***the representational rule.***

When I reflect back on how that representational strategy came so naturally to me, I feel shame and guilt. My beliefs functioned to Other those with diabetes who did appear to meet expectations of a stereotypical diabetic body, in effect legitimizing the stereotypes wrapped around diabetic embodiment. I look back to my old writings on social media and feel somehow betrayed by the versions of self I have been. However, I have come to understand that my historical response to fatphobic comments like "you don't look diabetic" are representative of a particular stage in my development and integration of ***diabetes identity.*** Early on in my life with diabetes around the age of 12, I made sense of my disease by distancing myself from it and its representations. Excruciating as it is to admit now, it took several years of reflective writing and reading disability studies literature to learn that my approach to stigma was destructive to the diabetes community. Looking back and seeing my own conditioned prejudices is painful. Yet, there is something generative about it too. What can I learn from digging deeply into the internalized ableism of my past life with diabetes? How can I use this discomfort to read today differently, to reimagine what being diabetic means, to embody a diabetes identity that doesn't rely on individualism and ableist ideologies? How do I use the self-observations that now weigh me down to create a different mode of being, one that doesn't rely on the rule/exception dichotomy?

In this chapter, I explore the process of *self-exceptionism*—where it comes from, how it manifests, and the tensions it draws forward as a discursive tool. Self-exceptionism means understanding oneself as an exception to the stereotypical rule, believing that the so-called rule does generally apply to others in the group. Using autonetnographic methods, I analyze 138 posts I wrote on the, now retired, diabetes blog I kept from 2012–2016—called *Unexpected Blues* (Kozinets 2015). At the outset, the purpose of the blog was to chronicle experiences that reminded me I had diabetes when I wasn't thinking of it; moments in which the world magically and poetically justified the conditions of my existence. I'd later describe my writing in the blog as *poetic prose*. In hindsight, blogging gave me exposure and access to others who shared the parts of diabetic experience that left me rattled or unsure. By writing it publicly, I slowly found others who felt judged like I did, who experienced diabetes trauma, who cried on the phone with insurance companies, and who rationed insulin out of necessity like I did.

Within my writings on *Unexpected Blues*, I locate evidence of shifting identity constructions and self-concepts that revolve around various versions of self-exceptionism. I contend with tensions that shook and shifted my sense of self with diabetes and disability as they appear in my writings. In so doing, I situate my experience within normalized narratives and representations of diabetes in broader American culture. I also contextualize my own experience within diabetes identity scholarship I have published and researched previously.

Here, I make a case for reading identity *in* diabetes and *diabetes identity* differently; the former being based within an individualized lens, and the latter within a claimed collective minority identity. I argue that diabetes identity formation, within American culture, involves a cyclical process of recognizing and rejecting patterns of self-exceptionism. I unpack moments of reckoning where I observed liberation from self-exceptionism in my blog. And, finally, I use frameworks of disability identity formation as described by disability studies scholars like Ellen Samuels, Carol Gill, Brenda Brueggemann, and Heather Evans to build a case for an opposing force to self-exceptionism: *radical trust*. As a generative and liberating framework, *radical trust* allows us to contest the dichotomy between rule and exception. I end this chapter with a discussion of the power that radical trust may have on diabetes identity.

Both in the blog and in this chapter, I make use of the proverbial "we," positioning myself as within the diabetic population—subjected to the same stereotypes and stigmas that I argue form so much of diabetes identity. With that said, my reflections are shaped and limited by my white, cis-gendered, straight, middle-class upbringing and experiences. It wasn't until I was diagnosed with a stigmatized chronic illness that I noticed overt discrimination. Considering my narrow set of experiences, what this chapter can offer, too, is limited.

Ascribed Identity in Diabetes

Dominant social and cultural representations of diabetes show the diabetic as an apathetic, fat, gluttonous person who chooses indulgence over health (Walker and Frazer 2021). Diabetes makes a person a monstrous Other, the abject with compromised agency (Fahey 2015). Stereotypical formulations of diabetes such as these center on lifestyle and character flaws (Bock 2017). This blame-laden *ascribed identity* is what we have to work with at diagnosis, us diabetic people. We are blamed regardless of context. My uncle said that despite "knowing better now," when he heard I was diagnosed with diabetes in 2001, he thought it was because I had eaten too many Cheetos—an indulgence I had been known to enjoy. And I remember having a similar thought. Wondering, what did I do to cause this?

Bringing diabetes into my self-concept has been a political act requiring unlearning and deconditioning. *Unexpected Blues* was my public outlet for unlearning pieces of ascribed identity in diabetes. I often offered justifications or apologies for what I perceived at the time to be poor diabetes management, accompanied by promises to do better, to *be* better than popular representations of diabetes said I would be. My promises extended to my personhood, implicitly conveying the idea that *being better at diabetes* would also make me a better person. In 2013, in a post about revealing secrets, I wrote:

> *being honest means giving something away. it means exposing what is underneath the parts of you that you actively work to show. it means not showing the parts of you that you like. it is like taking apart a mosaic, a beautiful crafted art piece to reveal concrete below …*

saying to someone who loves you, "sometimes i choose to not take care of myself" is really difficult. there is a moment of loss and sorrow. i had to say out loud this terrible thing about ME. this gray as concrete thing, that i hate to face anyway. this thing that makes me feel pain and shame and guilt and tragedy. this thing that swells up in me, trying to get out, trying to get attention. i am never ready to give it away.

but i didn't want to take it back. i wanted to find warmth. i wanted to change something in the universe as a result.

i don't know if i changed something, but i did get the warmth. i lost a secret.

What this post makes evident, is the explicit way I tied my sense of self and of self-worth to compliance. Said another way, I felt I was worth the amount of complying with diabetes management behaviors I was doing at any given time. I so deeply internalized the ableism saturating the medical establishment that I was absolutely convinced that by not doing diabetes tasks, I was purposely neglecting my body. I likened non-compliance with ugliness and blandness, a departure from the version of myself I crafted for the public—the one that appeared healthy. I unknowingly subscribed to the subtexts of social abuse and exclusion that stereotyped diabetic people as lazy and unwilling to do what it takes to see species-typical blood glucose levels.

Now, having had entrance into the theories and languages of disability studies, I realize that I was reckoning with ableism and diabetes stigma—trying to locate my self within or apart from *them*. I was trying to understand my relationship to non-compliance and the diabetic people the media and medical establishment identified as "truly" non-compliant. I remember feeling at the time at least I was aware of myself, and that my self-awareness set me apart. I felt as though my awareness made me the exception—with the rule being that most diabetic people didn't know themselves enough to understand their own lapse in compliance. It is only now, in the pauses I've taken to write this chapter that I see how profoundly my self-exceptionism functioned to de-politicize diabetes within my own narratives, and my reflections of my lived experience. As I mentioned before, though, self-exceptionism does not form in a vacuum.

In line with medical and psychological research into diabetes identity, diabetic people learn from medical professionals that accepting diabetes into one's self-concept is valuable insofar as it improves willingness and ability to self-manage (Walker and Litchman, 2021). We are told that accepting diabetes is an individualistic pursuit as if the impact of our identification stops, too, at the bounds of the individual. I argue, then, that the medical establishment medicalizes identity by individualizing it. Because medicalizing identity in diabetes also de-politicizes it, it takes much deconditioning and unlearning to be liberated from identity in diabetes as a framework of identification. Between internalizing ascribed identity in diabetes and claiming diabetes identity, the diabetic must reckon with the history of abuses others with diabetes have faced.

Identity in Diabetes and Self-Exceptionism

Diabetes identity is not bestowed upon a person at diagnosis, although contending with a life-altering diagnosis like diabetes can shake one's sense of self. While accepting diabetes into one's self concept has merit as a strategy to potentially improve mental health and diabetes self-management, it does not necessarily acknowledge a collective diabetes identity. At diagnosis, my healthcare team said I would live a "normal life" without complications from diabetes until I was 35—a falsehood that haunted me for nearly two decades.[1] They told me that I was the same Heather, but I would *simply* need to do a few more things to be healthy like my [non-diabetic] friends. I was told that while it was not clear why my body had turned on itself, that I would be *okay*. I was told I was lucky because I did not go into a coma before my doctor figured it out and because a scientist had discovered how to make synthetic insulin.[2] Overall, the healthcare team gave me narratives about an identity based in normalcy, not diabetic embodiment, and not disability. That is, I was not *a diabetic*, I was a *person who happened to have diabetes*—the latter of which

[1] As a young child, I interpreted the healthcare provider's comment as a signal of my end. I thought they were telling me I would die at the age of 35. Now, having processed that memory with my parents, who were also there at the time, I realize I was told that if I kept my blood sugars in range, I could expect to reach at least age 35 before seeing complications (like kidney disease, blindness, or amputations).

[2] These messages are likely type-specific. I was not blamed, shamed, or belittled for my diagnosis—an experience many with type 2 diabetes have described (Liu et al. 2017), especially those with fat embodiment (Rogge et al. 2004; Teixeira and Budd 2010). On the contrary; I recall hearing many times that I was "innocent". These welcome to type 1diabetes narratives set the groundwork of a diabetes identity built upon self-exceptionism. And my self-exceptionism was taught by my medical team, authenticated by comments I heard first-hand, and affirmed by popular media. By the age of 20, then 9 years post diagnosis, I had firmly internalized the idea that the diabetes stereotype (the rule) did not apply to me, nor to most others with type 1 diabetes (the exception).

was a rallying cry in many diabetes groups I would later join. And for my first 10 years with diabetes, I held that such person-first language was the only just approach to identification. I believed I could and should minimize the trauma diabetes brought to my life because I thought that appearing "normal" meant I was *doing* diabetes right. I did not have diabetes identity. But rather, a tight hold on a narrative rooted in ableism—an identity built upon distance from stereotypical representations of diabetes and toward able-bodied normative ones. In my experience, the desire to accentuate or highlight that distance is what self-exceptionism thrives upon.

My early blog posts (2012–2014), suggest that self-exceptionism was my primary tool for making sense of how diabetes fit within my self-concept. By 2014, I would reckon with the self-exceptionism that I had used to make sense of my identity in diabetes, calling it out for what it was: an internalized form of *defensive othering* (Ezzell 2009). Throughout this chapter, I provide examples of how self-exceptionism manifested in my own experience and identity with diabetes. I explain that my self-concept has historically involved thin embodiment, emotional self-awareness, and willingness to activate (i.e. perform diabetes behaviors). These attributes did not develop in a vacuum, they developed directly in response to the stereotypes of diabetes I felt oppressed by. Like the external process of defensive othering, I based my internal sense of self around how far I was from those stereotypes. That is, I was deciding who I was against the way the news media, public service campaigns, movies, and the like were representing diabetic people.

Self-exceptionism and diabetes identity are intimately tied. In her articles about making disability legible, disability studies scholar—Heather Evans, describes the process of un/covering as a mechanism of complex embodiment for folks with chronic illnesses (Evans 2017, 2019). Building on Tobin Siebers' theory of complex embodiment (Siebers 2008), Evans argues that "complex embodiment takes on a more nuanced dimension for those living with non-apparent impairment, as their membership (and associated stigma) must be established and reestablished in an ongoing process of identity assertion" (Evans 2017). I argue that the diabetic condition further complicates Evans and Siebers' theories of complex embodiment. Not only do people with diabetes have to manage stigmas associated with disability, but also of blame and shame. To use Erving Goffman's terminology, disability is considered a "discrediting attribute," meaning that those who are disabled are seen as discredited because of their impairments (Goffman 1963). In diabetes, however, the diagnosis is just the marker of that identity spoiling attribute. It is not only diabetes that spoils an identity, but also the imagined (mis)behaviors that brought the diabetes on. The genetic makeup of a person is not blamed by mainstream culture, but rather the choices and willpower that expressed their genes.[3] I argue that this distinction is what turns so many diabetic people toward a pathway of identity integration that leans heavily on stigma management strategies. Rather than identifying against non-diabetic people, the diabetic identifies against other diabetics—whereby creating an identity based on self-exceptionism.[4]

Moments of Reckoning

The cyclical process of claiming diabetes as a minority identity likely involves moments of reckoning. In several posts, I talk about how conversations and events challenge my relationship to diabetes (see for example: Walker 2014a, b). I call reflections of such events and conversations *moments of reckoning* because they have the power to create shifts in self-concept in relation to diabetes, disability, and one's place in the social world. *Moments of reckoning*, for me, occurred alongside emotions as divergent as grief, loss, feelings of inadequacy and empowerment, righteousness, and pride. For example, in 2014, I wrote about an experience I had while bartending (Walker 2014b). I was in conversation with another diabetic person when his non-diabetic friend expressed knowing little about the disease. The other diabetic launched into self-exceptionism-based education—spelling out the so-called behavioral differences between Type 1 and Type 2 diabetics. Recognizing his approach, I reflected in the post,

[3] Racism and classism are two factors impacting the way mainstream media portrays diabetes as well. While it is not within the scope of this paper to fully unpack these factors, they will be mentioned herein.

[4] In U.S. culture, self-exceptionism can also be interpreted as a function of whiteness because it centers the ideals of individualism and subscribes to a belief in meritocracy (see: Sumerau and Grollman 2018; Nakayama and Krizek 1995; Meeuf 2014; Jin and Ball 2018; Lardier et al. 2019; Ellis 2017). Hiding behind these ideals can stall social justice and policy reform that would make for a more just and equitable society. Similarly, hiding behind self-exceptionism or using it to form identity in diabetes works to maintain the splintering of diabetic groups by type, race, and class.

> i was there once. i was the PWD patron about three years ago, truly believing that i was educating my peers by drawing a harsh and finger pointing distinction between my obviously more challenging disease and the disease of someone who 'did it to themselves.'

After being vulnerable with readers about my past oppressive behavior, I shared how I responded in real time to this fellow diabetic and his non-diabetic friend. I offered a counter-narrative to his self-exceptionism. I said:

> actually ... no one is to blame for their body malfunctioning. no one caused their own suffering, and even if they did, who is helped by being told they are the reason they are sick ... i didn't stop there. i talked and talked until i was nearly in tears telling them that diabetes is severely misunderstood and misrepresented by the media, by healthcare professionals, family and friends, and even sometimes other people who have diabetes.

My reaction demonstrated growth toward a collective diabetes identity. Rather than representing myself as an ideal exception to the stereotypical rule, my approach worked to dismantle stigma the diabetic people of all types face.

Diabetes is with you for life. Even those with metabolic forms of diabetes, who are in remission, will always live a life that is adjusted to the threat of its return. In other words, you cannot have diabetes and then get rid of it and go on living like it was never there. It is there. It is with you in every micro-decision for the rest of your life. Throughout a long life with diabetes, there are moments in which the realities of living forever with this stigmatized disease must be reckoned. Living with diabetes not only eventually requires some form of internal acceptance of this new way of living,[5] but also of acknowledging the harm diabetic people have experienced in the past by way of stereotypes and discrimination.

Moments of reckoning involve internalizing and then rejecting the stigma that has kept diabetic people from power. For example, disability studies scholar Alison Kafer writes about this same phenomenon in disability identity. She says that claiming disability identity requires, "a reckoning, an acknowledgement, of the cyborg's history in institutionalization

[5] This argument may not apply to people who were diagnosed so early in life that they do not remember what life without diabetes was like. With that said, I would argue that even those diabetic people who do not remember non-diabetic life go through periods of asking "why me?".

and abuse" (128). Considering diabetes is a leading cause of institutionalization in skilled nursing facilities in the United States (Travis et al. 2004; Holup et al. 2017), and structural and institutional racism have led to worse health outcomes for Black, Indigenous, and people of color (BIPOC) in the United States (Golden, Joseph, and Hill-Briggs 2021; Spanakis and Golden 2013), the harm diabetic people reckon with stems from both institutionalization, stigmatizing stereotypes, and for BIPOC with diabetes, medical racism. As Kafer articulated, accepting diabetes on an individual level does not propel you into a future in which you are free from what has come before, and it does not necessarily build toward critical consciousness for the broader diabetes community. I argue that reckoning with the history of pain diabetic people have traversed as a result of stereotypical formulations of the disease is a required step in the process of claiming and integrating a collective diabetes identity.

Claimed Diabetes Identity

Through social and political actions, some diabetic people have begun to claim diabetes as a collective minority identity. For example, diabetic people on Twitter have collectively carved out a space on the platform they call Diabetes Twitter. Many of those people identify as activists and tweet about insulin affordability and recognize the ways in which society creates disablement for them. Their collective approach speaks to identity theories specific to minority groups. According to Asafa Jalata, "Collective identities are not automatically given but are essential outcomes of the mobilization process and crucial prerequisites to movement success" (Jalata 2002, 87). While Twitter is but one space where a particular collective diabetes identity may form, the ideological shifts toward a critical consciousness of diabetes experience seems to be catching in other stretches of the internet and beyond.[6] Disability studies scholar Tobin Siebers theorized disability as a minority identity stating that, "tired of discrimination and claiming disability as a positive identity, people with disabilities insist on the pertinence of disability to the human condition, on the value of disability as a form of diversity and on the power of disability as a critical concept for

[6] I make this observation noting that my research in this area primes me to attend to such ideological shifts in community narrative. Skeptics might argue that such a statement is a sign of confirmation bias. However, I argue that it is more attributable to priming and insider knowledges of where to look than bias.

thinking about human identity in general" (Siebers 2008, 3). Not only is disability identity as a minority identity about pointing out structural and systemic areas of exclusion and inequality, but about reclaiming value in human variation. And diabetics who claim diabetes identity, I argue, are getting closer to formulating diabetes as a minority identity in this way.

Advocates and activists who claim diabetes as a collective identity use it as a representational strategy and device to shift public thinking about diabetes. By sharing personal stories, narratives, and perspectives, people with diabetes counter oppressive, reductive, and stigmatizing stereotypes. Packaging their counternarratives in "I" statements conveys authority through experiential and epistemic knowledge. For example, an activist on Diabetes Twitter shared:

> "wrote an email to my new supervisor to let her know i'm diabetic. caught myself and changed "condition" to "disability" because im done downplaying this shit!!"—@sh1tpr1nce

This activist shared a personal story that demonstrates what unlearning the rhetoric that the medical establishment offers diabetic people can look like. By describing this moment, they offer a counternarrative as well. Rather than acquiesce to the minimizing metanarrative that diabetes is a *condition* that can be easily managed if the diabetic follows a few simple rules, this activist exclaims that diabetes is a serious debilitating disease. What's more, their tweet is bi-directional. That is, their counternarratives are directed toward non-diabetic audiences, but also toward those within the community—to other diabetic people. In my blog, the majority of posts did the latter. They spoke to others with diabetes. I used insider knowledges and languages to illustrate events and experiences in my diabetic life in hopes of connecting with others like me. I did this, in part because I believed I could offer counternarratives that could help others shift toward a more critical self-concept.

On November 17th, 2015, I wrote one of the last ever posts on *Unexpected Blues*, entitled, "*i'm coming out, i want the world to know, gonna let it show.*" The piece came three months into starting coursework in disability studies, which I say in the opening of the post (Walker 2015). I used repetition in the post for style, but also because I felt at the time I was saying what I figured many in my community were not ready to hear. I repeat the lines, "i'm disabled and i'm not sorry about it" throughout to signal my integrated disability and diabetes identity. The post then turned to a series of statements describing how society makes diabetes a disablement. For example, one statement reads,

> i am disabled by the pirate-like business the healthcare system has become. i'm made to spend my money on maintaining what physiologically doesn't work in my body. i can't decide to travel with the money i have to use for insulin, for pump supplies. what i can do out in the world is limited by the country i live in—who punishes me for my disease by making me pay for it. (Walker 2015)

In this excerpt, I paint debilitating aspects of diabetes onto external structures, rather than my perceived internal failings. I do not talk about how diabetes is for me, but how systems create disablement for diabetic people in general.

Diabetes and Disability Identity

Disability studies' advanced conceptualizations and formulations of group identity outpace that which is currently found in the diabetes space; however, I argue that diabetes identity is moving toward a more critically progressive self-concept. According to disability studies scholar, Carol Gill, disability identity development "affirms the disability experience as a positive and important feature of our identities" and affords disabled people the opportunity to "reclaim our disabled parts and become emotionally whole" (1997, 44). According to Gill, doing so requires "at least temporary relinquishment of former attachments, redefinition of self, and reconfiguration of relationships to others and society" (1997, 42). In diabetes, such redefinition would require forging diabetes identity against structures and institutions of oppression, rather than against the stereotypical representations of diabetes. What took me years of public emotional processing and readings of disability theory is coming to other diabetics much quicker. Other chapters in this volume, as well as work I've previously published confirm this (see chapters by Jeffrey Bennett, Lora Arduser, Valentina Sturiale and Guido Anselmi, and Clair Irwin; Walker and Litchman 2021).

As diabetic people are starting to claim disability identity, this unfolding drama is slow and, in some cases, still greatly leans into self-exceptionism. In her discussion of *Betweenity*, disability studies scholar, Brenda Brueggamann, contemplates a disabled existence that moves away from linguistic limitations and metaphorical dividing borders (Brueggemann 2009). She argues that it is within liminal spaces that we find the room, time, and deliverance to "create a new geometry," a new space to explore identity. While it is beyond the scope of this chapter to create a new geometry around diabetes identity entirely, this chapter can be a starting place for doing so in future work. For now, I propose an opposing force to self-exceptionism: *radical trust.*

Radical Trust

On the surface, *radical trust* is as it sounds: offering trust liberally and without limits. To use colloquialisms, it looks like giving the benefit of the doubt; like assuming the best. However, as a construct and analytical tool, radical trust functions best when applied at a systems, rather than individual level. The idea behind *radical trust* is similar to a construct from Psychology called *unconditional positive regard* (UPR) developed by Carl Rogers, an American Psychologist. First described by Rogers, UPR is an experimental therapeutic technique to establish rapport with clients (Rogers 1961). The explicit goal of UPR from a therapeutic sense is to create an environment where a client feels free from judgement and as a result has the freedom to locate and understand their inner strengths and resources (Lietaer 1980; Wilkins 2000). The UPR model, then, signals the locus of change as within the individual. Taken another way, with UPR, the client is assumed to be unable to locate and use the resources and strengths they have. It is up to the client to do the work and change themselves. On the other hand, radical trust intervenes at and identifies the locus of change within the systems and structures that constrain people's ability to use the resources and strengths they already have.

Radical trust means forgoing the way we imagine we would act if faced with a new disability or chronic illness. For example, you might imagine that if you were diagnosed with heart disease, you would stop eating fried food. You imagine that you would simply transform because your health called for it. Would you really though? And if you would under those conditions, why would you not just make those lifestyle changes now? Why does it take an actual threat instead of a hypothetical one, to transform habits and routines—if such transformation is even possible? I argue that imagining a future marked by stigmatization fails because it does not deal in complexity. That is, imagined futures are simplified and focused; they forget about the messiness of human nature and the structures and institutions that make transformation illusive.

Disability studies scholars like Alison Kafer have theorized how imagined futures, which are normatively deployed, constrain the complexity of disabled existence (Kafer 2013). When the futures of disabled persons are imagined, they are reduced and rendered illegible because they are imagined "in service of able-bodiedness and able-mindedness" (Rice et al. 2017). When non-disabled people imagine acquiring disability for themselves or a loved one, they see pain and suffering, not adaptation or growth. They see failed potential, rather than gain. In the case of diabetes, however, imagined futures are tinted with blame and shame—making them co-dependent with judgments of the present and past. That is to say, imagined futures of diabetic people come with an assessment of deservedness. So, we are getting minimized from two temporalities because the metanarrative of diabetes is so calcified (Walker and Frazer 2021). American culture[7] is too convinced that a diabetes diagnosis and or complications that arise from it are deserved. Trust of any magnitude, in any temporality, is radical in the diabetes space.

It seems, for the general public, giving diabetic people trust without limits is difficult to do. I would guess, that right now, most readers agree with my argument in principle, but are also thinking about a parent, sibling, child, cousin, grandparent, friend, or significant other who is struggling with some kind of illness. It probably hurts to see this person feeling unwell, and it probably hurts worse to feel like they could be doing more to be healthier. It hurts to imagine their life as less meaningful or impactful because they could or would not "do what it takes." It hurts. As a person who has lived with diabetes, I have heard the line "they don't take care of themselves like you do" from strangers and friends too many times to count. This line feeds on the metanarrative of diabetes and stems from the pain of seeing a loved one struggle. Radical trust does not require we abandon that hurt, but that we remedy it with a new narrative, one that is liberating and generative. Radical trust gives us the narrative that all people with diabetes are doing everything they can with the physical and emotional energy and material and mental resources they have available. Yes, every single person. There are no exceptions. If the person in your life who is struggling could be doing more, they would be.

[7] This cultural tendency can likely be found elsewhere. However, it is not within the scope of this chapter to explore global perspectives. Future research from countries outside of United States where the particularities of diabetes experience differ is warranted.

Radical trust is the far-reaching temporality—spanning past, present, and future—that signals a new kind of future for diabetic folk and diabetes identity. This is our first analytical, metaphorical, and literal move away from the metanarrative of diabetes as a disease deserved for the lazy, for the fat, for the unwilling, for the grotesquely indulgent. Radical trust is our first move away from self-exceptionism and toward a new geometry of diabetes identity.

References

Bock, Sheila. 2017. Contextualization, Reflexivity, and the Study of Diabetes-Related Stigma. *Journal of Folklore Research* 49 (2): 153–178.

Brueggemann, B. J. 2009. Introduction: The Deaf Subject Places Herself. In *Deaf Subjects: Between Identities and Places*. New York, NY: NYU Press.

Ellis, Christopher. 2017. Social Class, Meritocracy, and the Geography of the 'American Dream'. *The Forum* 15 (1): 51–70. https://doi.org/10.1515/for-2017-0004.

Evans, Heather D. 2017. Un/Covering : Making Disability Identity Legible. *Disability Studies Quartly* 37 (1): 1–29.

———. 2019. 'Trial by Fire': Forms of Impairment Disclosure and Implications for Disability Identity. *Disability and Society* 34 (5): 726–746. https://doi.org/10.1080/09687599.2019.1580187.

Ezzell, M.B. 2009. 'Barbie Dolls' on the Pitch: Identity Work, Defensive Othering and Inequality in Women's Rugby. *Social Problems* 56: 113–131.

Fahey, Tracy. 2015. Blood Sugar: Gothic Bodies and Diabetes. *Gothic Studies* 17 (1): 92–103. https://doi.org/10.7227/gs.17.1.7.

Gill, C.J. 1997. Four Types of Integration in Disability Identity Development. *Journal of Vocational Rehabilitation* 9 (97): 39–46. https://doi.org/10.1016/S1052-2263(97)00020-2.

Goffman, Erving. 1963, 1986. *Stigma: Notes on the Mamnagement of Spoiled Identity*. Simon & Schuster.

Golden, Sherita Hill, Joshua J. Joseph, and Felicia Hill-Briggs. 2021. Casting a Health Equity Lens on Endocrinology and Diabetes. *The Journal of Clinical Endocrinology and Metabolism* 106 (4): e1909–11916. https://doi.org/10.1210/clinem/dgaa938.

Holup, Amanda A., Katherine Hyer, Hongdao Meng, and Ladislav Volicer. 2017. Profile of Nursing Home Residents Admitted Directly From Home. *Journal of the American Medical Directors Association* 18 (2): 131–137. https://doi.org/10.1016/j.jamda.2016.08.017.

Jalata, Asafa. 2002. Revisiting the Black Struggle: Lessons for the 21st Century. *Journal of Black Studies* 33 (1): 86–116. https://doi.org/10.1177/002193470203300105.

Jin, Jin, and Stephen J. Ball. 2018. Meritocracy, Social Mobility and a New Form of Class Domination. *British Journal and Sociology and Education* 41 (1): 64–79. https://doi.org/10.1080/01425692.2019.1665496.

Kafer, Alison. 2013. *Feminist, Queer, Crip*. Indiana University Press.

Kozinets, Robert V. 2015. *Netnography: Redefined*. 2nd ed. SAGE Publications.

Lardier, David T., Katherine G. Herr, Veronica R. Barrios, Pauline Garcia-Reid, and Robert J. Reid. 2019. Merit in Meritocracy: Uncovering the Myth of Exceptionality and Self-Reliance Through the Voices of Urban Youth of Color. *Education and Urban Society* 51 (4): 474–500. https://doi.org/10.1177/0013124517727583.

Lietaer, G. 1980. Unconditional Positive Regard: A Controversial Basic Attitude in Client-Centered Therapy. In *Client-Centered Therapy and the Person-Centered Approach: New Directions in Theory, Research, and Practice*, ed. R.F. Levant and J.M. Shlien, 41–58. Greenwood Publishing Group.

Meeuf, Russell. 2014. The Nonnormative Celebrity Body and the Meritocracy of the Star System: Constructing Peter Dinklage in Entertainment Journalism. *Journal of Communication Inquiry* 38 (3): 204–222. https://doi.org/10.1177/0196859914532947.

Nakayama, Thomas K., and Robert L. Krizek. 1995. Whiteness: A Strategic Rhetoric. *Article in Quarterly Journal of Speech* 81 (August): 291–309. https://doi.org/10.1080/00335639509384117.

Nancy F., Liu Adam S., Brown Alexandra E., Folias Michael F., Younge Susan J., Guzman Kelly L., Close Richard, Wood. 2017. Stigma in People With Type 1 or Type 2 Diabetes. *Clinical Diabetes* 35 (1): 27–34. https://doi.org/10.2337/cd16-0020

Rice, Carla, Eliza Chandler, Jen Rinaldi, Nadine Changfoot, Kirsty Liddiard, Roxanne Mykitiuk, and Ingrid Mündel. 2017. Imagining Disability Futurities. *Hypatia* 32 (2): 213–229. https://doi.org/10.1111/hypa.12321.

Rogge, M. M., Greenwald, M., and Golden, A. (2004). Obesity, Stigma, and Civilized Oppression. *Advances in Nursing Science* 27 (4): 301–315.

Rogers, Carl R. 1961. *On Becoming a Person: A Therapist's View of Psychotherapy*. Houghton Mifflin Company.

Siebers, Tobin. 2008. *Disbaility Theory*. University of Michigan Press.

Spanakis, Elias K., and Sherita Hill Golden. 2013. Race/Ethnic Difference in Diabetes and Diabetic Complications. *Current Diabetes Reports* 13 (6): 814–823. https://doi.org/10.1007/s11892-013-0421-9.

Sumerau, J.E., and Eric Anthony Grollman. 2018. Obscuring Oppression: Racism, Cissexism, and the Persistence of Social Inequality. *Sociology of Race and Ethnicity* 4 (3): 322–337. https://doi.org/10.1177/2332649218755179.

Teixeira, M. E., and Budd, G. M. (2010). Obesity Stigma: A Newly Recognized Barrier to Comprehensive and Effective Type 2 Diabetes Management. *Journal of the American Academy of Nurse Practitioners* 22 (10): 527–533.

Travis, Shirley S., Robert J. Buchanan, Suojin Wang, and MyungSuk Kim. 2004. Analyses of Nursing Home Residents With Diabetes at Admission. *Journal of Medical Directors Association* 5 (5): 320–327. https://doi.org/10.1016/S1525-8610(04)70021-3.

Walker, Heather R. 2014a. *Bother Me Tomorrow, Today, i'll Buy No Sorrows*. Unexpected Blues. https://unexpectedblues.com/2014/12/28/bother-me-tomorrow-today-ill-buy-no-sorrows/

———. 2014b. *Ground Control to Major Tom*. Unexpected Blues. https://unexpectedblues.com/2014/10/23/ground-control-to-major-tom/

———. 2015. *I'm Coming out, i Want the World to Know, Gonna Let It Show*. Unexpected Blues. https://unexpectedblues.com/2015/11/17/im-coming-out-i-want-the-world-to-know-gonna-let-it-show/

Walker, Heather R., and Bianca Claire Frazer. 2021. The Metanarrative of Diabetes: Should You Be Eating That? In *Metanarratives of Disability: Culture, Assumed Authority, and the Normative Social Order*, ed. David Bolt, 156–168. Routledge Taylor and Francis Group.

Walker, Heather R., and Michelle L. Litchman. 2021. Diabetes Identity: A Mechanism of Social Change. *Qualitative Health Research*, January. https://doi.org/10.1177/1049732320984740

Wilkins, Paul. 2000. Unconditional Positive Regard Reconsidered. *British Journal of Guidance & Counselling* 28. https://doi.org/10.1080/030698800109592.

"Especially Made for Them": Summer Camps for Diabetic Children

Kirsten E. Gardner

Why come to camp? I come to camp to have fun to learn how to do things that I have never done before. Camp is fun, camp is serious. Camp is the place to learn to draw up your own insulin. Camp is the place to learn how to swim good so if someone is drowning you could help them. Camp is a place you can meet new friends and be with old friends. To learn about diabetes so if I eat too much I know how much insulin to take to control myself. To be away from home for at least 2 to 4 weeks. To learn to help others when they are sick. To learn to live with different people. To meet people from different states. To learn to be together.

—Lori, Clara Barton Camper, 1975

Camp to me means LOVE, friendship, togetherness, willingness, and getting along with people. It is trying new things and making new friends. Camp to me means trying to pull myself together and have a fun time and get away for awhile. Camp is someplace to come to relax

K. E. Gardner (✉)
University of Texas San Antonio, San Antonio, TX, USA
e-mail: kirsten.gardner@utsa.edu

B. C. Frazer, H. R. Walker (eds.), *(Un)doing Diabetes: Representation, Disability, Culture*, Palgrave Studies in Science and Popular Culture, https://doi.org/10.1007/978-3-030-83110-3_19

and enjoy yourself. You enjoy wildness and the outdoor life. Camp is a place to take care of yourself and your diabetes.
—Maureen, Clara Barton Camper, 1975

I come to camp to have fun and to learn about diabetes and how to control myself from eating too much. To take the right amount of insulin to keep my blood sugar down. To be in good control. Camp is a place to go to get away from home for awhile.
—Eileen, Clara Barton Camper, 1975

Written half a century ago, Maureen, Eileen, and Lori's voices still carry meaning today. Camps for children with diabetes, which served a few children as early as 1925 attract more than 30,000 children per year today. Summer camps for children with diabetes are deliberately constructed spaces designed to provide a diabetes-friendly environment for campers to experience all the promises of residential camping including new friendships, fun, and outdoor recreation.[1] The goals articulated by the earliest camp founders, "to give a genuine camping experience to children with diabetes" still resonate and many campers with diabetes express great appreciation for these spaces.[2] Recent media like the award-winning documentary *Crip Camp* has brought representations of summer camp experiences for people with disabilities to the public eye. *Crip Camp* specifically emphasizes the revolutionary power of community such teenagers discovered at summer camp.

This essay examines the construction of camp spaces to better understand how the experiences of children living with diabetes intersected with those working on diabetes programming. Contemporary camps build on the goals created nearly a century ago. As one brochure reads, "These camps provide a fun, safe, educational and diabetes-friendly environment for children with Type 1 diabetes and their families where youth gain the confidence, skills and knowledge to achieve their full potential."("Type 1 Diabetes | Finding the Right Summer Camp" 2020) In other words, the creation of summer camps for children with diabetes started nearly a century ago in an effort to build diabetes-centric communities.

Here, I provide a historical analysis of camps for children with diabetes that allows us to interrogate how campers, counselors, medical specialists, and philanthropists all engaged with ideas of living with diabetes. I argue

[1] (Association 2012) See p. S72.
[2] John Papers, "The Camp," p. 1.

that camp spaces for children with diabetes nurtured a sense of community built around notions of fun, friendship, mentoring, practice, and knowledge, while also relying on charity and medical models of disability to garner public and financial support. As the American Diabetes Association (ADA) explained, camps for diabetes children shared the goal of facilitating "a traditional camping experience in a medically safe environment" and enabling "children with diabetes to meet and share their experiences with one another while they learn to be more responsible for their condition."(Association 2012, 72) I conclude that many campers loved these experiences and benefitted from the programming, while recognizing that some campers did not enjoy camp nor benefit from its stated goal. For others still, it may have been a nightmare. Some campers left evidence that the experience had been difficult in the form of short stories that had eerie elements including death, dark nights, and rippling water and identifying as someone who "didn't want to come to this crummy camp anyway" (Priscilla White Papers 1913–1989).[3]

Extending the questions raised by the comment above, this analysis also uses disability studies to critique the unforeseen impacts of these founders' goals. For example, diabetes camp was segregated from non-disabled camp. Disability activists and scholars recognize the benefits of such a "crip camp," but it is worth noting that the world of camping did not have to make any changes to accommodate diabetic kids and their needs. Instead, this new diabetes-only space created a temporal accessibly built environment apart from the world that often ignores bodies disabled by chronic illness or defined by nonvisible disability. While summer camps for children with diabetes provided a pathway for thousands of campers who never considered that diabetes would make them less of a camper, what would a world built for people with diabetes look like? Summer camps, though segregated from the wider population, offer one model.[4]

(Un)doing Diabetes: Representation, Disability, Culture embraces disability studies as a way to re-frame challenges faced by those living with

[3] Priscilla White Papers. Correspondence and Related, 1947–1989. Joslin Diabetes Foundation camp: camper-created activity flyers and related, 1975, n.d. MC 997, folder 1.10. Schlesinger Library, Radcliffe Institute, Harvard University, Cambridge, Mass. See Seq. 1 and 3.

[4] Ibid. See also *Report for 1931*, p. 2. In this report, John imagines a future with more diabetes incidence which would "ultimately be handles by the state rather than by private individuals or corporations." John had a very clear focus on the need for diabetes-friendly environments.

diabetes, reconsidering narratives of progress or deficit, and instead offering an interdisciplinary framework that allows for deeper analysis on how diabetes, often a nonvisible disability, informs our communities and lives. This theoretical framework insists that we disrupt progressive timelines like the one outlined above, rejecting a story limited to medical advancement and triumph, in favor of a more useful analysis asking *why* bodies with diabetes are too often deemed problematic, faulty, atypical, or "fixable." While I apply disability studies theories throughout the chapter, I confess that in many ways, this perspective even challenged how I have viewed my own story.

I have lived with Type 1 diabetes for 36 years, and while I never attended diabetes camp, I have long been intrigued by such spaces. When I reflect on my experiences of living with diabetes, I frequently turn to a timeline that starts with my diagnosis as a teenager who hated injections. Trained as a historian, perhaps I am working to track change and continuity in this relatively linear space. My timeline is then marked by medical transformations in diabetes care that shifted my daily routines. For instance, the early years of my timeline include performing urinalysis over a bathroom sink, while more recent years include the addition of continuous glucose monitoring (CGM) and the adoption of some diabetes apps on my telephone. The timeline charts four decades of medical innovation—from multiple injections to pumping technology, from reliance on pork insulin to synthetic insulin, from urinalysis to CGM. I rarely, if ever, include in my diabetes timeline the terrifying moments of living with the disease, such as the summer I started drowning due to low blood sugar or the ten-week hospital stay when I prayed that my daughter would make it to viability as my body struggled with severe pre-eclampsia (a higher risk in pregnancy with diabetes). Perhaps my focus on progress and improvement guides my daily coping mechanisms and reflects my tendency to deflect the challenges posed by living with diabetes.

In my own life, I resisted labeling diabetes as a disability for many years, so my contribution to this collection is curious—even to me. As Alison Kafer makes clear in *Feminist Queer Crip*, popular notions of disability speak to a deficiency mindset, a missing part, and dysfunctional whole. I suspect this deficit model informed my own resistance to the identity. As I examined my archival sources through the lens of disability studies however, I was struck with the stated objective of many camps for children with diabetes to provide the disability-related accommodations unique to diabetes. Realizing that children with diabetes could not participate in the American Camp movement, Henry J. John built a camp for them. As he recalled in 1930, "In-as-much as no ordinary camp can provide these facilities and assume the responsibility for the weighed and carefully calculated diet, the administration of insulin and the daily emergencies which can arise in the case of any child who is taking insulin, this camp was constructed"[5](Henry John Papers 1903–1971). Thus, even in his time, authorities making these camp spaces did not deny that campers with diabetes have disability-related experiences that cannot be ignored or denied.

In order to understand how places, such as diabetes camps, aimed to create transformative space for campers with diabetes, I analyzed the history, trends, and practices within various camp settings with a particular focus on Camp Ho Mita Koda and Clara Barton Camp.[6] Started in the 1920s, diabetes camps opened with explicit goals: to offer recreation, to foster a supportive community, encourage peer-to-peer mentorship, sponsor educational programming, and encourage youth to develop a sense of independence. These spaces, grounded in shared and experiential youth knowledge, created a foundation for the breadth of diabetes spaces today that range from campgrounds to conference centers to online virtual communities—all designed to create "a potential site for collective reimagining."(Alison Kafer 2013, 9) No space is perfect, and many camps relied on philanthropy that patronized the campers, relying on a charity model that frames people with disabilities, in this case diabetes, as helpless and in need of financial support. Additionally, many camps designed medical programs that centered disease, surveillance, and even collected medical data to inform new therapeutic models. Still, I argue that only by examining these spaces through multiple lenses will we better understand the tensions evident between expert driven goals, self-determination among campers, and how these groups envision the potential futures of people with diabetes.

[5] Henry J. John Papers, The Western Reserve Historical Society, Cleveland, OH. Container 3, Collection #3621, Board Vol. 2, *Report for 1930 of the "Ho Mita, Koda, Inc." (Summer Camp for Diabetic Children)*, p. 1.

[6] Both CHMK and CBC have extensive archival records which allows for greater analysis of the intentions of camp founders, and reflections of campers.

Transformation with Assistance: The Beginning Stages of Building Summer Camps for Children with Diabetes

American Summer Camps emerged in the late nineteenth-century as youth spaces that offered rustic settings, back-to-nature activities, and organized fun (Huizinga 2016). Camp's focus on fun and play offers a lens to consider the power of play, defined by Johan Huizinga as a critical element in society whereby "… free and meaningful activity, carried out for its own sake, spatially and temporally segregated from the requirements of practical life, and bound by a self-contained system of rules that holds absolutely."(Rodriguez 2006) Overnight summer camps had the added bonus of offering youth a sense of independence, a life away from home, and new camp friendships. As Abigail A. Van Slyck has argued, "Among social institutions, only public schools have touched the lives of more youngsters."(Van Slyck 2006, xxiii-xxvii.) The creation of summer camps for children with diabetes expanded on the model of organized fun by incorporating medical services and laboratory spaces for children with diabetes. In this more complicated version of summer camping, children with diabetes gained tools for efficacy. One camper who later served as counselor and then trained to become a nurse explained,

> My camp experience taught me that I could see the good in my disease and that it wouldn't define me. It encouraged me to take the best control of my health (for me that meant switching to an insulin pump like my smart cabin mate Emily) so that I would have the chance at life I deserved! It taught me lessons they just don't have time for in the clinic setting.[7]

At the same time that camp proved positively transformative for some campers, camp founders and supporters often portrayed children with diabetes through a lens of medical abjection, charity, and deficit. Over time, the camps emerge as a space of contradictions—often fostering independence and confidence for campers, but perhaps implicitly amplifying notions of pity.

[7] "A Diabetes Camp Love Story," July 19, 2012. https://www.medtronicdiabetes.com/loop-blog/a-diabetes-camp-love-story/.

The Development and Intentions of Camp Ho Mita Koda (CHMK)

In 1925, a few years after the discovery of insulin, Dr. Leonard F. C. Wendt opened an early camp for children with diabetes and by mid-century nearly two dozen such camps had opened throughout the United States (Marble 1952; Association 2012). When diabetologist Dr. Henry J. John opened a camp in 1929 he noted, "The problem of diabetic children is a difficult one. They can't go to any camp."[8] Collaborating with his wife, Betty John, and several philanthropists in the Cleveland, Ohio area, John located the camp on 48 acres with more than 24,000 pine trees. Camp Ho Mita Koda (CHMK) included 26 buildings, a large outdoor stage, a tennis court, baseball diamond, a wading pool, and a limestone bust of the discoverer of insulin, Dr. Charles Banting.[9] Like many camps for children, CHMK offered a variety of activities including "swimming, tennis, baseball, archery, badminton .... crafts, painting, sculpture, woodcraft, nature, hiking (both short and overnight), cookouts, square dancing, dramatics, stunts, singing, other campfire activities, hayrides, carnivals, puppetry and the camp newspaper."[10] In addition to recreation, CHMK offered campers diabetes education, lessons of disease management, an expert medical staff, and it encouraged peer-to-peer mentorship among its campers and counselors with diabetes.

CHMK founders described a mission centered on building accommodation for the child with diabetes and fostering a youth community:

> At camp, for the first time in his diabetic life he sees others in the same boat as himself. He finds out how much each has adjusted to his own problems. He soon learns how little a problem it need be if he can only think of the onerous routine to which he is subjected as JUST ANOTHER PHYSICAL FUNCTION IN HIS OWN LIFE WHICH RENDERS HIM AS NORMAL AS ANY OTHER CHILD.

By naming diabetes as "just another physical function in his own life," this camp offered an alternative framing to medical discourse that frequently focused on the *fixability* of diabetes through behavior modification. Instead of focusing on behaviors, camp founders imagined diabetes as part

[8] John Papers, Container 2, "The Camp," 1. See also, John Manuscript/Diary, p. 4.

[9] In its first year, 1929, the camp hosted 6 children. Camp attendees increased dramatically in the ensuing years. See 1932 report, p. 1. The name of the camp honored the Sioux and "Ho Mita Koda" translated into "Hail, my Friend." The camp also included a totem pole.

[10] John Papers, "The Camp," p. 4.

of the child's world through modification of ***attitude***. In this sense, their thinking still fell in line with medical and cultural discourse that favors "normal" able bodies over disabled ones. It seemed, then, that a goal of the camp was to train youth to see diabetes as non-disabling, as non-limiting. CHMK nurtured the creation of a community of campers living with diabetes and promoted these attitudinal shifts as ***positive ideas*** about living with diabetes. And it seemed like campers saw this mission as favorable. One camper's definition of what diabetes means to her demonstrates this trend. As Maureen wrote, "***To me diabetes means not really having a disease but having something sort of healthy happen to you. Diabetes means having to watch what you eat, and watch your weight.***" Here, Maureen minimized the chronic stresses and discomforts that diabetes brings to the body and presented an attitude of diabetes almost as a gift. Her thinking conforms to cultural expectations of overcoming disability, a narrative that disability studies scholars have problematized for decades (Bloom 2019). For many camp founders and campers, summer camps could provide solutions by creating more accessible youth experiences for children with diabetes navigating the path to adulthood.[11]

At CHMK, campers published a newspaper that chronicled camp experiences, ranging from the results of sporting competitions to descriptions of camping. The newspaper, *Needle Point News*, offered the voice of children who centered their recreational experiences when describing camp. In 1939, one camper wrote:

> To almost all of us camp was a departure from the life we lived back home. We slept close to the trees towering majestically above our heads whle the stars beamed down and fresh clean air filled is with a desire for joy and laughter. In tennis and baseball, we learned to train out eyes and muscles so that we improved our game. Swimming has taught us not to fear the water. The publishing of the Needle Point News was the combined effort of all the campers because it was they that brightened its pages from cover to cover.[12]

[11] (Erevelles 2014; Alison Kafer 2013) Erevelles offers a political/relational model of disability that locates the built environment as a focal point for disability studies. Likewise, Kafer reminds us that, "In imagining more accessible futures, I am yearning for an elsewhere—and, perhaps, an 'elsewhen'—in which disability is understood otherwise: as political, as valuable, as integral." (See p. 3) See also Lennard Davis, *Enforcing Normalcy*. Leonard critiques of the cultural construction of "Normal" (as used above in the CHMK mission statement) and its scientific claims about the human body.

[12] *Needle Point News*, 1939. See "Ever Onward" on p. 3.

The 1941 newspaper cover of *Needle Point News* also captures vivid imagery of active and healthy campers. The front piece, a black and white wood cut portrays fifteen campers in different poses, with the majority engaged in activity. Several campers play tennis, others hike, and a few campers create music and art. This cover depicts diabetic campers as active, productive, non-disabled children. The cover highlights the skills of athletes, musicians, carpenters and more. Perhaps most strikingly, campers are all engaged in recreation and a sense of joy is evident in the woodcut. Because this newspaper was written by and for campers, it offers unique insight to their perception of the camping experience. Overwhelmingly, campers chronicled the friendships, fun, and recreation formed at camp, rarely published stories in *Needle Point News* on their identities as children with diabetes.

Camp founders continually expressed their intention that campers would gain more independence at camp. However, the stories outlined in *Needle Point News* suggest that campers often followed a schedule outlined by staff, ate from limited selection diet, and consulted with experts for their medical needs. As camp founder Henry John wrote, "I feel that we should aid them so that they can reach maturity in as good physical condition as possible. With a sound physical constitution, they can become self-supporting and self-respecting citizens instead of charges incumbent on their families or communities."[13] Conflating ideas of productivity with value, John's focus on improving campers' lives was constructed through a deficit lens. His views assumed people with diabetes would have problems with independent living, economic productivity, and general livelihood if and only if their bodies decayed as a result of diabetes complications. Yet at the same time, his careful camp design built an environment that responded to the world of diabetes, allowing campers to experience camping, sports, crafts, and the outdoors, in a space prepared to address medical needs.

John also designed programing that fostered friendship and support among people with diabetes. Many campers noted the powerful friendships that camp forged. As one young camper wrote in 1975, "Camp is for fun and games, for laughing and crying, with old and new friends. Camp is like one big family to you and me."[14] Another camper recalled the

[13] Ibid.

[14] Priscilla White Papers. Correspondence and Related, 1947–1989. Joslin Diabetes Foundation camp: camper-created activity flyers and related, 1975, n.d. MC 997, folder 1.10. Schlesinger Library, Radcliffe Institute, Harvard University, Cambridge, Mass. Seq. 38.

significance of her camp experience as follows, "Camp HMK was great to teach me that not only was i NOT the only one, but after we all took our shots and blood sugars, it was time to have fun and in a way, forget that you were the only one and here we're all alike. I have to say that Camp HMK was single-handedly one of the best experiences in my childhood."[15] Camps for children with diabetes offered confounding narratives, filled with camper's stories that captured a new sense of independence and joy, while often framed by experts who designed a space informed by medical and charity models that centered on children living with diabetes.

The Development and Intentions of Clara Barton Camp

In Boston, diabetologist specialist Elliot P. Joslin imagined a summer camp for children with diabetes that would serve as an "island of safety" for youth seeking outdoor summer camping opportunities. Upon hearing about this idea, members of the American Universalist Women (AUW) donated the historic space of the Clara Barton Birthplace and committed financial support to open such a camp. The AUW wanted to build an "island of safety," while simultaneously embracing a charity model of disability that allowed them to serve this youth population. Since the early 1920s, the AUW had been considering how they might repurpose the Barton space. When Joslin presented his camp idea, AUW members imagined innocent and underprivileged children in need. Their donation provided economic stability for the camp, although also included frequent references to the humanitarian mission of serving children with diabetes.[16] This rhetoric was not unique to Camp Clara Barton. Dr. John presented a charity model of diabetes when he explained the purpose of CHMK as a space ".... to care for a group of unfortunate children afflicted with an incurable condition, 'diabetes', to give them during the summer the advantage of outdoor life in the form of a vacation and also to relieve the

[15] See "Latest Comments" in "A Diabetes Camp Love Story," https://www.medtronic-diabetes.com/loop-blog/a-diabetes-camp-love-story/.

[16] Association of Universalist Women. Records 1869–1957. https://id.lib.harvard.edu/ead/div00181/catalog Accessed March 17, 2021. The Clara Barton Camp also garnered financial support from the Unitarian and Other Liberal Christian Women. (White and Waskow 1947).

mothers."[17] Identifying the campers as needy and unfortunate, and implying that their family are burdened by care, functioned to dismiss the agency so many campers displayed within camp, such as their success in recording their stories in a camp newspaper.

By 1932, the Clara Barton Camp opened its overnight youth camp located in North Oxford, Massachusetts—approximately 50 miles from Boston, Massachusetts where the world-renown Joslin Diabetes clinic stood.[18] In its first year, it welcomed 56 girls, organized into four groups of fourteen. Each group visited the camp for two weeks. AUW supporters felt their work, which now explicitly supported the creations of a camp for girls with diabetes, fulfilled a humanitarian mission. With a clear purpose of service, AUW members worked to provide an "... opportunity for diabetic girls up to 15 years of age to receive essential medical supervision while enjoying a happy camping experience."[19] Although children living with diabetes are not painted as victims per se, philanthropic support for this camp and many others seems dependent on those who perceive the audience as desperate.

In a parallel vein, medical experts also felt working at the camps fulfilled a professional mission, and medical information was gleaned, shared, and often the subject for medical journals. In the early decades of the insulin-era, diabetologists sought diabetes protocols that served children with diabetes. As Camp Clara Barton medical director Dr. Priscilla White explained, "The purpose of the camp as an adjunct to the treatment of juvenile diabetes is only partly recreational, designed largely to serve the child by permitting a period of adjustment and training in an environment normal for the age, to give relaxation for the worried and tired parents and to reduce the cost of medical care." While diabetologists debated insulin doses, best diet plans, the significance of medical data, and the expectations set on people living with diabetes, campers with diabetes provided evidence for emerging theories. As one journalist unapologetically

[17] See Henry J. John Papers, *report of 1930 of "Camp Ho Mita Koda, Inc.," (Summer Camp for Diabetic Children,* p.1.)

[18] Priscilla White Manuscript Collection, Schlesinger Library, Box 91-M113. Document undated but likely penned in the 1970s.

[19] The AAUW bought the land in 1921 to commemorate the birthplace of Universalist member and American Red Cross founder Clara Barton. AAUW members built a camp for children with diabetes as a way of dedicating the special space to humanitarian work that built national character. Unitarian Universalist Women's Federation. Camps Committee. (1904). Records, 1904–1967 (inclusive).

described, "These camps are also a valuable means of learning for medical students, house staff, and paramedical personnel and are a perfect setting for scientists studying the medical and psychological problems of the diabetic child."(Klam and Silver 1975, 80) The medical data, described at the time as being harvested from children, reified a conversation about the diseased body of the campers and campers had a clear sense that their bodies produced data, measurements, and medical insight.

As a rule, the Clara Barton Camp served girls with diabetes aged seven to eleven years, hoping to serve underprivileged girls in particular. Camp promotional material promised that all campers were welcome, regardless of class, race, religion, or ethnicity. Although camp records offer limited information about the demographics of campers, historical records suggest campers came from a variety of backgrounds—a stark contrast to camp demographics today which are predominantly white and upper-to-middle-class (Valenzuela et al. 2020). Clara Barton Camp welcomed international campers from Argentina and Venezuela as early as the 1940s; Spanish-speaking sisters from Syracuse, New York; and identified several campers by faith including Jewish campers, Roman Catholic Campers, and Protestant campers. The Clara Barton Camp garnered financial support from New England Deaconess physicians, members of the AUW, and other supporters. This unique collaboration served many audiences, each of whom perceived diabetes differently: those living with diabetes, those designing camps for children living with diabetes, and those who perceived their support for such spaces as benevolent and altruistic. ***Looking Back at the Foundations of CBC and CHMK.***

Both the Clara Barton Camp, Camp Ho Mita Koda, and dozens of other diabetes camps throughout North America opened with and depended upon the generous support of philanthropic organizations. For some, such as the American Universalist Women, their support of the camp represented "humanitarian" service, while for others, such as the Ho Mita Koda supporters, the camp's promise to create productive citizens seemed to fill a moral imperative of the era. Regardless of the specific nature of the bequest, diabetes camps set up pathways for financial support that targeted diabetes care and programming.[20] Philanthropic collaboration of church and science, cooperation between medicine and the public, and alliances of professional and lay audiences, revealed how

[20] Abigail A. Van Slyck in *Campfire and youth culture*. See also Abigail A. Van Slyck, "Kitchen Technologies and Meal Time Rituals."

essential such partnerships could be in advancing new ideas and projects. Diabetes camp allowed medical professionals to intervein in the lives of children with diabetes—in the form of camps, supportive community, and education—aiming to prioritize the value of community and confidence to do diabetes self-care.

As I've discussed herein, the metrics of success measuring camp and camper outcomes within it depended on language of normalcy and ideas of conquering the disease. A narrative of overcoming gave life to the camp and camper's philosophy of health. As Betty John wrote in 1957,

> Diabetic children have come a long way toward living a nearly normal life since those early days of spindly legs and potbellies back in the late '20s. Those campers are today's counselors, doctors, nurses, dieticians. They are tennis champions, sea captains, Fulbright scholars, food experts, lawyers, industrialists and fathers and mothers of healthy children. There are good reasons for sending diabetic children to the camps especially planned for them. (19)

Betty John's statement articulates a further friction that Disability studies scholars have identified, theorized, and problematized throughout its history as an academic field: the supercrip narrative (Schalk 2016). According to Disability studies scholars Gerard Goggin and Christopher Newall, the supercrip narrative is a representational troupe that relies on a cultural myth that in order for disabled people to live full lives with disability, they, "need to come to terms with [the] bitter tragedy [that is disability], and show courage in heroically overcoming their lot while they bide their time for the cure that will come" (Goggin and Newall 2004, np). Further, Goggin and Newall argue that the "crucial function that the trope of the super-crip plays [is] the policing of people with disabilities in contemporary culture and society ... the figure of the super-crip is also very much bound up with the construction of the 'normal' body, a general economy of representation that affects everyone" (Goggin and Newall 2004, np). Supercrip narratives seem to have not only been emblematic of the time when diabetes camps first came into being, but only recently begun to shift across varying disability communities. Advances in thinking and theorizing disability is relatively new, even more new are such advances in theorizing diabetes as a state of disablement. It is by looking at camp founders' and campers' stories and thoughts that we can see these shifts in thinking and conceptions of what it means to live with diabetes today.

Technology, Medicine, and Care: Day to Day Experiences at Summer Camp

Diabetes camps explicitly redefined recreational space to accommodate the medical needs of children living with diabetes. When camps for children with diabetes opened throughout the United States in the early twentieth century, they pulled on many conventions evident in America camping culture, including a belief that children prospered in the rustic outdoors, enjoyed outdoor games, and benefited from sports and recreation. While traditional overnight summer camps tended to be anti-modern and "devoid of modern technologies of comfort," (Van Slyck 2006, xxiv) diabetes camps centered technology by building medical laboratories in the wilderness. The medical clinic, accessible to all campers, promised nursing care, insulin, and diagnostic technologies for diabetes care. As Dr. White explained in 1947, "In addition to the physical requirements of any summer camp, a camp for diabetic children must provide a laboratory and must include a plan for weighed diets. Essential tests include those for acetone, quantitative and qualitative tests for sugar, capillary blood sugars and white blood counts." (White and Waskow 1947, 435) The medical resources and specialized staff served a dual role of medical care and assuring parents a safety net as they sent young children with diabetes into the wilderness.

By 1957, *Diabetes*, a publication of the American Diabetes Association, established four central standards for diabetes camps: (1) campers needed physicals and medical notes before camp started, (2) medical laboratories needed to be located on camp grounds, (3) sanitation procedures needed to be in place, and (4) all camp staff needed to be trained in diabetes management. As one example of recruiting expert staff trained in diabetes management, the Clara Barton camp included medical staff, a head nurse, two assistant nurses, a laboratory technician, and a dietician.

Surveillance, Food, and Weight Monitoring at Camp

While access to medical care in the built environment functioned as an accommodation, the material culture of a clinic in the wilderness also reminded children that their lived reality required constant medical surveillance. In a conscientious effort to build a diabetes friendly space, diabetes camps reified the centrality of medical evaluation in the life of a child with diabetes. In creative and imaginative ways, summer camps for children with diabetes transformed space to both fulfill the needs of its community and perhaps to affirm the centrality of technology, medicine, and care as children shaped an identity around living with chronic illness.

As Dr. Priscilla White, the medical director at CBC published in 1947, "a camp for diabetic children must provide a laboratory and must include a plan for weighed diets. Essential tests include those for acetone, quantitative and qualitative tests for sugar, capillary blood sugars and white blood counts." She then described the food service, based on a medical model perspective that failed to recognize and legitimize the children's expertise (or perhaps emerging expertise) in food selection. White said, "Errors were minimized by weighing the hot foods at the table. This task is done by a regular counsellor. Cold foods are weighed and served at each child's place before the meal."(White and Waskow 1947, 435) Such careful weighing and counting of food in front of children provokes yet another critique: how does such a process impact a child's relationship with food? Is this level of self-surveillance the lesson intended for children with diabetes to learn, given the founder's goals to foster independence? And if yes, is this hyper-vigilant process encouraging disordered eating that may create or amplify future complications? What role do new technologies, like CGMs, play in the area of food quantification for children with diabetes?

Furthermore, camp records capture the centrality of diet and the desire to avoid obesity among campers (as, it is assumed within the medical establishment, it would make disease management more difficult). References to "ideal weight," celebratory banquets stripped of special foods and desserts, and keeping a nutritionist on staff reflected the ways in which diabetes camps made diet and integral part of diabetes management and camp culture. Scholars in fat studies have articulated a need for the use of standpoint theory when analyzing cultural representations of fatness and its assumed counterpart: diabetes (Stoll and Thoune 2020). Standpoint theory emphasizes insider situated-knowledges, and argues that knowledge created about marginalized populations needs to be not only informed by, but also led by insiders to the population of study. Centering the perspective and experiences of children with diabetes at camp, then, would have inherently introduced considerations of power and power dynamics. Standpoint theory, then, urges "scholars to pay attention to the relationship of power as a distinctive kind of obstacle to the production of scientific knowledge" (Rolin 2009, 222).

There can be little doubt that the facilities, expertise, and community of summer camps for children with diabetes allowed the creation of a powerful space. The absence of parents and caregivers allowed campers to gain independence and express leadership. While the structured and surveillant environment ensured the children with diabetes were safe medically, they did little to consider the potential long-term psychological ramifications stemming from such surveillance. If research at the time the camps began had used analytical frameworks and study designs that centered the voice of children with diabetes themselves, as would be possible using standpoint theory, what we know about the experiences of diabetes camp might vary dramatically.

Lasting Impacts: Diabetes and Independence as Identity

Despite its methodological flaws, a historical analysis of camps for children with diabetes throughout the past century opens a window for understanding the intersecting and overlapping identities of youth and disease (Walker and Litchman 2021). Early twentieth century medical spaces, whether they be found in the hospital, clinic, home, or a rustic camp setting, allowed for practices of self-care. In this case, young campers became increasingly proficient at independent diabetes self- management. Camps promised to promote independence and confidence and allowed children with diabetes to imagine a future without parental guidance and oversight.

CBC collected several projects completed by campers in the mid-1970s including a project that invited campers to imagine a future and record it. One camper. Cathi, created a document entitled "Future's of America" where she listed fifteen campers by name and then predicted each camper's future career. Cathi clearly envisioned professional career paths for many of her peers, listing nurse, ballet dancer, writer, professional swimmer, lab technician, psychologist, hair dresser, chocolate baker, gas station attendant, doctor, teacher, secretary, and pediatrician as future careers.[21] Another camper, Teresa, offered a futuristic vision entitled "Prophesy." In her article, she too imagined an independent future with little medical

[21] Priscilla White Papers. Correspondence and Related, 1947–1989. Joslin Diabetes Foundation camp: camper-created activity flyers and related, 1975, n.d. MC 997, folder 1.10. Schlesinger Library, Radcliffe Institute, Harvard University, Cambridge, Mass. See Seq. 18.

surveillance and oversight. She wrote futuristically, imagining fellow camper Sue had entered the 2000 Olympics and "raced against Mark Spitz in a mixed competition. She came in first and made him look like a fool." Yet another example, camper Diane had become "a pro at stunts," who taught trampoline lessons, and served as a nurse in the infirmary.[22] The futures children with diabetes imagined for themselves did not center around diabetes.

Diabetologist, Dr. Henry J. John, also focused his research on identity formation in his campers' world. As he explained in his 1934 diabetes manual, campers "see some fifty children with a condition just like his own, having the time of their lives. No one to remind him of his diabetes, no one to pity him, because all his companions are in the same boat." John concluded that, a camper, "goes back home a different boy, imbued with a spirit of accomplishing things in life."(John 1934, 80–81) John and other built diabetes camp to accomplish their vision of helping each child with diabetes become an informed person living with diabetes who could make independent decisions about medication, measuring sugars, and monitoring diets.

Dr. John believed that children with diabetes experienced some cultural dissonance. He perceived the late 1920s as an era when "discipline at large in our social system is lax." He added that children with diabetes grew up under a system of, "severe discipline, (for only by such is their survival possible)." He further elaborated his ideas about identity formation in youth with diabetes, arguing that camps helped, "diabetic children to regain self-confidence of having an incurable condition." He observed a change in the psychology and attributed this emerging self-confidence to peer modeling and more. "Through their close association in camp the younger children see the older ones progressing in school, going to college and accomplishing something in life and this is a stimulus for them to do likewise." (Report of 1931, p. 1).

Dr. John brought a missionary zeal to his work in this camp, often referring to the work within the camps as "rehabilitation" as campers discovered an independent identity distinct from their parents who cared for them. In annual reports, he referred to the ever-expanding population of

[22] Priscilla White Papers. Correspondence and Related, 1947–1989. Joslin Diabetes Foundation camp: camper-created activity flyers and related, 1975, n.d. MC 997, folder 1.10. Schlesinger Library, Radcliffe Institute, Harvard University, Cambridge, Mass. See. Seq. 24

children with diabetes, labeling this population a "tremendous army." (The Annual Report 1932, p. 1) In his view, camp offered a space for campers to acquire skills (confidence, support networks, medical education) that would ensure fiscal and social independence into adulthood and beyond. Embracing an economic model of disability, he explained to donors, "The final reward ... will come when we shall see these children, as they grow up, rehabilitated to useful occupations, to independence and self-sustainance, as useful members of our social structure. Only then will the final goal be reached." (Report of 1931, p. 7).

John's description of diabetes care as self-reliance within a broken social contract captures a representation of diabetes that still seems prevalent today: that diabetes, when not managed by the individual, is a drain on society. He encouraged children with diabetes to embrace diabetes and the work involved with individualized diets, adjustable insulin dosages (with injections up to four times a day), caring for insulin reactions like hypoglycemia, while also embracing entertainment, exercise, and recreation in general. He hired people with diabetes as staff who promised to mentor others and hoped to recruit campers to join camp staff in the future.[23] There are many points to criticize in John's approach that can be linked with cultural expectations of what living with diabetes *should* look like. Regardless, John did initiate the creation of a built environment that gave (and still today gives) children with diabetes a glimpse into what it would be like if the world accommodated their needs. Diabetes camps are not without problems, but I argue, based on the records I examined here, that they do more good than harm.

Concluding Thoughts: Imagining Diabetic Futures through Summer Camp

People with diabetes occupy liminal spaces where a largely invisible disability may go unnoticed. I think of countless moments when I find myself in a public space witnessing someone across the room testing their blood sugar, wearing an insulin pump, or sporting a CGM on their arm. Instantly, I know I share an intimate experience with this stranger. At times, I act on

[23] Ibid., p. 5. The bust of Dr. Banting was added in 1932 during the 10th anniversary of the discovery of insulin. Modeled by Cleveland sculptor, Joe Motto and carved with Indiana limestone. Motto donated his time throughout the summer, teaching the campers art. Likewise, the wading pool was added in 1932. See pp. 3–4 of 1932 report.

this shared experience of living with diabetes and begin a conversation, and yet just as frequently I will observe the other person with diabetes from afar, noting their habits and presentation.

In a parallel vein, beginning nearly a century ago, camp spaces for children with diabetes opened as segregated and safe options where campers lived in environment with medical support and often made instant connections with peers. For many, camps for diabetic children offered a fun environment that fostered learning about diabetes and built networks of support unimaginable in alternative non-diabetic youth spaces. As Kafir reminds us, community building offers a path to re-imagining social, cultural, and political barrier-free environments. Camps for diabetic children created spaced for collective re-imagination and transformation.

In the twenty-first century, such collective and collaborative spaces exclusively for people with diabetes have become more extensive. Digital spaces designed by people with diabetes—Facebook groups, Twitter feeds, and established subscription-based online communities such as *TuDiabetes*—have fostered dynamic communities of people. Unlike the camps examined within, many of these forums now recognize and grapple with the significance of intersecting identities of class, gender, sexuality, race and ethnicity. Locally, public health agencies organize community meetings, YMCAs host programming about diabetes, and philanthropic groups including the American Diabetes Association promote community-building projects for people with diabetes. Such community building enterprises recognize the value of the lived experience and the expertise of those within these communities.

The creation of recreational spaces designed for children with diabetes in the early twentieth century allowed campers and their parents to imagine a different world, at least for a few weeks. It demonstrated how material surroundings can change to serve the community and all those who live in it. Rural outdoor locations can be redesigned to include accessible and affordable technology and medical needs. Diet could be re-imagined to include nutritious food selections and measurement devices. Communities can be built with intention and evolve to consider the expertise of those living with disability. Camp designs included plenty of flaws, and programming and services could have benefitted from more camper expertise. Likewise, some campers enjoyed the experience far more than others. Regardless, summer camps for children with diabetes engaged the imagination to create a parallel space, both emotional and material, designed for children who lived with diabetes.

References

Alison Kafer. 2013. *Feminist, Queer, Crip*. Bloomington: Indiana University Press.

Association, American Diabetes. 2012. Diabetes Management at Camps for Children with Diabetes. *Diabetes Care* 35 (Supplement 1): S72–S75. https://doi.org/10.2337/dc12-s072.

Association of Universalist Women. Records. 1869–1957. https://id.lib.harvard.edu/ead/div00181/catalog. Accessed 26 April 2021.

Bloom, Molly. 2019. Liminal Spaces, Titanium Braces: Narrative Tropes of Competence Among Wheelchair Basketball Players. *Journal of Linguistic Anthropology* 29 (1): 119–137. https://doi.org/10.1111/jola.12214.

Camp Ho Mita Koda library. 1929–present. Newbury Township, OH.

"Diabetes Identity: A Mechanism of Social Change—Heather R. Walker, Michelle L. Litchman, 2021". n.d.. https://journals.sagepub.com/doi/10.1177/1049732320984740. Accessed 26 April 2021.

Erevelles, Nirmala. 2014. Thinking With Disability Studies. *Disability Studies Quarterly* 34 (2). https://doi.org/10.18061/dsq.v34i2.4248.

Goggin, G., and Newell, C. 2004. Fame and Disability: Christopher Reeve, Super Crips, and Infamous Celebrity. *M/C Journal* 7 (5): https://doi.org/10.5204/mcj.2404

Huizinga, Johan. 2016. *Homo Ludens: A Study of the Play-Element in Culture*. Angelico Press.

John, Henry Jerry. 1903–1971. Henry Jerry John Papers. http://catalog.wrhs.org/collections/view?docId=ead/MS3621.xml.

———. 1934. *Diabetic Manual for Patients*. St. Louis: The C.V. Mosby Company.

Klam, W.P., and A.A. Silver. 1975. Camps for Diabetic Children. *Pediatric Annals* 4 (6): 80–87.

Marble, Alexander. 1952. Summer Camps for Diabetic Children. *Diabetes* 1 (3): 245–251. https://doi.org/10.2337/diab.1.3.245.

Priscilla White Papers. 1913–1989. Schlesinger Library, Radcliffe Institute, Harvard University, Cambridge, MA. https://id.lib.harvard.edu/ead/sch01670/catalog. Accessed 26 April 2021.

Rodriguez, Hector. 2006. The Playful and the Serious: An Approximation to Huizinga's Homo Ludens. *Game Studies* 6 (1). http://gamestudies.org/06010601/articles/rodriges.

Rolin, Kristina. 2009. Standpoint Theory as a Methodology for the Study of Power Relations. *Hypatia* 24 (4): 218–226.

Schalk, Sami. 2016. Reevaluating the Supercrip. *Journal of Literary & Cultural Disability Studies* 10 (1): 71–86. https://doi.org/10.3828/jlcds.2016.5.

Stoll, Laurie Cooper, and Darci L. Thoune. 2020. Elevating the Voices and Research of Fat Scholars and Activists: Standpoint Theory in Fat Studies. *Fat Studies* 9 (2): 93–100. https://doi.org/10.1080/21604851.2019.1629812.

"Type 1 Diabetes | Finding the Right Summer Camp". May 1, 2020. Diabetes Self-Management. https://www.diabetesselfmanagement.com/about-diabetes/diabetes-kids/type-1-diabetes-summer-camp/. Accessed 26 Feb 2021.

Valenzuela, Jessica M., Sam E. Records, Kelly A. Mueller, Megan T. Martin, and Risa M. Wolf. 2020. Racial Ethnic Disparities in Youth with Type 1 Diabetes Participating in Diabetes Summer Camps. *Diabetes Care* 43 (4): 903–905. https://doi.org/10.2337/dc19-1502.

Van Slyck, Abigail Ayres. 2006. *A Manufactured Wilderness: Summer Camps and the Shaping of American Youth, 1890–1960*. Architecture, Landscape, and American Culture Series. Minneapolis: University of Minnesota Press.

Verschueren, Margaux, Leen Oris, Laurence Claes, Philip Moons, Ilse Weets, and Koen Luyckx. 2020. Identity Formation in Adolescents and Emerging Adults with Type 1 Diabetes. *Psychology, Health & Medicine* 25 (5): 519–529. https://doi.org/10.1080/13548506.2019.1653482.

White, Priscilla, and Eleanor A. Waskow. 1947. Summer Camps for Diabetic Children. *Medical Clinics of North America* 31 (2): 435–444. https://doi.org/10.1016/S0025-7125(16)35845-X.

Troubling Cure and Cripping Futurity: Queering Narratives of Diabetes

SK Sabada

Introduction

Among the swarm of parents, endocrinologists, nurses and dieticians gathered in clusters lamenting the ghosts of futures not meant for us, we bowled. Children, mostly white, mostly "juvenile" diabetics, filled the bowling alley to the brim. We laughed and played under the JDRF[1]

[1] JDRF, formally an acronym for Juvenile Diabetes Research Foundation, is a nonprofit organization that claims to provide research and support to the type one diabetes community but mainly just works to serve the medical establishment. I consider JDRF to be a detriment to collective building among diabetics namely because it operates from the medical/tragedy model of disability, situating diabetes as a condition that needs to be contained and cured, when this is not what most diabetics, particularly within the United States, have been asking for. Namely, what diabetics, myself included, actively advocate for, are financial and medical support.

SK Sabada (✉)
York University, Toronto, ON, Canada
e-mail: sk97@yorku.ca

B. C. Frazer, H. R. Walker (eds.), *(Un)doing Diabetes: Representation, Disability, Culture*, Palgrave Studies in Science and Popular Culture, https://doi.org/10.1007/978-3-030-83110-3_20

banners, mindful of the cords of our insulin pumps so as to avoid the dreadful tearing of our sites. We darted around the endocrinology teams with sugar on our tongues; an enjoyment for which they would have otherwise scolded us. After all, it would not exactly make for good optics in the bowling alley to shame the very poster children whose disability gave them their careers. That kind of behavior was reserved for the clinic.

I can recall, at the time, feeling displaced. On the one hand, I felt the joy my diabetic friends and I shared, while I also observed the performative grieving the adults in the room partook in. At the time, I remembered thinking that though they likely had legitimate and complicated feelings about the diagnoses of the children in the room, their behaviors appeared insincere. I figured their sorrow was likely rooted in heteronormative ideals of a successful life that they could no longer imagine for us. One minute they lamented a future they did not want for us—which was also the cause for such fundraising events—yet in the next, they had drifted onto other conversations which ended in laughter. It was disconcerting to see them wishing away the very disease that had brought my friends and I such joy through our shared experiences while attending an event aimed at raising funds for a cure. That some diabetics wish for a cure is not of consequence here. What is of consequence are the ways in which we reduce the burden of diabetes by living with it on our own terms, how we want to, not how the medical establishment says we should. This chapter provides a starting point for the development of critical diabetic embodiment and is commited to unpacking and upholding diabetic desires. Diabetic desires are expansive. Diabetic desires find their roots in the politics of disability justice and critical disability studies theory. Our desires are self-determined.

To develop a critical articulation of diabetic embodiment as part of the tapestry of disabled subjectivity, we must deeply interrogate how and what we desire outside of our biomedicalization. This may manifest in the ways diabetics choose to engage with each other and our non-diabetic allies, and what spaces we choose to cultivate such relationships in. What possibilities do a diabetic-led space outside of biomedical institutions engender? In what ways do we hold space and care for each other as we experience diabetes, beyond what we have been conditioned to do by the medical establishment and ableist ideologies at large? To begin this work, it is helpful to read diabetic desire in tandem with the emancipatory project of crip futurity.

Crip futurity is a rejection of the hegemonic concept of time, which insists upon structuring life around non-disabled embodiment (Kafer 2013, 27). In its rejection, crip futurity functions as an emancipatory project. This project allows for us to grow into our disablement by rejecting the external influences that disorient our growth. Consider the figure of the queer child who haunts the peripherals of the imagined and acceptable (coded for cisgender and heterosexual) childhood. In similar ways, because diabetic childhood is marked by illness and constant medicating, we are likely to not be seen by parents as meeting conventional markers of childhood development (Edelman 2004, 3). Because diabetic children are read by society through such harsh biomedicalization—which portrays our existence in opposition to desirable normative bodies—our growth is systemically sideways. Describing sideways growth of diabetic childhood is aided by borrowing from Kathryn Bond Stockton's work on the sideways growth of the queer child (2009). In examining the complexities involved in defining childhood development, Stockton suggests that the idealized growth pattern expected of children is vertical: to grow up is to grow "toward full stature, marriage, work, reproduction and the loss of childishness." (4) This configuration bears particular importance for diabetic children, because the constructions of their childhood, much like the queer child, is marked by perceived delays. Diabetic children, whose childhoods emerge in perpetual states of physical impairment and social disablement, grow sideways, parallel from the non-queer, non-disabled childhood of their peers. In this chapter, I use the framework of Crip futurity to trouble what it means to grow sideways. Crip futurity challenges the futures imagined for us by our non-disabled parents, friends, and healthcare providers. It disrupts the confining constructs that implicate the diabetic experience as central to all future endeavors—successes or failures. The Crip futurity framework takes back diabetic futures and desires and encourages us to rearticulate diabetic embodiment, itself, as desirable.

Positionality

As a queer, nonbinary, diabetic scholar and former child, I am quite familiar with bring Othered. I remember those around me who did not share in my identities, creating my otherness in ways that countered my own desires. The SKs that were designed, made, and set out for me were largely SKs that I did not know, nor ones that I wanted. Counter to cultural preferences that favor able-bodiedness, I did not lament over the loss of a "normal" future because I did not care for one. In fact, I recall wondering as a child, why I would want to be able-bodied when that meant I would no longer feel part machine (e.g. I wore an insulin pump). Looking back, it is clear that I was claiming a cyborg identity, though at the time I didn't have that liberating terminology. I remember wondering: Why would I want to be a girl and grow up to date boys, when I could be myself and love fluidly? To be SK, diabetic and strange (coded here for queer and nonbinary) was to be free in ways my peers were not. I felt liberated when I rejected the futures imagined for me based around my marginalities.

These childhood self-actualizations turned out to drastically inform my politics as I grew into a queer nonbinary diabetic scholar. I position my research within Alison Kafer's political/relational model of disability, which recognizes the ways disability is both a body of politics and a tangible experience of moving through the world in a body that is impaired (Kafer 2013, 6–7).

Autofiction as Methodology

This paper employs autofiction as its primary methodology, with further theoretical groundings in the political/relational model of disability. I utilize autofiction as a method of engaging in critical disability discourse because the knowledge that I bring forth in this work is embodied. My experiences as a queer nonbinary diabetic inherently shape the ways in which I approach the conversations surrounding queer/crip futurity, disabled childhood, and narratives of diabetes. Autofiction enables me to revisit select moments of particular affective and ephemeral significance. Stemming from the tradition of autoethnography, autofiction is a methodology that more directly allows for a reflexive engagement with discourses of power (Gingras 2012, 72). By reflexively examining moments in my childhood where I lacked the language to effectively communicate my experience of ableism and disability, I use autofiction as a means of calling upon my past in order to move toward my desired future. Temporally, I live a future that my child-self did not anticipate. My child-self imagined a future where I could be free to be diabetic and disabled without the constraints of ableism and queerphobia. Now, as an adult, I have terminology to name what I was desiring: a full crip future (Sandahl 2003). It is through autofiction that I reveal my child-self's affective responses to their ableist experiences as a means to queer and crip diabetic desire and futurity.

Outwardly, the diabetic body almost parallels our non-diabetic counterparts. Charities like the JDRF and current clinical diabetes and endocrine care practices perpetuate the conceptualization of diabetic life as 'normal'—as non-disabled. The rhetoric, then, that diabetics are exposed to through non-profit messaging expresses medical paternalism, medical moralism, and healthiness as an indicator of "capacity" to function on par with our non-diabetic counterparts. Medical paternalism and moralism function dually for diabetics (child and adult alike), particularly in clinical settings. Given how the treatment and management of our care often emerges out of medicine's overemphasis on the management of patient behavior, we are often disavowed of having agency over the direction and method in which we receive care. We are told that as long as a diabetic follows the rules set forward by the medical establishment—continues to self-monitor, to take insulin when appropriate, to eat "healthily" (coded here for not consuming carbs or sugars), and to exercise regularly—then truly, a diabetic can be "normal" like their non-diabetic counterparts. Further extending this cultural logic, diabetics who adhere to these demands are seen as moral for they willfully comply with the rules that the medical establishment says earn health. On the other hand, simple refusals like choosing not to weigh oneself might be read by non-disabled people as an act of non-compliance, which is then attributed to the diabetic patient's character. The patient is vilified. This vilification has grave consequences for the development of a critical diabetic embodiment. It means that our behaviors are being read through a false dichotomy of compliance and defiance, our complexity stripped away by largely non-disabled onlookers.

Diabetics, similar to others with invisible or episodic disabilities, are expected to meet the demands of compulsory able-bodiedness (McRuer 2006, 2). We are expected to appear non-disabled and achieve species-typical functioning as often as possible. In the case of diabetes, this means performing behaviors like checking blood sugar, giving insulin shots, etc. Doing these behaviors, even if in secret, maintains the diabetic maintains the ability to not only "pass" as non-disabled (Goffman 1959), but also casts the appearance of a life without limits. As Robert McRuer identifies, these passing behaviors are evidence that our culture believes, "... able-bodied identities, able-bodied perspectives are preferable and what we all, collectively, are aiming for" (9). For diabetes, we can pass as non-disabled because our impairments are internal. Yet, we also perform disability in a way that contributes to the spectacle of diabetes monstered and villainized by the medical industrial complex in our capitalistic society. Diabetics often serve unknowingly as agents of what I call, "endocrinological ableism,". ***Endocrinological ableism*** is a form of ableism specific to the violence enacted by clinicians and caregivers under endocrinology as a discipline. This kind of ableism speaks to the ways in which people who rely on endocrinology for care (like diabetics and trans folks) are disproportionately surveilled and policed by clinicians for perceived "bad" behavior regarding their treatment.

The Symbolic Child

In order to understand this deployment, we must first note the way western ableist culture theorizes the symbolic Child. The symbolic Child exists as a symbol of childhood that cannot be parsed from futurity: "[the] Child remains the perpetual horizon of every acknowledged politics, the fantasmatic beneficiary of every political intervention" (Edelman, p. 3). The symbolic Child is a political one. Its power hinges on being a formulation of desirability. As Edelman argues, the symbolic Child "authenticate[s] social order" (p. 3). This figure assumes only qualities that reaffirm the significance and power of idealized normative embodiment. It is structured by upward development, moving toward the supposed future, "toward full stature, marriage, work, reproduction, and the loss of childishness" (p. 4). Edelman argues that for the queer child, growth is always sideways, marked by their delay and perceived inability to meet heteronormative conventions. The disabled child also undergoes a sideways growth pattern. Doctors, parents and advocates articulate disabled childhood as a child's inability to meet developmentalist conventions, while also fixating on the ways in which the disabled child requires support (Castañeda 2001).

The Symbolic Diabetic Child

Because diabetes can be so episodic, diabetic children are often treated as disabled subjects who are not entirely disabled at all times, but are still subjected to the full-time ramifications of ableism. When I was a child, I attended a summer camp meant for Type 1 diabetic children. One of the major selling points that a nurse frequently used to entice me was the promise that this camp was like any other camp, "just with diabetics." At the time, this promise was appealing because I craved a space meant for people like me. I imagined a place where I could have fun without being disrupted by non-diabetic authority figures who seemed to believe they knew my body better than I did (e.g., asking if my blood sugar is low because I was cranky or hostile). As a child, I was aware of and sensitive to the ways in which my body and behavior toward my diabetes were being surveiled by paternalistic medical authorities. I saw through the doctors who told me to log blood sugars on a sheet of paper that did nothing to help me, but gave them ammunition to prove I wasn't doing as I was told. I hoped that camp would be a space where this kind of surveillance and medical invasiveness would be absent.

Unfortunately, like most spaces meant for diabetic youth, being at camp turned out to be just as heavily regulated, if not more so, than regular life. Although diabetes camps have mainly diabetic children in attendance, these spaces seem to be managed by non-diabetic staff from large charities like the JDRF.[2] Although the counsellors were mainly comprised of diabetic teenagers, these counsellors also worked under the authority of medical staff who in turn got to regulate nearly every aspect of camp life. Camp was also a heavily gender-segregated space, which unnerved my queer sensibility. The time we spent doing activities was organized around medical procedures and was decided by the medical team. For example, before and after going swimming, canoeing or rock-climbing, we were all instructed to check our blood sugars.

Unsurprisingly, we were further regulated during mealtimes: for the first three years of my experience as a camper, our food was regulated in terms of type and quantity. We were expected to eat only the foods that we were given—which had been decided by both the medical team and the external requests of our parents. If the camper's meal card listed three servings of starch, then that camper had no choice but to eat three servings of starch. No more, no less. I remember campers arguing with counselors that their diet capacity fluctuated and they did not always want to consume the regulated amounts assigned to them. Counsellors, at the behest of the doctors, levelled these arguments and cited that they had already been given their insulin (under supervision…yet another level of surveillance) and that this could not be changed. These arguments were

[2] In my own experience at a camp that was first only funded but later owned and operated by the JDRF, while junior counsellors and senior counsellors were often diabetics who were former campers at the same camp, those involved in the management of non-cabin spaces, like the arts, water, climbing and horseback riding programs were largely not diabetic. Nobody on the medical staff was diabetic.

further intensified by "casual" reminders (coded for threats) of the consequences: "if you don't eat, your blood-sugar will go low, you don't want that to happen, do you?" and "if you eat more than that, your blood-sugar will be high and you will feel sick," and my personal favorite, "you are not leaving until you finish your meal." In this way, the structures of food and eating at camp leveraged camper's disability against them. It is not as if the consequences could not be avoided. A child who did not wish to consume, for example, an extra serving of vegetables, could have done so at little risk to their health. It was not as if these supposed "healthy meals" were dripping in sugars, but because these children experience episodic disability, disability that is inherently temporal, the threat of illness is always underscored by personal accountability. When a kid would go low or high after resisting compliance, their failure to comply was weaponized. The threats of futures filled with diabetes-related complications linger in conversations and structures of food and eating at diabetes camp in a way that further moralizes diabetic behaviors. Not only are we darkening our future by failing to comply with the rules of medical compliance, but we are bad people if we accept the looming possibility of bodily decay in the future. In other words, the prospect of a dark (coded for disabled) future is used to compel diabetic children to do as they are told under the assumption that the individual who misbehaves is reprehensible. In turn, the more the threat of disability emerged as I grew, the more my own identification of a positive future seemed incompatible with the ableist logics undergirding endocrinology.

The Narrative and Optics of "Good" and "Bad": Moralizing Diabetes Behaviors

Authority figures, like parents and doctors, who moralize the choices of children with diabetes suggests that on some level, diabetic kids deserve episodic disability. They judge how much the diabetic child fails to match up to the figure of the symbolic Child. If the symbolic Child is a figure that illuminates the most utopic ideals of our culture in the United States, then the figure of the queer/crip child signals to "a future that bears too many traces of the ills of the present to be desirable…a future with disability is a future no one wants, and the figure of the disabled person, especially the disabled fetus or child, becomes the symbol of this undesired future" (Kafer, p. 2). Kafer's critiques concepts of futurity reaffirm the position of queer/crip children as spectres, whose very existences reaffirm ableist and queerphobic beliefs about what the future should be. Through the refusal to follow meal plans made by adults, diabetic children fail to align with the symbolic future all children are supposed to represent. What's more, the existence of a diabetic child is proof enough of failure: disability cannot be constructed as anything other than failure because able-bodiedness is not only compulsory but is also the defining concept through which disabled embodiment often emerges (Davis 2006, 8). A disabled child who resists ableist domination is a child that threatens ableist fragility.

Disruption and refusal are more deliberate forms of rebellion against compulsory ableism. When a diabetic child refuses to comply, the complexity of non-figurative, non-symbolic children becomes apparent. That complexity presents a representation of diabetes embodiment and lived-experience that cannot be erased or over-simplified. Unlike the figurative, symbolic Child, the "real" lived experiences of queer and crip trouble the constraints set upon them.

Children, both disabled and non-disabled, are conceptually messy. They constantly trouble the constraints set upon them, they rupture and agitate covert and insidious structural and individual experiences of oppression. For instance, in primary school, I knew my teachers were not well-versed enough in diabetes care to be able to tell when I was having an episode of hyper- or hypo-glycemia (i.e. being *high* or *low*). Knowing this, a few times in my third-grade math class I said I was low when I wasn't in order to avoid being scolded for not understanding multiplication tables quickly enough. After being told by that teacher that I couldn't get external educational support, I relied on diabetes to get the support and extra time I needed. I played on my teacher's ignorance of diabetes and framed my math comprehension level as an episodic issue of disability. The way I strategized was possible because of the messiness of my crip childhood. Without my diabetes, the teacher likely would not have helped me but at the same time, this meant that I had to use my diabetes in a way that suggested I was a "bad" diabetic. She perceived my use of blood sugar as a "lack of control" over my disease, and this manifested in poor grading on the "self-regulation" section of my progress report cards, even when she was aware of my needs on my Individual Education Plan.

Authority figures often moralize children's health choices. When these figures frame the episodes as caused by the diabetic's behavior, it becomes an extremely common form of ableism that diabetic children experience.

This moralizing also works in tandem with the logic of compulsory ableism. "Good" diabetics are those who experience disability less visibly and are only good because they contribute to the medical industrial complex's "unwavering […] commitment to cure's ultimate goal—ensuring that body-mind trouble no longer exists as if it had never existed in the first place" (Clare 2017, 76). Good diabetics act as a kind of proof that there is possibility for non-visible (coded for better) experiences of disability. Good diabetics are used as agents of endocrinological ableism. While proponents of compulsory ableism may still view the mere existence of "good" diabetics as a failure, authority figures use the existence of the "good" diabetic to justify shaming and antagonizing "bad" diabetics.

The privileging of "good" versus "bad" diabetic children permeates diabetic youth culture. Just as disability functions as a form of marginalization, diabetic children are also marginalized in ways not apparent to the adults around them. Non-disabled adults reaffirm structural ableism through continuous verbal and non-verbal reminders that normality and rejecting diabetes-related limits are the ultimate goals when living with diabetes. Whether silent or spoken, these ableist proclivities pass onto both disabled and nondisabled children around them as internalized ableism.

As someone who already felt ostracized for reasons I could not yet name, I struggled with developing a willingness to comply with the demands of ableism that my cisgender diabetic friends subscribed to. I already held transgressive thoughts about diabetes. For example, I proclaimed myself the "diabetic kid" when surrounded by non-diabetic peers, a move that would later influence my sense of self as a closeted child both in terms of my sexuality and my gender. My feelings of ostracization led me to believe I was failing at times to hide either my cripness or my queerness and sometimes both at the same time. This occurred most often when I felt I could not hide the ways my body differed from my non-disabled, non-queer peers. When, as a ten-year-old tomboy with short hair, I needed new insulin pump to be sent to me, I was horrified to learn that the replacement pump would be pink. I felt anxious at being exposed by such a bright color (my previous pump had been grey) when I had often kept my pump hidden in a black pouch on my belt. I did not want to be outed or laughed at.

The Symbolic Non-Binary Diabetic Child

When I was around 12 years old, I observed my diabetic friends shifted the expectations they held for themselves in terms of diabetes management. Having been socialized and misgendered a girl, I noticed when the other girls I knew fixated on measuring and controlling their diets. It no longer seemed to matter that the point of carb-counting was aimed at the better control of blood-sugars. Instead, it appeared as though these friends had entered a competition to see who ate the healthiest and the least. This behavior proved to exacerbate the pressure amongst other multiply marginalized diabetic girls at camp. Suddenly, friends who experienced poverty were subjected to scrutiny for eating "unhealthy" food that may have consisted of high-carb, high-sodium and high trans-fat. We had no reason to regard fatness[3] with cruelty, but the internal fatphobic structures that informed (and continue to inform) our biomedicalized, ableist culture made it easy to do exactly that. So, most fat kids claimed that their fatness was caused by lipohypertrophy, too ashamed to accept fatness without medical justifications. As I witnessed this culture of fatphobia and body-shaming develop, I felt a need as a closeted non-binary queer child to hide the body I was growing into. I did not want to eat less but at the same time, I did not want to acknowledge the existence of my body at all. To engage in the conversations that my diabetic peers were having meant that I would have to acknowledge that I had a body that was changing in ways I felt sick over. Regardless of what I did or did not do, I felt like I too was at risk of experiencing judgement.

For the most part, it seemed like the non-diabetic adults around us maintained and encouraged moral judgement of our bodies. It became clear to me that health moralism and fatphobia were being taught to diabetic children by the adults who occupied our disabled spaces. Several of my friends and my own brother had diabetic adulthood leveraged against them as a threat by healthcare providers and even friends and family. Pictures of amputations were presented to us as consequences of bad diabetes management. We were being threatened with the possibility of

[3] I reclaim the language of fatness here, not in an attempt to echo the fat positivity movement, because I do not recognize being fat positive as doing enough to dismantle fatphobia and especially how fatphobia relates to ableism. I situate fatness alongside the ways I situate disability: we cannot construct or identify fat embodiment as being a counter-construction of non-fat embodiment. Fatness, beyond its physical manifestation, is a political orientation and one that I use here to resist fatphobia as it relates to this discussion on diabetes.

developing comorbid complications in future adulthood. The intention of showing such images was likely to encourage us to "take care" of our bodies. It was as if the diabetic people in these images did not care, but we could. Or perhaps, it was the intention of the adults around us to imply that these diabetic adults had not cared enough. Either way, the adults applied ableist and micro-aggressive logic to these images. Regardless of whether the action was based in fear, love, or disgust, the fact was that the experience of diabetic adults in health crisis were being co-opted and used as a means of manipulating us into being compliant with diabetes self-management

Positioning the lived experience of diabetic embodiment—including caring for oneself, as something someone simply does or does not do enough of is truly insidious because it not only blames and shames people for their impairment, but also demonizes the natural unruliness of bodies. People can do everything "right" in terms of their diabetes management and still end up developing complications. Complications are not evidence of flawed behavior. Complications are conditions that happen because a body, existing in for-profit systems of care wrought with capitalism-based inequities and racism, is sick and ages. So many external factors rooted in our social, cultural, and political environments complicate the ways we come to care for ourselves. What of the inaccessibility to healthy food, the expense of medication, the precarity of occupations with or without insurance benefits, stable housing? We rely on these and other external factors to continue living, doing what we can to survive. The representation of diabetes maintained by the medical establishment does not favor survivorship though, it rather favors a form of thriving that closely mimics able-bodiedness. Further, I speculate that the shame and blame associated with fat and disabled bodies has so been internalized in people with diabetes that we cannot imagine a reality in which it is worthwhile to invest in and care for ourselves. We cannot image a reality in which it is worthwhile to care for each other. In this way, the narrative of shame and blame is a callous means of affectively and effectively disenfranchising disabled people, diabetics especially. For me, being shown pictures of diabetic adults with amputations by non-diabetic adults flattened all the complexity of diabetic experience. Their photos were co-opted, used as fear tactic—compulsory ableism in the form of emotional and psychological manipulation.

Liberation From Moralizing Health & Diabetes

I recall being expected to feel a sense of repulsion and fear of the dark future that able-bodied adults imagined for me. The tricky thing about assuming a child's loyalty to an ideological framework of control over disablement, is that one would have to also believe that children are not capable of having critical thinking and power of their own.

As a child, I knew when I was being emotionally manipulated and denigrated by non-diabetic adults based on my diabetes. How could I have possibly been conditioned to comply with these systems of oppression into my adulthood, as if my diabetes was not intrinsically a part of me? I did not want the future that they had made for me and even when I did comply, I was given very little stake in engendering new possible futures. For that reason, it seemed more important to me to pursue my relationship with diabetes as one in which we were prepared for all possible futures—more disabled or less. If I did not have the resources to meet the standards of endocrinological ableism, I could at least begin to think about how I might function in a future where my body was further disabled by complications. Here, the construction of childhood, both symbolic and real, cannot be separated from a childhood ability to perceive, interpret and account for the world around them. As a child, outside of disability, I outrightly knew what made people decidedly "good" and "bad." I knew, even if I could not yet name them, that my trajectory would not match with the hallmarks of a cisheteronormative able-bodied life. I knew I was queer before I had the language to describe my experiences as such, just as my brother knew of his neurodivergence before receiving a diagnosis.

As much as compulsory ableism underpinned my existence, I was aware of the startling difference between "real" (coded for non-famous) diabetic adults experiencing complications and the shiny, athletic diabetic adults (coded for famous) that appeared on ads for the latest sensors and insulin pumps. How could it be that the people and organizations that supposedly represented and advocated around our shared condition, could feel so much pity and desire to help and to save and to protect, also be the very organizations who stratified our diabetic elders? How could we, as diabetic youths, possibly trust them? How could we trust those who shamed us regularly for our lack of control, who raised money through carefully constructing and conditioning whole generations of youth to hate the bodies allowed us to live—albeit with the addition of needing medication on a daily basis?

As I grew older, I began to realize that my experiences of diabetes in social settings were a series of complicated illusions to secure a sanitized and acceptable portrayal of diabetes. These portrayals had previously lulled me into a false sense of security with medical authority. These portrayals convinced me that the medical system would not denigrate me if I performed well and that my future would be the same as my non-diabetic peers. Using disgust and revulsion to manipulate people into changing their behavior only works as intended if it can be rationalized as an appropriate response to the behavior in question (Knapp 2003, 254). Disgust is rationalized as a response to diabetics with complications precisely because we use language as a pedagogical tool to condition ourselves to think of further debility as inherently bad. The truth is, any diabetic can be a "bad" diabetic. In fact, on the hours spent outside of the clinic, I would wager that most of us are, or at least participate in behaviors we have conditioned ourselves to feel shame for. The joke of it all rests in the optics. Diabetes care primarily functions not as an apparatus of medicine to support diabetics in their care, but to shame those who cannot lead lives that make our disability unapparent.

One way to strategize resistance to compulsory ableism is in embracing disability as a form of human variation. As my friends and I came into the twilight of our youth, we began to embrace the very thing that made us feel so ugly to begin with. By the time I hit my teens, I had long let go of the hopes of cure and advancements in endocrinological technology that would supposedly allow me to live a "normal" life. Regardless of what one does to manage diabetes, of how much one can hide, one cannot erase disablement from their existence. Non-disabled adults offering normalcy is not an acceptable response to disabled folks in need of support. Instead, I offer this: it is paramount that disabled people acknowledge their own desirability. Normalcy will offer us nothing if we are not normal to begin with. As I argued at the outset of this chapter, diabetic adults who were diagnosed in childhood have likely been forced to grow sideways instead of upward and with that, we have left many developmental milestones unmarked. We have survived because of our sideways growth; we have learned what works best for our bodies and we have met milestones non-diabetic people are incapable of imagining. We have been inherently shaped by the contexts in which we live as diabetics (good and bad, child and adult) and to turn our backs on the knowledge we have gained as we experience diabetes in favor of meeting the standards of a healthcare system that would quicker see us dead than thrive, is to lose all sense of compassion for oneself and for each other.

Desiring disability, to use a colloquialism, is easier said than done. For diabetics, it is crucial to situate our existence as both desirable and vital to dismantling internalized and institutionalized ableism. To be transgressive, we have to choose to love diabetes and how it brings us into being. We have to actively denounce systems of healthcare and capitalism that berates, shames, and encourages us to antagonize each other based on supposed health maxims (e.g. eat well, exercise, and lose weight). This is not to say that there is no place for frustration or anger. Diabetes can be challenging, exhausting, debilitating, but it is as much as us as we are it. Here, let us turn to the concept of access intimacy. Mia Mingus suggests that access intimacy is a fluid and elusive concept which describes the building of relationships through mutual care (2011). It is showing up in tangible ways when possible for each other. To hold each other accountable. To show radical compassion and care for each other in ways that go beyond traditional care work, beyond just meeting needs. It can be found in friendships, in familial relations, in total strangers. It is choosing each other and ourselves every time, even when wrought with the complexity of all the facets of our identities and experiences. This concept is particularly important because of the potential it offers in terms of diabetics learning to foster communities beyond the horror we have been told to expect for ourselves. Access intimacy eats away at that which has degraded us by allowing us to hold space for ourselves, each other and the inherent messiness of being disabled.

Conclusion

I began this chapter with a scene from my childhood in a bowling alley at a JDRF fundraiser. I asked us to consider what it means to develop a critical diabetic embodiment through the examination of diabetic desire and crip futurity. This examination was made possible through an autofictive approach that recounted my experiences growing up as a queer nonbinary diabetic child. In order to move beyond the imagined futures set for diabetics by non-diabetic authority figures, I insist we begin to articulate and interrogate what diabetic desire and embodiment look like. For myself, the process of liberation from the constrained futures given to me by largely non-diabetic world I live in, remains ongoing. It is hard to say exactly what my own liberation might look like, even now, as I do the work of examining diabetic embodiment. I wonder often, if my child self would be pleased to know that our politics largely remained the same. Or perhaps they would be disappointed that we still looking for futures that are not based on ableism and heteronormativity and cisnormativity. Even though this liberation has yet to happen for us, I see more possibility as diabetics increasingly collectivize public forums like social media. When we are one of the elders of our diabetic community, we will reach out to those younger than us so that they know there is more to being diabetic than what the medical establishment and cultural ableism has convinced us there was. To do this, it is crucial to examine collective diabetic embodiment as a relatively untapped resource of knowledge and culture, to fully embrace our power as disabled people capable of destabilizing ableism precisely through our experiences of episodic disability.

References

Castañeda, Claudia. 2001. Developmentalism And the Child in Nineteenth-Century Science. *Science as Culture* 10 (3): 375–409, Routledge. *Taylor and Francis+NEJM*, Sept. https://doi.org/10.1080/09505430120074145.

Clare, Eli. 2017. Structure of Cure. In *Brilliant Imperfection: Grappling with Cure*, 76. Durham and London: Duke University Press.

Davis, Lennard J. 2006. *Disability Studies Reader*. Routledge.

Edelman, Lee. 2004. *No Future: Queer Theory and the Death Drive*. Duke University Press.

Gingras, Jacqui. April 2012. Embracing Vulnerability: Completing the Autofictive Circle in Health Profession Education. *Journal of Transformative Education* 10 (2): 67–89. https://doi.org/10.1177/1545968312460632.

Goffman, Erving. 1959. *The Presentation of Self in Everyday Life*. Anchor Books. New York, NY: Bantam Doubleday Dell Publishing Group.

Kafer, Alison. 2013. *Feminist, Queer, Crip*, 6–7. Indiana University Press. Accessed September 16, 2020. http://www.jstor.org/stable/j.ctt16gz79x.

Knapp, Christopher. 2003. De-Moralizing Disgustingness. *Philosophy and Phenomenological Research* 66 (2): 253–278. Accessed September 15, 2020. http://www.jstor.org/stable/20140536.

McRuer, Robert. 2006. *Crip Theory: Cultural Signs of Queerness and Disability*. New York: New York University Press. 6 × 9. 281 pgs. 0-8147-5712-X.

Mingus, Mia. 2011. Access Intimacy: The Missing Link. *Leaving Evidence* (blog), May 5. https://leavingevidence.wordpress.com/2011/05/05/access-intimacy-the-missing-link/.

Sandahl, Carrie. April 2003. Queering the Crip or Cripping the Queer?: Intersections of Queer and Crip Identities in Solo Autobiographical Performance. *GLQ 9* (1–2): 25–56. https://doi.org/10.1215/10642684-9-1-2-25

Stockton, Kathryn Bond. 2009. *The Queer Child, or Growing Sideways in the Twentieth Century*. Duke University Press.

Diabetes Advocacy: Many Voices, One Message

Stephen Shaul

MAY, 2014: It was a beautiful late spring day in Baltimore, and I'm at work downtown. Since we don't get many sunny, not-too-hot, not-too-cold days in the city, I decided to take my lunch down to the promenade by the harbor next to where I worked. After a long winter, I was looking forward to soaking up the sun for an hour.

I was feeling pretty good about things generally. Work was good, and I had been writing a blog for a little over two years on a variety of diabetes topics (http://happy-medium.net). I was glad to have an outlet to talk about my life with diabetes and the issues that were important to me. Though many of my friends and none of my co-workers knew about the blog, I felt that my voice was growing and I could see myself reaching even more readers as the months went on. I couldn't really understand what that meant at the time. I didn't think of myself as a diabetes advocate, but somewhere in my mind I believed I could eventually become the

S. Shaul (✉)
Baltimore, MD, USA

B. C. Frazer, H. R. Walker (eds.), *(Un)doing Diabetes: Representation, Disability, Culture*, Palgrave Studies in Science and Popular Culture, https://doi.org/10.1007/978-3-030-83110-3_21

well-spoken man who righted all the wrongs and solved all the problems, whatever I thought the problems were at the time.

Meanwhile, despite managing my diabetes fairly well for a few years, I had resisted wearing a continuous glucose monitor (CGM) because I was already uncomfortable with wearing the insulin pump that had been part of my life for four years. On that day, as I headed downstairs for lunch, I knew my blood sugar was going low, but without a CGM, I didn't know how close to danger I really was. I thought I could get to my lunch destination before it became more than just a minor nuisance.

But in the time it took for me to head downstairs from the office, walk around the corner and go about a hundred yards to a nearby bench by the water, I was sweating, shaking, and losing my balance. In the shadow of my workplace, my hypoglycemia caused me to fall on the ground in one of the most visible parts of the city.

There were many people passing by on their way to or from lunch. What did they do? What else? They got out their cell phones and started shooting video of me desperately reaching for the lunch I dropped, where there was an orange that I needed to consume immediately. A few of the passerbys conversed among themselves about what my issue might be. At the time, I remember thinking they probably thought I was on some kind of drug. I still wonder if they were perfectly happy letting me struggle on the ground so I could be the subject of their social media post that afternoon.

Eventually, one kind soul helped me, and I recovered enough to eat my lunch and work the rest of the day. In this instance, just shaking off the haziness of hypoglycemia wasn't enough. I was stung, shocked, even angered at the lack of empathy shown for someone trying to save himself during a life-threatening hypoglycemic event. But I also saw something more clearly than I had ever seen it before. I wish I had had an advocate, or someone who would have been on my side in the public sphere to support me. I wondered how I might have been my own advocate. What might that mean for me deciding to wear a CGM, taking up space at work with diabetes needs, or boldly asking for help in an emergency?

One Destination, Many Avenues

There are many people living with diabetes, which suggests that we need all the advocates we can get. There are thirty-one million people living with diabetes in the United States alone (International Diabetes Federation

2019), and this statistic represents more than just a number. These are thirty-one million individuals with complex needs, stories, and varying degrees of access to vital knowledge, technology, and support. In fact, many people face barriers to the health care and health information that makes living with diabetes easier. Many lack the time, the resources, or the knowledge to effectively advocate for their needs on their own behalf. To, me, it has seemed like a great many advocates do not actually have diabetes themselves (e.g. parents of children with diabetes). However, as disability consciousness grows in the diabetes community, more and more people with diabetes align with the popular disability rights slogan, "nothing about us without us" and fight for a seat at the table. James Charlton's book of the same name, *Nothing About Us Without Us: Disability, Oppression, and Empowerment*, does a great job of explaining why this has become a popular theme among advocates. Likewise, there are already many voices out there in the advocacy space. Those voices advocate for a great many things. But in my advocacy journey, I found out that one goal holds true for every advocate: better lives for everyone living with diabetes.

This one overarching goal shapes the variety of messages in support of people with diabetes who are affected by policy decisions. Advocacy in diabetes looks like voices in support of those who deserve to be treated with respect by health care professionals and indeed, others living with diabetes. For a long time, I had the fantasy that a diabetes advocate was like a superhero, fighting for the "little guy" by giving grand speeches and truly living and breathing advocacy in every moment of my life. Diabetes advocates are people who step in where others can't, in service to all this and more. Knowing this, and considering my own experiences, I realized I didn't need to become the Singular Important Voice for diabetes advocacy. Instead, I could share my voice on a number of levels and now I focus on showing others how they can do the same.

Getting started with advocacy was neither easy nor fast. I often found myself wondering how and where I might start at all. I realized I was facing both internal and external hurdles. In my case, I needed to start with an admission: I needed to say, "I will be an advocate," and then, "I am an advocate." Earlier that year, I was invited to attend a clinical diabetes conference as a representive of the patient perspective. Some people might identify being invited to such a conference as something that only happens to advocates, but at the time I didn't yet see it that way. While there, I met a friend who was working with a small, now dissolved, advocacy group. I remember telling him that volunteering for the group would be great, but

I didn't think of myself as an advocate yet, and they probably needed "real advocates," whatever they are. He told me that advocacy is more about inclusion than exclusion, and we need all the advocates we can get. That exchange gave me the confidence to be able to say, "I am an advocate."

It became clear to me that I couldn't start by waiting for someone to declare me an advocate, because even in the best of circumstances, it doesn't happen in the way you'd expect. Before this moment, it had not occurred to me that advocacy is as you make it. I, like many fellow advocates I've come to know, have been swept up in the image of "an advocate" that some large advocacy organizations portray. The portrayal of an advocate they put forward looks like Miss America or Nick Jonas in a Superbowl ad. If that is what an advocate was, it certainly wasn't me. So, in my experience, transforming and expanding my ideas about what an advocate is and does was necessary to move forward. Thanks to that friend, I got the nudge I needed to do just that.

Often, I hear similar stories from others who feel that their voice is small, so they don't believe they can have a big impact. It's almost as if we're afraid to call ourselves an advocate, like that term should be reserved for celebrities or non-profit leaders. Nothing could be farther from the truth. In reality, if you are helping to make life better for even one person with diabetes you are making a huge impact in that one life, and you deserve to call yourself an advocate. For me, in order to get others to believe in my advocacy, I had to be comfortable thinking of my own efforts as being worthy of that definition. I needed to see the act of, for example, telling a neighbor what an insulin pump was, as an act of advocacy. Take it from me: I didn't need to move mountains. I just needed to move a couple of rocks here and there to begin making a difference. Mountains could be climbed and moved later.

Next, I had to find my advocacy perspective. Some folks advocate for lowering the cost of prescription medications. Others for fair treatment of kids, adults, or seniors living with diabetes. There are those who petition the U.S. Food and Drug Administration to speed up approvals of new devices or drugs. Still others advocate by sharing what they discover about living with diabetes in the most inclusive way they can.

The First Step and the Lesson It Taught Me

I pause to confess here that I wasn't sure exactly where my advocacy would start or what it would lead to. As I mentioned before, I had bought into the fantasy of what "the advocate" was supposed to look like. To me, the fantasy of advocacy looked like sales, and I'm no salesman. I didn't like the idea of selling someone on my idea of better access to analog insulins like they were the latest coffee maker, for example. So, I thought this wasn't an area in which I was going to excel.

But, I surprised myself. I was happy to start by speaking up at a public workshop at the U.S. Food and Drug Administration in November 2014. The subject of the meeting was interoperability of diabetes devices, or in other words, how our glucose meters, continuous glucose monitors, insulin pumps, or even our smart phones work to share information and even help two or more of these devices work better together. Here was something that I knew was important to everyone living with diabetes. There were presentations by FDA staff, researchers working on code and conducting clinical trials, and industry representatives. As is the case in these public workshops, there was also a time for public comment, where anyone could share their views on the subject at hand. That was the opening I was looking for.

I signed up to comment during this part of the proceedings, prepared some remarks, and got up to speak when my name was called. I was a bit shaky in the beginning, but I made it through my almost four allotted minutes and shared what was important to me about interoperability in diabetes device development. That last part is really important to remember. As I wrote at the time: "I understand that companies want to advocate for what's in their best interest. Well, that's what I was doing too. Advocating for what is best for me as a patient." That lesson, that patient priorities should always be part of the discussion, that I learned that cold day in 2014, is one I would share with others years later.

The Importance of Social Media

Social media plays a big part in diabetes advocacy, and for me, it was a great place to learn from others. Whether it's through organized advocacy under the banner of a nonprofit or independent advocacy groups, through Twitter, blogs, Instagram, podcasts, or just about any other social media platform you can name, there are so many avenues of advocacy to employ. There is no shortage of ways for people to begin sharing their voice for change. It is a terrific way to meet others who advocate, and as I mentioned, to learn more about advocacy itself. While individual opinions can vary widely, it is a sure way to say what you want to say the way you want to say it, knowing that this form of advocacy will be useful to advocates trying to make change in the future.

In my case, while I didn't know much about advocating to begin with, I was lucky enough to be in places where information was being shared: in public meetings held by nonprofits, in symposia, or at the U.S. Food and Drug Administration. Those public gatherings allowed for a two-pronged approach to my early years of advocacy. First, I could ask questions and use public comment time in the meetings to share my own feelings and perspectives. Second, I could disseminate the information I was learning in real time via social media, so others would be able to access the same knowledge.

Using your voice and amplifying the voice of others is one of the most powerful forms of advocacy. It was an easy way to advocate since nearly every gathering I attended in those days was free to the public. With virtual presentations becoming more commonplace these days, it's even easier to advocate this way. And, because diabetes communities are not monolithic, there is no way one person can represent the intersectional oppressions faced by all people with diabetes. In other words, we really do need to support all the new and diverse advocates coming into the community who are sharing their stories.

The Power of Yes

As time went on, I made acquaintances and became involved in advocacy initiatives led by others. For me, there was nothing so easy as saying "Yes" when someone asked for help with something I believed in. In the process I was able to learn more from people who have been advocating much longer than I have. Helping others with their own projects has allowed me to speak before organizations that wanted to know more about life with diabetes in the twenty-first century. I didn't always speak before big crowds, but that didn't matter. I was changing. My relationship to diabetes was changing. And so, to me, advocacy was like throwing a pebble in a pond. While what I was doing may have seemed small, I hope and believe the effect may have rippled out in a way that created bigger impact.

In 2015, I was also lucky enough to be asked by a grassroots community organizer to help facilitate sessions at the Diabetes UnConference, where adults living with diabetes gathered to discuss diabetes-related topics that were decided on the spot. These discussions took place at gatherings where the agendas were driven by the attendees and covered a wide variety of questions, answers, advice, and soul searching. For example, a session on language and diabetes got us all talking about diabetes identity and how hard it can be to accept this part of ourselves we didn't ask for. I'd been blogging about diabetes for some time at that point, but opened up more in those sessions than I had in years. The discussions weren't always easy, but the results were magnificent.

Opportunities like this eventually led to Washington, where on several occasions I got to advocate in front of members of Congress and their staff. While talking with a Senator or member of the House of Representatives may seem daunting, I just remembered what I was there for, that for the most part they want to hear what I'm advocating for, and to tell my story because no one knows it as well as I do.

Those last two points are the hallmarks of effective advocacy. No one is going to help you with your issue if you don't tell them what you want. I will note that it is surprising how many times people have a great story to tell without getting to the point of what they really wanted in the first place. Also, whether you're weaving in the story of how it affects you (or a parent or a child or a spouse or a friend), making your advocacy message reflect your own lived experiences makes it tangible to non-diabetic audiences. It makes it easy for the listener to understand why your message is important and worthy of consideration. For the listener, it is far more difficult to ignore a person and their story than it is to ignore a complex policy issue.

Coming Full Circle

At that FDA workshop in 2014, I learned a powerful lesson that advocacy has to be personal. And finally, I got a chance to pass along that lesson when I went to Washington, D.C. four years later as part of a non-profit group of advocates to speak one-on-one on important diabetes issues before members of Congress and their staff. In this case, the team I was leading was meeting with a Legislative Assistant for a U.S. Senator. The legislative assistant kept peppering the advocates on my team about how the Senator's support might hurt business interests in his state. What could we do to assure him that those business interests wouldn't be affected?

That's when I stepped in and reminded him that the business interests he was concerned about have plenty of lobbyists meeting with him and his Senator on a regular basis, and I'm sure they do a great job. But we were there on behalf of patients (and in this particular instance, elderly diabetes patients), and we were going to advocate on behalf of what is important to the people we represent. That ended the repeated questioning.

People in the Room Make the Decisions

Eventually, I found ways to advocate on my own. When my state developed an advisory council on health and wellness, I volunteered and wound up as the lone patient advocate in the group. The committee I worked on developed the state's first Diabetes Action Plan (Maryland Diabetes Action Plan 2020) that describes standards of care, measurement benchmarks, and other criteria that can help states manage how they consider diabetes within the overall health care landscape. Without advocate perspectives in the room, these plans might lack the depth, empathy, and even common sense required for them to be truly effective.

In all of my efforts, there were ups and downs and personality conflicts. There were times when it seemed like progress was moving at a snail's pace. Hardly anything happens exactly like you imagine it will. Yet there were moments of triumph and a sense of accomplishment whenever I remembered that one overarching goal: better lives for everyone living with diabetes.

I think one of the reasons people take to diabetes advocacy so well is that people with diabetes in their lives already possess the two most important qualities needed to advocate: perseverance and empathy. Time and again we've shown the ability to persevere through the most difficult challenges, diabetes-related and otherwise. And knowing what it takes, we have the empathy to understand what it's like for someone else to go through similar difficulties. These qualities make advocacy feel more meaningful. It reminds us that we are not the only individuals who will benefit from any changes that come from this work. It is the ripple.

Taken as a whole, it might seem like advocacy efforts are mighty. But the truth is we all advocate where think advocating is welcomed, in the time we have available, in the forms where we work best. We might not all make big speeches or raise millions of dollars in donations.

Being your own advocate can even mean not answering a question, or disengaging—like an act of radical self-care. I could have been my own advocate back in 2014 by just wearing a continuous glucose monitor—because that in and of itself, is a form of advocacy. It is bringing diabetes out of hiding. But in the process of advocating in the way we can, we are able to form networks of friends and acquaintances who entrust us to share the most important aspects of our lives with diabetes in order to help make life for the next generation of those diagnosed better than ever before.

In my case, I didn't imagine it and hope and wait for it to happen. I used my voice where I could use it, when I could use it. I will never forget my lunchtime experience all those years ago, and in remembering it, I can't help but continue to advocate for a world in which my experience doesn't ever again happen to anyone else.

* * *

An Open Letter to Almost-Advocates

Dear reader,

Let this chapter be your call to action. You may already be advocating, and you don't know it. Claim it, own it, wear it. You are an advocate. Even in the moments in which you need to be silent, you are advocating for your needs and what you need in that moment. Everyone has barriers of some kind, and it's okay to only do what you can. Tell your story when you can and how you can. Each moment is yours and every part of your story matters. It is my hope that my chapter, and this book, will expand your thinking on advocacy. It is going to take all of us to make life better for everyone living with diabetes.

Sincerely,
A fellow Diabetes Advocate

References

International Diabetes Federation. 2019. *IDF Diabetes Atlas.* 9th ed. Brussels, Belgium: International Diabetes Federation. https://diabetesatlas.org/upload/resources/material/20200302_133351_IDFATLAS9e-final-web.pdf

Maryland Diabetes Action Plan. 2020. https://phpa.health.maryland.gov/CCDPC/Pages/diabetes-action-plan.aspx.

Afterword

Therese (Tess) Jones

In the United States, diabetes has become so familiar that it is now necessary to defamiliarize it, to make it strange in order to trouble our assumptions, perspectives, and constructions of it. In Bianca C. Frazer's and Heather R. Walker's words, what is needed is an opportunity to offer diabetes as a *new case study*, and with this edited collection of original work, they not only disrupt our blithe notice of diabetes as it is performed in the popular imaginary but also our automatic assumption that we know what it is, how it is theorized, and how it is experienced. In fact, as they note in the Introduction, diabetes has become so commonplace, so comfortable that we often employ it handily as a moral and medical rhetorical device: both to destigmatize certain conditions such as substance abuse disorder and to normalize once lethal illnesses such as HIV/AIDS, which, like diabetes, is now a "manageable chronic disease."

T. (Tess) Jones (✉)
Arts and Humanities in Healthcare Program, University of Colorado Anschutz Medical Campus, Aurora, CO, USA
e-mail: therese.jones@cuanschutz.edu

B. C. Frazer, H. R. Walker (eds.), *(Un)doing Diabetes: Representation, Disability, Culture*, Palgrave Studies in Science and Popular Culture, https://doi.org/10.1007/978-3-030-83110-3_22

The theoretical concept of defamiliarization was first articulated in 1920 by the Russian formalist critic, Victor Shklovsky, to describe the essentially estranging purpose and effect of art. All human perception, according to Shklovsky, involves an inevitable habituation to the familiar; gradually that which is familiar fades away, and perception becomes automatic. Art (and I would add radical and transformative critical inquiry such as what we have here) forces us to look at the familiar with new eyes and in new ways through a process that he calls *estrangement* (*ostranenie*).[1] Integral to this disorienting and disquieting state is an opportunity to encounter and examine taken-for-granted assumptions, unconscious biases, and unquestioned attitudes by posing provocative questions, paradoxes, contrasts, and contradictions. Thus, this collection challenges what we know or think we know about diabetes and confronts us with the unknown—what Frazer and Walker describe as the "undoing" of diabetes. This, in turn, prompts reflection and action—the "doing" of diabetes in imaginative and activist representations created by community members themselves.

The critical questioning of assumptions, biases, and attitudes that can distort and dehumanize relationships in medical care has long been a goal of health humanities and disability studies educators like myself who introduce learners to counter and resistive narratives. Take, for example, Peggy Ornstein's contrarian view of the "pink movement" of breast cancer awareness. What many health professions students and working clinicians would likely describe as an effective public health advocacy strategy to reduce stigma and break silence around the disease can be seen, instead, as alienating and dehumanizing to someone living with it. Ornstein disrupts the taken-for-granted and asks readers to look for assumptions and motives that underlie common constructions and stereotypical depictions: "A funny thing happened on the way to destigmatization. The experience of actual women with cancer...—women like me—got lost. Rather than truly breaking silences, acceptable narratives of coping emerged, each tied up with a pretty pink bow."[2]

During my own reeducation and reorientation to diabetes in light of this work, I found myself reviewing the contradictory and charged

[1] Lemon LT and MJ Ries (trans). *Russian Formalist Criticism: Four Essays* (Omaha: U of Nebraska Press, 1965).

[2] Ornstein P. "Think about Pink." *New York Times Magazine* (12 November 2010): http://www.nytimes.com/2010/11/14/magazine/14FOB-wwln-t.html.

responses to the $5.6 million Dexcom GS CGM Super Bowl ad with Nick Jonas, something that would not have caught my attention in the past. On one side were the swooning fans who refer to Jonas as their "dia-crush," thrilled with the interest in and even the glamorization of diabetes and especially about continuous glucose monitoring with posts such as "Be cool. Like Nick." On the other side were serious and intense critiques about the morality of such a huge expenditure (including Nick's fee) during an insulin pricing crisis *and* a pandemic in which access to basic health care and life-saving medications have become front and center issues in our reckoning with racial and disability injustice in America.[3]

Shlovsky warns that if our whole complex lives go on unconsciously, it is if our lives have never been. As we walk along mechanically, it is the unexpected stone in the middle of the path that trips us, forcing us to look up, to pause, perhaps to change direction. This collection does that, and I am grateful for the interruption and the disruption.

[3] Hoskins M. "Mixed Reactions to Dexcom's Awareness-Raising Super Bowl Ad" (10 February 2021): https://www.healthline.com/diabetesmine.

Index[1]

[1] Note: Page numbers followed by 'n' refer to notes.

B. C. Frazer, H. R. Walker (eds.), *(Un)doing Diabetes: Representation, Disability, Culture*, Palgrave Studies in Science and Popular Culture, https://doi.org/10.1007/978-3-030-83110-3

M

The manufacturer's authorised representative in the EU is Springer Nature Customer Service Centre GmbH, Europaplatz 3, 69115 Heidelberg, Germany. If you have any concerns regarding our products, please contact ProductSafety@springernature.com

Printed and bound by CPI Group (UK) Ltd, Croydon, CR0 4YY
30/09/2026
02225327-0013